THE
COMPLETE DOCTOR'S
Healthy
Back Bible

A Practical Manual
for Understanding,
Preventing and
Treating Back Pain

Dr. Stephen Reed, MD, FRCSC
and Penny Kendall-Reed, MSc, ND

with Dr. Michael Ford, MD, FRCSC
and Dr. Charles Gregory, MD, ChB, FRCP(C)

Robert
ROSE

The authors would like to thank the following for sharing their knowledge and expertise during the writing of this book: Dr Michael Ford, Dr Charles Gregory, Dr Anthony Mascia, Helen Razmjou, Sabine Stojanovich, Amanda Webber, Lynn Kendall, and Fred Antwi-Nsiah.

The nutritional, medical, and health information presented in this book is based on the research, training, and professional experience of the authors, and is true and complete to the best of their knowledge. However, this book is intended only as an informative guide for those wishing to know more about health, nutrition, and medicine; it is not intended to replace or countermand the advice given by the reader's personal physician. Because each person and situation is unique, the authors and the publisher urge the reader to check with a qualified healthcare professional before using any procedure where there is a question as to its appropriateness. A physician should be consulted before beginning any exercise program. The author and the publisher are not responsible for any adverse effects or consequences resulting from the use of the information in this book. It is the responsibility of the reader to consult a physician or other qualified healthcare professional regarding his or her personal care.

National Library of Canada Cataloguing in Publication

Reed, Stephen Charles, 1961–
     The complete doctor's healthy back bible : a practical manual for understanding, preventing and treating back pain / Stephen C. Reed, Penny Kendall-Reed, Michael H. Ford.

Includes index.
ISBN 0-7788-0091-1 (bound).— ISBN 0-7788-0090-3 (pbk.)

1. Backache. 2. Back—Care and hygiene. I. Kendall-Reed, Penny II. Ford, Michael H. III. Title.

RD768.R43 2004   617.5'64   C2003-906527-8

Edited by Bob Hilderley, Senior Editor, Health.
Design and page composition by PageWave Graphics Inc.
Exercise and posture illustrations by Kveta.
Back cover photograph by Helen Tansey.
Functional Spinal Unit illustration from *Orthopaedic Knowledge Update: Spine 2*.
Causes of back pain illustration courtesy of Searle Arthritis Care.

The publisher acknowledges the financial support of the Government of Canada through the Book Publishing Industry Development Program.

Published by Robert Rose Inc.,
120 Eglinton Ave. E., Suite 800,
Toronto, Ontario Canada M4P 1E2
Tel: (416) 322-6552.

Printed and bound in Canada.

1 2 3 4 5 6 7 8 9 CPL 12 11 10 09 08 07 06 05 04

Contents

Preface 5

Quick Reference Guide to
Back Pain Symptoms, Diagnosis,
Treatments & Prevention 8

Back Anatomy and
Pain Pathology
Illustrations 10

Back Questions and Answers

Should I See a Doctor? **18**
Naming Your Pain 19
Guidelines for Seeking
  Medical Care 24

Who Treats Back Pain? **26**
Emergency Care 26
Family Doctor 27
Naturopathic Doctor 27
Orthopedic Surgeon 28
Rheumatologist 29
Physiotherapist 30
Occupational Therapist 31
Chiropractor 31
Osteopath 32
Massage Therapist 33
Acupuncturist 33
Chronic Pain Specialist 33

How Is Back Pain Diagnosed? **34**
Benefits of Diagnosis 34
History 35
Examination 36
Classifications of Symptoms 38
Diagnostic Tests 47

What Causes Back Pain? **60**
Spine Anatomy 60
Spinal Cord and Nerves 69
Pain Sensation and Control 72
Specific Origins of Back Pain 81

Back Pain Treatment Strategies

Physical Treatments for Back Care **110**
Non-Invasive Treatments 110
Hands-On Physical Treatments 120

Exercise Treatments for Back Care **135**
Exercise Basics 136
Stretching 137
Strengthening 140
Cardiovascular Exercise 141
Specific Back Exercises 144
Cardiovascular Fitness Exercises . . . 154
Sexual Intercourse 156

Weight Management for Back Care . . . **158**
Ideal Weight 158
Diet Trends 161
Naturopathic Diet 163

Natural Supplements for Back Care . . **169**
Selecting and Combining
  Supplements 171
Minerals 172
Supplements 176
Herbs 181
Vitamins 188
Essential Fatty Acids 192
Additional Supplements for Stress,
  Anxiety, and Depression 195

Medications for Back Care **200**
  Painkillers (Analgesics) 200
  Muscle Relaxants 205
  Anti-Depressant Medication 205
  Medicinal Treatment of
    Inflammatory Arthritis 207

Injection Therapy **208**
  Epidural Steroid Injections 208
  Facet Joint Injections 211
  Medial Branch Neurotomy 212
  Botulinum Toxin (Botox)
    Injections 213
  Sacroiliac Joint Injections 213
  Chemonucleosis (Chymopapain
    Injections) for Disc Herniation 214
  Intradiscal Electrothermal
    Coagulation (IDET™) 216

Spinal Surgery **217**
  Back Surgery Basics 217
  Surgical Techniques 221

Chronic Pain Management **234**
  What is Pain? 234
  Pain-Tension-Anxiety (PTA)
    Cycle 241
  Multi-Disciplinary Treatment 244
  Self-Help 248

Practical Treatment Manual

Sudden Onset Back Pain **252**
  Lumbar Strain 252
  Disc Herniation and Sciatica 260
  Fractures 264
  Osteoporosis 267

Recurring Back Pain **271**
  Symptoms 271
  Treating the Individual Episode 272
  Preventing Recurrence 274

Persistent (Chronic) Back Pain **279**
  Degenerative Disc Disease 279
  Osteoarthritis (Degenerative
    Joint Disease) 284
  Spinal Stenosis 286
  Instability from Arthritis
    (Degenerative Spondylolisthesis) . . 288
  Rheumatoid Arthritis 289
  Ankylosing Spondylitis 290
  Psoriatic Arthritis 291
  Psoriatic Arthropathy 292
  Other Types of Lumbar
    Spine Instability 293

Glossary 295

Selected References 305

Index 312

Preface

A friend of mine once suggested that all doctors should experience, at least once, the illnesses and treatments they see and prescribe. With reference to low back pain, they may have had a point!

Last summer, following a particularly rigorous landscaping endeavor, I awoke with low back pain. I am a fairly fit 40-year-old man who works out at the gym, three or four times a week; I run, I cycle, and I play soccer on a Sunday morning. I am pretty much used to the aches and pains that follow an overzealous bench press or a vigorous defensive tackle. The adage that "after 40 the pain really never goes away, it just changes location," seems ever more true, a reality softened by the occasional anti-inflammatory, savior of the masters athlete. However, nothing could have prepared me for the shock of not being able to move or even cough without tear-inducing pain from my back. I see patients with all kinds of orthopedic injuries and was aware of the impact of back pain on patients' ability to function even remotely close to normality. I was aware of the difficulty in gaining pain control in low back pain, its intractability and emotional connotations, far more than many other conditions considered 'more serious'.

Yet here I was, barely able to make it to breakfast (a meal I consider most vital to daily survival), half crying, half laughing at the severity of the discomfort emanating from some ill-defined area called my 'low-back'. And what was worse was the fact that I had not even sustained a sympathy-worthy injury to cause all this. I had simply moved a little dirt to provide space for some new hostas!

Not to be defeated by this simple 'muscle inflammation', as I had clinically determined it to be, I put the 'practice what you preach' plan into action. Ice packs, Tylenol, an anti-inflammatory, and a couple of simple stretches and I should be out planting by noon, I reassured myself. But an hour later I'd made it no farther than the bathroom, more out of dire necessity than by overcoming discomfort. I was getting a little annoyed. After all I had an awful lot of things to do and a barbeque to attend that evening. My wife Penny (and co-author of this book), as always, was very supportive and understanding, offering a never-ending supply of ice/heat packs, massage, acupuncture, and other naturopathic remedies — even a trip to the pharmacy to find something 'stronger'. This last offer may have been her chance to escape my increasing and inexcusable grouchiness, a perfect example of the emotional aspect of severe, yet inexplicable pain.

Well, the hostas never got planted — but I did make it to the barbeque. A man in pain has to establish priorities! And I did indeed improve and become more mobile. The acute discomfort subsided as quickly as it had arisen. However, 4 weeks later I was still feeling the occasional twinge, continued to be a little stiff, and woke once or twice at night with an ache in my low back. Did I reassure myself that this was quite typical for a 'lumbar strain', that there were no concerning features in my symptoms, and that overall I was gradually getting better? Of course not! I conjured up every serious back condition ever reported in the medical literature and managed to fit the symptoms to my discomfort. Doctors indeed make the worst patients.

Needless to say, by 6 weeks I was completely pain free and back to normal. My quite unnecessary X-ray, as I expected, showed not even a hint of anything abnormal.

Some individuals, however, have a different experience with their back pain. It may not resolve so quickly, it may persist or recur. It may be more disabling and disturbing to their daily lives, occasionally becoming chronic and threatening their overall mood and well-being.

We begin the book by answering the most pressing questions you may ask when you experience back pain: Should I See a Doctor? Who Treats Back Pain? What Are the Causes of Back Pain? We next provide full descriptions of treatments, from ice packs through medications to surgery. We then bring these treatment strategies to bear upon specific back problems, from acute lumbar strain through recurrent back pain to chronic arthritic conditions.

This book has been written for both kinds of back pain sufferers — those who suffer occasionally and those who suffer recurrently and chronically.

To orient yourself to the medical terms involved in describing back pain and back care, we recommend that you quickly glance through the Glossary at the back of the book and return to it whenever you encounter a term in the book that requires clarification. Similarly, we recommend that you glance at the Back Anatomy and Pain Pathology illustrations at the front of the book and bookmark this section for quick reference as you read further. Perhaps the best way to introduce you to the complex language of back pain and back care is visually through these simplified medical illustrations of the bones, nerves, muscles, and ligaments of the spinal column.

In the effort to make this book authoritative, we have based our information on current medical research. These sources are listed in the 'Selected References' section at the back of the book. And in the effort to be comprehensive, we have called on a team of expert consultants, namely Dr Michael Ford, a surgeon who specializes in back surgery; Helen Razmjou, a physical therapist who specializes in mechanical diagnosis and treatment of low back pain; Sabine Stojanovich, a certified personal trainer and rehabilitation conditioning consultant; and Dr Charles Gregory, a psychiatrist who specializes in chronic pain management. We bring to the book our own expertise, Stephen as an orthopedic surgeon, and Penny as a naturopathic doctor with special knowledge of nutritional supplements and weight management. We are also the co-authors of *Healing Arthritis: Complementary Naturopathic, Orthopedic, and Drug Treatments* as well as *The Complete Doctor's Stress Solution*. Penny is also the author of *The Naturopathic Diet: A Guide for Managing Weight, Preventing Illness, and Achieving Optimum Health*.

We trust the comprehensive information presented in *The Complete Doctor's Healthy Back Bible* will lead to a speedy recovery and to the prevention of this most common ailment in the future.

— Stephen Reed, MD and Penny Kendall-Reed, ND

The third section of this book serves as a practical treatment and recovery manual. Some readers may choose to begin reading this manual, then move back through the book for more comprehensive explanations.

Quick Reference Guide to Back Pain Symptoms, Diagnosis, Treatments & Prevention

This chart provides a brief summary of the symptoms, diagnosis, treatment, and prevention of most common back conditions. After reading further in this book, you may find it helpful to highlight or circle the symptoms that correspond to your back pain and use this information to chart a course for recovery, ideally in consultation with your family doctor.

'Red Flags'
Indications of Potentially Serious Causes of Back Pain

- Significant injury
- Symptoms of cauda equina syndrome
- Severe, unremitting night pain
- Fever
- History of cancer
- Rapid and unexplained weight loss
- History of osteoporosis or steroid medication

Back Conditions	Sudden Onset Back Pain Lumbar Strain	Disc Herniation/ Sciatica	Compression Fracture
Symptoms	• Rapid onset (within 36 hours) • Often related to injury • Back pain dominant • No numbness/weakness • No "Red Flags"	• Rapid onset (within 36 hours) • Common in men age 30–60 • Often related to injury • Predominantly leg pain • Possible numbness/ weakness • No "Red Flags"	• Immediate or rapid onset • Often related to fall • Back pain predominant • History of osteoporosis/ steroids • Pain at rest • Elderly patient
Diagnosis	• Clinical history/findings • Tests not indicated	• Clinical history/ findings • Cat scan/MRI • EMG tests	• Clinical suspicion • X-rays • Bone scan • Cat scan/MRI

Treatments	Acute (first 48 hours)
	• Ice
	• Reduced activity (not bed rest)
	• Comfortable postures
	• Gentle stretching
	• Analgesics/NSAIDS
	• Water, Ca/Mg, EFAs, Zinc
	• Manipulation/ Acupuncture
	
	Subacute (first 48 hours)
	• Heat and ice
	• Increase activity (not bed rest)
	• More stretching
	• Yoga/Thai Chi
	• Manipulation/Massage/ Acupuncture
		• Reduced activity (not bed rest)
		• Ice
		• Comfortable postures
		• EFAs, B-vitamins, Manganese
		• Analgesics/NSAIDS
		• Injection therapy
		• Surgery
			• Emergency spine precautions
			• If fracture stable:
			  - Analgesics/NSAIDS
			  - Mobilize +/- Brace
			  - Extension exercises
			  - Vertebroplasty
			  - Osteoporosis treatment

Prevention	• Core conditioning • Aerobic fitness • Correct lifting/ ergonomics • Improved posture • Weight management	• Core conditioning • Aerobic fitness • Correct lifting/ ergonomics • Improved posture • Weight management • CA/Mg, Manganese, GS/MSM	• CA/Mg, Vitamin D, Boron, Zinc

Recurrent Back Pain	Persistent Back Pain	Disc Degeneration	Spinal Osteoarthritis	Spinal Stenosis

• Recurrent back pain with pain-free periods
• Pain similar each recurrence
• Common causes:
  - Spinal deconditioning
  - Poor posture/ ergonomics
  - Inadequate training/strength
  - Overweight
  - Stress
	• Prolonged recovery from acute attack
	• Frequent recurrence
	• Limited or no pain-free periods
		• Age 20–50 years
		• Heavy lifting, vibration
		• 40% of persistent back pain sufferers commonly exist with no symptoms
		• Typically back-dominant pain
		• Pain worse with flexion
		• Overweight/Smoking
			• Common over age 50
			• Rarely symptomatic
			• Most arthritis on X-rays not related to pain
			• Aching back pain
			• Often worse with extension
				• Back pain increasing with walking
				• Leg pain/numbness associated with walking
				• Weakness/ clumsiness in legs
				• Symptoms eased by flexing forward

• Low likelihood of serious spine pathology • Clinical history/ findings	• Clinical history/ findings • X-rays • Bone scan • Cat scan/MRI • Discography • Facet blocks	• X-rays • CAT scan/MRI • Discography	• X-rays • CAT scan • Bone scan • Blood tests (inflammatory arthritis)	• Clinical history/ symptoms • CAT scan/MRI • EMG studies
• Each episode treated individually as per acute back pain	• Vary depending on cause • Fitness/core strengthening • Weight management • Acupuncture • Injection therapy • Surgery (rarely)	• Core conditioning • Aerobic fitness • Correct lifting/ ergonomics • Improved posture • Weight management • GS/MSM/ Anti-oxidants • Injection therapy • Surgery	• Heat/hydrotherapy • Lumbar support • Core conditioning • Weight management • GS/MSM/Ginger/ Devil's Claw • Analgesics/NSAIDS • Massage • Injection Therapy • Surgery (rarely)	• Postural adjustment • Exercise • Core strength • EFAs/B-vitamins/ GS/MSSM • Stop smoking • Injection therapy • Surgery
• Core conditioning • Aerobic fitness • Correct lifting/ ergonomics • Improved posture • Weight management • Yoga, Tai Chi, Alexander • Stress management	• Active treatment of acute phase • GS/MSM/HA • Fitness/core strengthening • Weight management • Stress management	• Stop smoking • Weight loss • Posture program • Core conditioning	• GS/MSM/HA • Weight management • Fitness/core strengthening	• Fitness/core strengthening • Posture training • Weight loss • Essential Fatty Acids • Stop smoking

Back Anatomy and Pain Pathology Illustrations

Perhaps the best way to introduce you to the complex language of back pain and back care is visually through the following simplified medical illustrations of the bones, nerves, muscles, and ligaments of the spinal column. As you read further in the book, you may find it convenient to bookmark these pages and return to them from time to time.

Vertebral Column

Lateral view of the vertebral column with hip bone and portion of the skull superimposed onto the human profile.

Anterior view of the vertebral column showing the cervical, thoracic, and lumbar vertebrae, and the sacrum and coccyx.

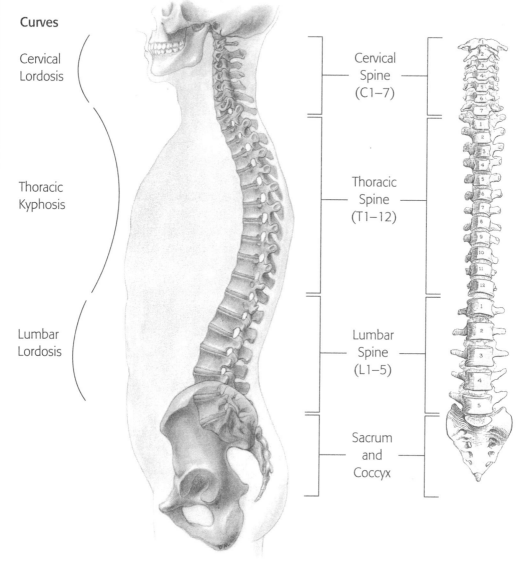

Curves

Cervical Lordosis

Thoracic Kyphosis

Lumbar Lordosis

Cervical Spine (C1–7)

Thoracic Spine (T1–12)

Lumbar Spine (L1–5)

Sacrum and Coccyx

Vertebral Column, Lumbar Region

Median section of the lumbar region of the vertebral column, with the image to the right indicating the orientation of the main illustration.

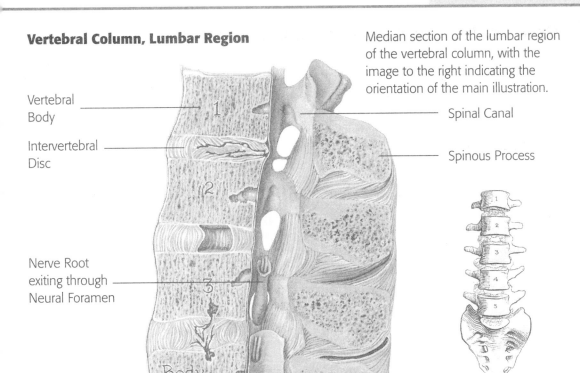

Vertebral Body

Intervertebral Disc

Nerve Root exiting through Neural Foramen

Spinal Canal

Spinous Process

Lumbar Vertebra

Lateral and superior views of a lumbar vertebra.

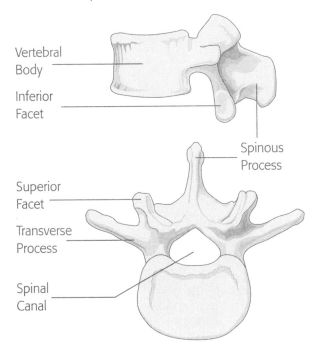

Vertebral Body

Inferior Facet

Spinous Process

Superior Facet

Transverse Process

Spinal Canal

Intervertebral Disc

Lateral view of the intervertebral disc, with sections removed to show direction of fibers and with the annulus fibrosus shown dissected.

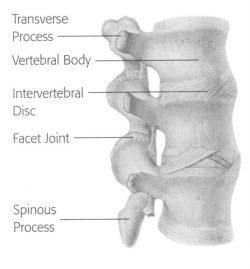

Transverse Process

Vertebral Body

Intervertebral Disc

Facet Joint

Spinous Process

Intervetebral Disc and Ligaments

Superior view of transverse section of the intervetebral disc and ligaments, with the nucleus pulposus removed and the epiphyseal plate exposed.

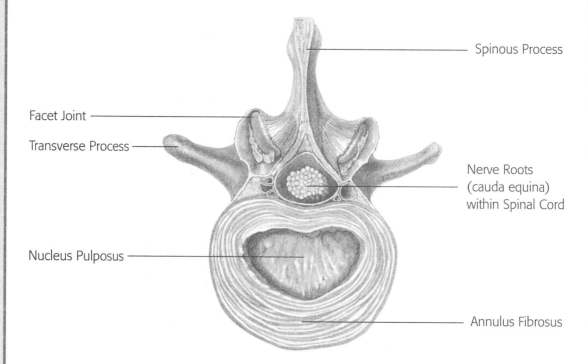

Spinous Process

Facet Joint

Transverse Process

Nerve Roots (cauda equina) within Spinal Cord

Nucleus Pulposus

Annulus Fibrosus

Functional Spinal Unit Ligaments

Diagram showing the various ligaments in the functional spinal unit. Two vertebrae with a disc between them and ligaments make up a functional spinal unit.

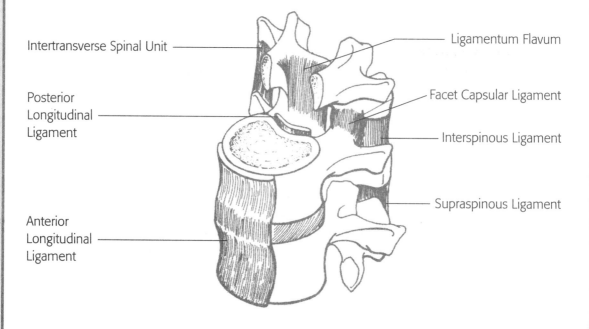

Intertransverse Spinal Unit

Posterior Longitudinal Ligament

Anterior Longitudinal Ligament

Ligamentum Flavum

Facet Capsular Ligament

Interspinous Ligament

Supraspinous Ligament

Back Muscles

Diagram showing extrinsic muscles of the back with the intrinsic muscles partly revealed.

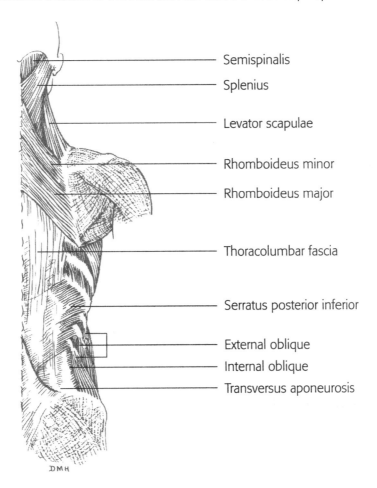

- Semispinalis
- Splenius
- Levator scapulae
- Rhomboideus minor
- Rhomboideus major
- Thoracolumbar fascia
- Serratus posterior inferior
- External oblique
- Internal oblique
- Transversus aponeurosis

DMH

Lumbar Back Muscle

Transverse section of back muscle at the lumbar spine level, showing muscles within sheaths/compartments (left) and empty sheaths (right).

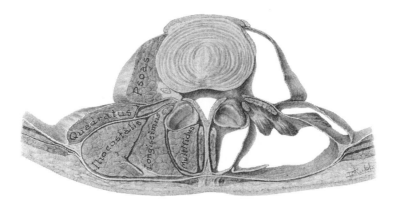

Spinal Nerve Roots

Lateral view of the spinal column with the brain silhouetted, showing the spinal cord origin of the spinal nerves.

Spinal Cord

Transverse section of the lumbar spine, showing left and right laminae behind the spinal cord.

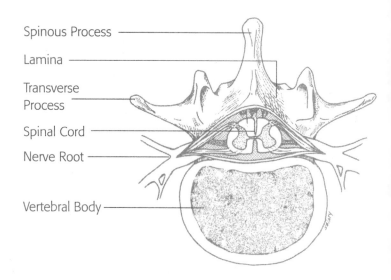

Spinous Process

Lamina

Transverse Process

Spinal Cord

Nerve Root

Vertebral Body

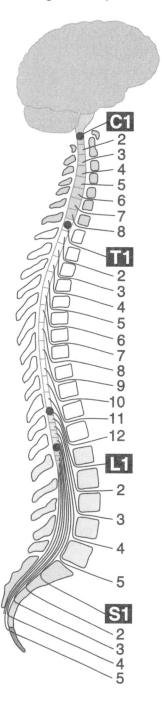

C1
2
3
4
5
6
7
8
T1
2
3
4
5
6
7
8
9
10
11
12
L1
2
3
4
5
S1
2
3
4
5

Spinal Nerves

Posterolateral view of a section of the spinal column, showing the vertebrae and their corresponding spinal nerves.

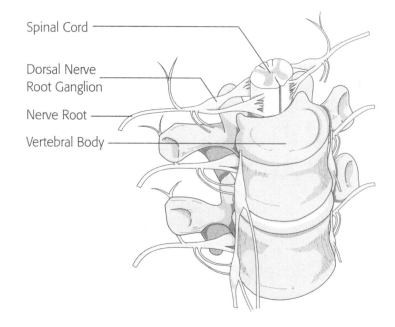

Spinal Cord

Dorsal Nerve Root Ganglion

Nerve Root

Vertebral Body

Sciatic Nerve

Posterior view of pelvic area, showing location of sciatic nerve and associated skeletal structures.

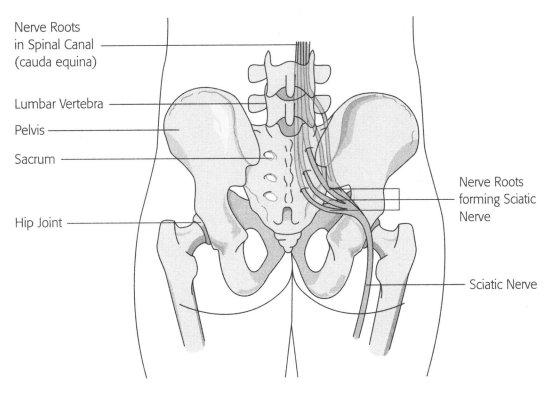

Nerve Roots in Spinal Canal (cauda equina)

Lumbar Vertebra

Pelvis

Sacrum

Hip Joint

Nerve Roots forming Sciatic Nerve

Sciatic Nerve

Anatomic Planes

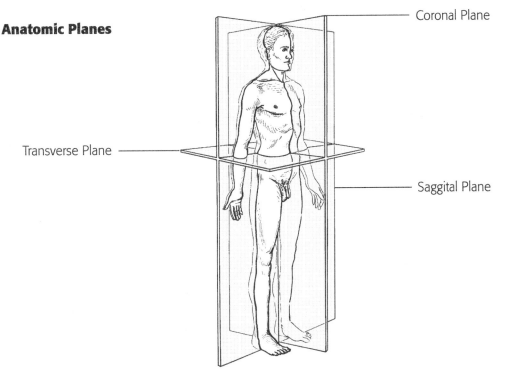

Coronal Plane

Transverse Plane

Saggital Plane

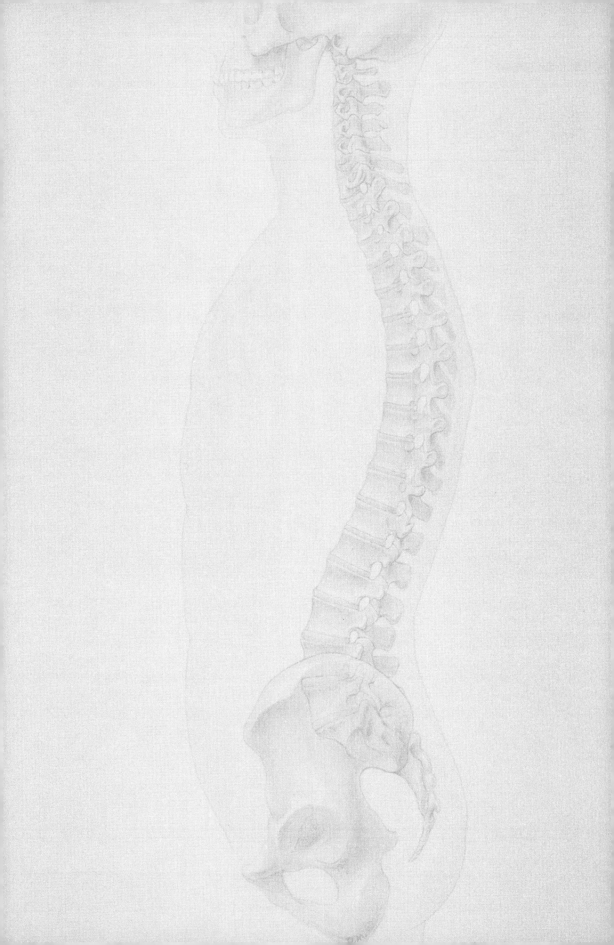

Back Questions and Answers

Should I See a Doctor?

Key Medical Terms

Be sure to bookmark the Glossary at the back of the book for quick reference to definitions of the key medical terms used for describing back pain and back care.

L ow back pain is an exceedingly common yet perplexing problem. Over the course of our lifetime, there is a 90% chance that we will suffer at least one bout of low back pain. Back pain represents the second most common cause of a visit to the doctor after colds and flu. The acute category of back pain, lasting 4 to 6 weeks, is the leading cause of disability under the age of 45 and responsible for billions of dollars spent in diagnosis and treatment.

Fortunately, only a small percentage of people who develop low back pain will have symptoms for longer than 2 weeks. Most back pain is harmless and self-limiting, a short but annoying hindrance to daily life that resolves as rapidly as it appears. Because back pain often comes and often goes, we have trouble determining if it is serious enough to warrant medical attention. If we just wait another day, the pain might go away, we reason.

However, for the novice sufferer, for the person with recurring bouts of pain, and for the small percentage of people with chronic pain, recovery statistics offer little reassurance. These people need to understand their pain and its cause, know when their symptoms indicate a serious problem that needs medical attention, and begin to plan their recovery. In the presence of 'Red Flag' indicators of potentially serious causes of back pain, emergency medical care, invasive surgery, or longer-term care may be needed.

✔ BACK FACTS

No doubt about it, back pain *is* painful! The single most important treatment of back pain is reliable information.

- 90% of us will experience an episode of low back pain at least once during our lives.
- 90% of acute low back pain will resolve within 4 to 6 weeks.
- 90% of low back pain cases will have no specific cause, such as disc herniation or arthritis. In most cases of low back pain, no specific injury or event is identified as a cause.
- Less than 1% of acute low back pain is due to a serious spinal condition, such as infection or cancer. The figure is even lower below age 50.
- Less than 2% of back pain patients end up needing surgery.
- Bed rest slows your recovery; staying active speeds up your recovery.

Naming Your Pain

Finding a way to describe your pain is the first step in understanding it. This helps in the mental process of rationalizing the pain and in the emotional process of coping with it. This information is also useful in diagnosing the cause of your pain and developing a treatment plan. Common to many medical specialties, such evaluation is one of the first clinical thought processes taught in medical school. Using these terms, you will be able to communicate symptoms to a healthcare professional, establishing the temporal and physical nature of the pain along with associated symptoms.

Key terms for describing back pain are *onset* and *duration*, *recurrence* and *persistence, location* and *movement, associated symptoms* and *intensity*.

Timeframe

The most common way to describe back pain is according to its temporal onset and duration and its pattern of recurrence and persistence.

Acute Onset Back Pain

Pain that comes on rapidly is generally called 'acute', although the definition of acute is somewhat vague. Acute 'onset' back pain means pain that has appeared quite suddenly, instantaneously, or over a matter of minutes or hours. This may happen overnight such that you go to bed pain free but wake with pain. Do not be confused by the term 'acute low back pain', a valid but somewhat misleading term that refers to back pain of less than three-month duration.

Clearly, if there has been an injury, the onset and severity of pain are likely to reflect the seriousness of that injury. A fall from height or serious motor vehicle accident with sudden and rapid development of low back pain is likely to indicate fracture, major ligament disruption, or acute disc herniation. A minor fall or accident with pain developing over hours to days more likely points to a muscle sprain or low-grade ligament injury.

Insidious Onset Back Pain

Pain that comes on insidiously may do so over a period of days, months, or even years. Insidious onset with rapidly progressing and unremitting pain usually indicates a serious medical condition either affecting the spine (infection, osteoporotic fracture, or malignancy) or non-spinal conditions such as stomach ulcer, inflammation of the pancreas, or an aneurysm of the aorta. Pain gradually increasing over a longer timeframe, often with variations in intensity, indicates a possible degenerative process such as arthritis or disc deterioration. Acute

'Red Flags'

Indications of Potentially Serious Causes of Back Pain

- Significant injury
- Symptoms of cauda equina syndrome
- Severe, unremitting night pain
- Fever
- History of cancer
- Rapid and unexplained weight loss
- History of osteoporosis or steroid medication

Key Back Pain Terms

- **Onset and Duration:** the timeframe of pain development
- **Recurrence and Persistence:** the pattern of repeat episodes
- **Location:** where the pain begins and where it spreads
- **Movement:** aggravating or easing positions
- **Associated Symptoms:** specific or general health issues
- **Intensity:** how serious does the pain feel

• Acute:
  onset of pain within the past 4 to 6 weeks

• Sub-Acute:
  onset of pain within the past 6 to 12 weeks

• Recurrent:
  episodes of pain lasting less than 12 weeks with significant pain-free intervals

• Chronic:
  pain lasting longer than 12 weeks

'Acute' and 'sub-acute' are often combined under the 'acute' heading, although the dividing line at 6 weeks proves useful when planning investigation and treatment.

development of 'new' pain in an individual with chronic low back pain should be considered independently as a potentially additional condition, although clearly this needs to be in the context of any existing diagnosis.

Duration

Pain duration is also an important consideration. Only about 10% of individuals with acute onset of low back pain will have symptoms that last longer than 10 to 12 weeks. Pain lasting longer than 4 weeks generally requires investigation regardless of whether there are suspicious 'Red Flag' symptoms or findings. Short duration pain usually indicates a muscular or ligamentous cause; over 90% will have no serious identifiable illness or spinal condition. Pain lasting beyond 4 to 6 weeks may indicate an underlying problem such as disc herniation or facet joint degeneration. Pain continuing for 3 to 6 months may indicate generalized arthritis, osteoporosis, or spinal deconditioning.

Pattern

Recurrence

'Recurrent low back pain' is defined as periodic episodes of 'acute' low back pain ('acute' being used in the 'less than three-month duration' sense) separated by pain-free intervals. The pattern of recurrence can help establish severity and point toward a cause. Rapid-onset, short-lasting pain recurring every few years would indicate a simple soft tissue strain, whereas episodes occurring every few months might indicate instability or degeneration. Even if the cause is repeated muscle strain, the more frequent and more disabling the pain, the more likely there is to be an underlying process that warrants investigation and treatment.

Persistence

Although not defined in the clinical setting, persistent back pain is used in the context of this book to describe low back pain that does not resolve within expected timeframes or becomes constant. While 'recurrent' back pain resolves completely between episodes, persistent pain is always there, albeit with varying degrees of severity. The clinical term 'chronic' might include both 'persistent low back pain' and 'chronic low back pain syndrome'.

Chronicity

The division between 'persistent' and 'chronic' may seem a little vague. However, we feel that the term 'chronic low back pain' should be assigned to the complex syndrome that includes mental and emotional factors and serious functional disability, along with back pain symptoms.

Location

Low back pain can be notoriously hard to localize, symptoms often being vague and diffuse. However, if the site of the most severe pain can be identified, the secondary or referred pain sources can be marginalized, allowing a more specific diagnosis and treatment. It is sometimes useful to divide pain into *central* (related to the spine and surrounding muscles) and *peripheral* (pain in the buttocks, thighs, or legs).

Central

Pain confined to the absolute midline of the spine, the area of those palpable bony prominences (spinous processes), suggests a problem within the bony elements, such as instability or localized arthritis. If the pain is not only midline, but specific to one level or location, it may represent, depending on the history, a fracture, infection, or malignancy. Pain worse on either side of the spine generally indicates muscular injury, particularly if it is predominantly to one side. However, this type of paraspinal muscle pain is so common to many low back conditions it may be difficult to isolate. Certainly, the more diffuse and widespread the pain, the more likely there is to be a generalized spinal problem, such as arthritis, multi-level disc degeneration, or muscular weakness.

Peripheral

Pain extending to the legs is frequently associated with low back disorders. The nature and distribution of this pain is important in determining its cause and the source within the spine. An important question to ask is whether the pain is worse in the back with secondary radiation to the buttocks and legs, or whether the pain is actually more severe in one or both legs. 'Leg pain' should be considered pain below the fold of the buttock in the thigh, lower leg, or foot. Leg pain is generally indicative of referred or radicular pain, secondary to nerve root compression or traction, and is commonly called 'sciatica'. Pain that is principally in the back with radiation to the buttocks and possibly the back of the thigh is more likely to be caused by facet or disc pain. The more specific the leg pain, the more specific the nerve compression. For example, a disc herniation with pressure on the right L5 nerve root will often cause right-sided, leg-dominant pain localized to the outside of the lower leg and foot. Spinal stenosis, a narrowing of the spinal canal secondary to degenerative change, causes pressure on a number of roots such that the leg symptoms are still dominant but in this case more diffuse.

Pain radiating to the legs may be associated with symptoms suggesting nerve dysfunction, such as numbness, pins-and-needles type tingling, or weakness in a muscle group. The

Back Pain vs. Leg Pain

Back-dominant Pain
- Worst pain is in the low back.
- Pain may radiate to one or both buttocks.
- Leg pain mild or intermittent.

Leg-dominant Pain
- Worst pain is in the legs.
- Leg pain is below the buttock as far as the toes.
- Back pain may exist but is less bothersome.

more specific and localized these symptoms, the more likely they represent true nerve damage. The exception to this is the serious condition called 'cauda equina syndrome', in which significant compression of the contents of the spinal canal results in generalized loss of power, sensation, and bowel or bladder control. This rapidly developing situation is considered an emergency.

Different locations of pain can, and frequently do, exist at the same time in the same person. Trying to establish the one or two principal sources and identifying secondary pain from radiation is a useful exercise in both the diagnosis and management of low back pain.

Associated Symptoms

Besides pain, low back disorders can be associated with a large number of other symptoms that often further help clarify the diagnosis. Sensory nerve dysfunction can lead to feelings of 'pins and needles', itching, tingling, burning, or frank loss of feeling over a specific area of the skin. The more localized and specific the area, the more likely a certain nerve root is compressed or damaged. Motor nerve dysfunction may be more subtle and hard to detect. However, when significant it may result in loss of the ability to move a joint (for example, lifting up the great toe) or weakness such as reduced strength to depress the break, clutch, and gas pedals of your car.

Loss of bladder control, either the inability to go or involuntary release of urine, is a serious symptom that requires emergency assessment. Loss of bowel continence

Movements and Positions

Perhaps the most useful descriptors of pain are those concerning aggravating or relieving factors. With regard to the low back, this predominantly involves movements and positions. These factors also provide the basis for some of the systems used to classify low back pain into diagnostic and treatment groups.

Bending, Lifting, Twisting, Vibration

Back pain that is aggravated by bending, lifting, twisting, and other such movements is generally considered 'mechanical' in nature. It is brought on by motion of the spinal elements during normal activities and relieved by lying down. Typically, pain that is worse with forward bending is considered to be arising from the disc. Disc pain is also aggravated by twisting or flexing sideways, as well as by vibration, caused by riding in a vehicle, for example.

Extension, Straightening, Arching

Back pain that is worse with extension is usually associated with the facet joints and is irritated by straightening up from a bent position, lying on your belly, or arching backward.

should be treated with similar concern. These symptoms indicate compression of the leash of exiting nerve roots at the bottom of the spinal cord and is termed cauda equina syndrome. This syndrome is also associated with weakness or numbness in both legs and loss of skin sensation over the 'saddle' area between your legs.

Other important symptoms include heaviness or fatigue in the legs with walking, or a feeling as if you are walking on cotton wool. This may indicate tightness in the spinal canal termed spinal stenosis.

While the majority of low back disorders are localized to the spine and produce no ill effects on the rest of the body, general health issues and systemic symptoms are important to assess as they may help with the diagnosis and unveil potentially serious conditions of the spine or other areas. For example, onset of back pain associated with fever or chills may indicate a spinal infection or an infection of the kidney. The two symptoms may be coincidental and unrelated (a back strain and a bout of the flu, for example), but they should be evaluated by your doctor. The same is true of nausea, vomiting, or dramatic change in bowel activity, such as constipation or diarrhea. In a woman, increased or irregular menstrual bleeding associated with back pain may indicate endometriosis, ectopic pregnancy, or fibroids. Rapid and unexplained weight loss, excessive sweating at night, or anemia points to a potentially serious problem such as malignancy and warrants full investigation.

Cauda equina Syndrome Symptoms ('Red Flag')

- Inability to pass urine.
- Full bladder with leaking.
- Loss of bowel continence.
- Loss of feeling or power in both legs.
- Loss of feeling in the 'saddle' area between the legs.

Catching
Sudden 'catching' pain on a certain motion suggests instability of one of the spinal segments.

Prolonged Posture
Pain associated with prolonged posture generally points to muscle fatigue or spinal imbalance.

Coughing, Sneezing
Most individuals will experience an increase in central back pain with coughing or sneezing, but this is due to sudden contraction of sensitive muscles. Increased peripheral or radicular pain with coughing, however, may indicate nerve compression within the spinal canal.

Peripheral Symptoms
Peripheral symptoms may also be aggravated by movement. Leg pain associated with prolonged extension of the spine during walking, for example, often indicates tightness or 'stenosis' within the spinal canal such as occurs with advanced degeneration. Patients with this condition also develop 'heaviness' or even numbness in their legs with standing. They often rest in a flexed position (sitting or leaning over a shopping cart) to relieve the discomfort. Some individuals with sciatica find their leg symptoms are worsened or eased by certain activities or positions, and this can have an important bearing on their treatment and outcome.

Intensity

Finding words to describe the seriousness of your pain is probably one of the hardest things to do. Pain is such an individual experience that the vocabulary required to explain it to someone else is often quite inadequate. Descriptions such as 'ache' or 'sore' are incomplete, while something as graphic as "it's like someone has taken a red hot dagger and twisted it into my spine" is not an experience many can relate to.

Nevertheless, the type of pain experienced can sometimes be helpful in working toward a diagnosis. A sharp, stabbing pain is often due to muscle injury, while a dull, burning ache suggests a possible degenerative disorder. Deep, gnawing, or boring, unforgiving pain may relate to stimulation of the sympathetic pain nerves. If this type of pain is continuous and unrelieved by rest or at night, it may indicate a more serious problem such as infection or malignancy.

Pain Scales

Intensity of pain is also difficult to describe and is best considered on a scale, numerically or visually on a color-coded scale.

Numerical Scale:

Zero "0" = No Pain ———— to ———— Ten "10" = Worst Pain Imaginable

Visual Analog Scale:

No Pain ———— to ———— Worst Pain Imaginable

Color Scale:

No Pain: Cool Blue ———— to ———— Worst Pain: Red Hot

Guidelines for Seeking Medical Care

Unfortunately, it is impossible to dictate strict rules as to when a patient with back pain should seek medical attention. Individual patients vary so much in their presentation and experience of symptoms that rules can never apply to everyone. We all have our own level of comfort with our health, some of us worrying too much, others not enough, so the final decision as to when to see a doctor will always reside with the individual. However, having said that, it is possible to set some guidelines to help in the decision-making process.

These guidelines apply equally to patients with new onset back pain, to patients suffering recurrent pain, and to chronic pain sufferers with sudden significant increase in symptoms. Without any of the 'warning' signs to indicate an emergency or urgent visit to the doctor, you may decide to follow some of the simple treatment guidelines presented later in this book and see if the pain settles down. Remembering that nearly 90% of individuals who develop low back pain will have recovered sufficient to resume most normal activities within 4 weeks, you should remain optimistic. This also applies to those with recurrent attacks, though timeframes and treatments may vary. If indeed your pain does subside, learn from the experience, start a preventive program, and be prepared should a further episode occur in the future.

The effort to determine the seriousness of your pain may have allayed fears or raised concerns, depending on your specific symptoms. If you feel you need to see a medical professional about your back pain, the next chapter will better prepare you to do so.

Chronic Pain

The causes of chronic low back pain vary considerably. Some people may do well with treatments such as exercise, diet and lifestyle changes, natural therapies, and supplements; others may require surgery. In some cases a 'cure' may not be possible, but controlling your symptoms and staying 'in charge' of your back will allow a normal lifestyle.

Seeking Medical Attention

Reasons to Seek "Emergency" (within hours) Attention:
- Significant injury, accident or fall with development of low back pain or sharp increase in pre-existing back pain.
- Symptoms of cauda equina syndrome.
- Rapid onset of back pain associated with high fever.
- Sudden development in back pain in the presence of osteoporosis.
- Rapidly worsening back pain unrelieved by rest.

Reasons to Seek 'Urgent' (within days) Attention:
- Associated unexplained weight loss.
- History of cancer.
- Severe unremitting night pain.
- Loss of feeling in one leg or reduced strength (unless associated with symptoms of cauda equina syndrome in which case it should be considered an emergency).
- Symptoms to indicate a 'non-spinal' cause of the back pain.

Reasons to Seek Attention within 4 to 6 Weeks:
- Back pain not resolving or getting worse.
- Persistent or progressive nerve dysfunction (numbness, weakness, etc)
- Symptoms suggesting 'instability' such as catching or locking.
- Back pain that improves with exercise, associated hip, heel, or foot pain (may indicate an inflammatory arthritis).
- Age over 50 years.

Who Treats Back Pain?

Despite preliminary efforts to determine the seriousness of your back pain, the severity of the discomfort, combined with poor localization and referral to other areas, makes it difficult to rationalize. Add to this problem the restricted mobility back pain often enforces, as well as the potentially strange associated symptoms such as numbness or nausea, and suddenly it becomes a frightening experience. If you pull a leg muscle it generally hurts in one area; there may even be some local bruising. It hurts when you press it or try to move or stretch adjacent joints. The problem is easy to understand and cope with. Rest, ice, and it will likely resolve in a few days. While the same may be true for the majority of back pain, the severity of the symptoms often frightens one into conjuring up a myriad of serious conditions as a cause. This inevitably leads to a visit to the doctor.

The decision to seek medical attention is not taken lightly by most people as it implies significant concern about the health issue. Who do you see? What kind of medical professionals diagnose and treat back pain?

Emergency Care

For symptoms needing emergency attention, the doctor of first contact will vary according to your circumstances, location, and medical system.

Ideally, an emergent visit to your family doctor is the best because your doctor has access to your medical history, including previous related tests, consultations, or surgeries, and can use this in formulating a diagnosis. You can then be referred, if appropriate, to a hospital for specialist assessment and investigation.

Unfortunately, this route is not always possible and a trip to the emergency department may be your only way of timely access to care. For symptoms of cauda equina syndrome in particular, time is of the essence and you should not delay treatment. Make your symptoms known to the admitting nurse so an informed decision can be made as to your triage status.

'Red Flags'

- Significant injury
- Symptoms of cauda equina syndrome
- Severe, unremitting night pain
- Fever
- History of cancer
- Rapid and unexplained weight loss
- History of osteoporosis or steroid medication

Family Doctor

With persistent or recurrent back pain, a visit to your family doctor will likely be the first step in the process of diagnosis and treatment. This may involve blood tests, special investigations, and referral to other practitioners for treatment or consultation.

While not a specialist in back pain, injury, or disease, your family doctor will be more comfortable treating certain back conditions than others, depending upon training and experience. Orthopedic training is sadly inadequate for most family doctors, dependant on individual post-graduate learning effort. Family doctors also often lack adequate time in their schedules to perform a complete diagnostic assessment. However, your doctor will be able to identify the 'Red Flags' indicative of more serious conditions and organize urgent or emergency referral. Your doctor will also be able to reassure you if you have interpreted some of your symptoms incorrectly and are concerned about some unpleasant underlying pathology.

Whatever your diagnosis and subsequent medical course, your family doctor should be able to provide a pivotal point around which management of your back pain should center. Whether you suffer a simple back strain that resolves with a few sessions of physiotherapy or a disc herniation requiring specialist assessment and surgery, it is invaluable to have one individual who coordinates care. This avoids missed diagnoses, duplication of tests, over- or under-treatment, multiple medications, and, above all, a confused and disoriented patient.

Family Doctor's Role

- Assesses presence of 'Red Flag' causes of low back pain.
- Puts your back pain in the perspective of your medical history.
- Coordinates care, referrals, investigations, and medications.
- Recommends non-surgical treatments.

Naturopathic Doctor

Naturopathic medicine is complementary to traditional 'allopathic' medicine. The symbiosis of naturopathic and allopathic treatments can often achieve a better outcome than either alone.

Naturopathic Doctor's Role

- Assesses presence of 'Red Flag' causes of low back pain.
- Offers advice on diet and natural supplementation.
- Recommends natural therapies such as massage and acupuncture.
- Organizes a preventive program.
- Provides support during traditional treatments (such as medication, injection therapy, or surgery).

Naturopathic doctors are trained in the use of clinical nutrition, botanical or herbal medicine, homeopathic medicine, traditional Chinese medicine and acupuncture, hands-on techniques, and lifestyle counseling. Training for naturopathic medicine is extensive. A three-year degree of pre-med study at university is followed by a four-year, full-time program at a naturopathic college. In all licensed provinces or states in North America, a naturopathic physician must also pass licensing exams (such as NPLEX in some states and provinces in North America) before being allowed to practice.

A naturopathic doctor uses natural substances and therapies to stimulate the body's innate healing response and thus to produce a therapeutic effect. Prevention of disease is a central concept within naturopathic medicine, which emphasizes patient education to reduce the incidence of disease and education of the physical body itself, strengthening its component parts to improve overall health and thus to resist disease.

Naturopathic doctors will evaluate not only your back, but also your entire health and lifestyle. In the event of potentially serious pathology, they will refer you to an appropriate specialist or suggest you contact your family medical doctor. If traditional treatment is required (surgery, for example), they can help prepare your body and then aid recovery. Naturopathic treatments for back conditions include dietary changes and natural supplementation (minerals, herbal medicines, etc.), physical therapies such as acupuncture and massage, and techniques for relaxation and stress management to help you cope with your back pain.

Orthopedic Surgeon

Orthopedic surgery is the medical specialty concerned with the locomotor system — the bones, joints, muscles, ligaments, and tendons of the body that provide support and allow movement. From the neck to the feet, orthopedic surgeons treat strains, fractures, dislocations, instabilities, and arthritis. Although they do perform surgeries, including joint replacement, arthroscopy, and fracture repair, they evaluate and coordinate many non-surgical therapies beneficial to the healing and repair of the musculoskeletal system. After medical school and internship, orthopedic surgeons generally train for four years in a residency program before spending one to two years in subspecialty fellowships, honing their skills in a particular field such as total joint replacement.

Orthopedic surgeons, as with many specialties, often have areas of particular interest or expertise. Although all orthopedists will have done some spine surgery during their training, only some will feel they have had sufficient experience to continue this in practice. They may have chosen to complete a fellowship program, working closely with a spinal surgeon as post-graduate specialty training. These individuals will generally concentrate on building a spine-based practice, seeing patients with spinal disorders and concentrating on spinal surgery.

While orthopedic surgeons specializing in other areas such as knee or shoulder reconstruction are equally as capable of assessing patients with back problems, they would not proceed with surgery if required, instead referring the patient to a spine specialist. This process inevitably results in greater delays for the patient, so seeing a spinal expert with a direct referral is best. Of course referral to an orthopedic surgeon or spinal expert does not mean you are going to have surgery. Apart from certain emergencies, such as cauda equina syndrome or a severe fracture, surgery remains a last resort. Your orthopedist will ensure that all other appropriate non-surgical therapies have been tried before recommending an operation. Even then, the decision to go ahead is yours. The orthopedic surgeon will explain the available options, benefits, and risks so you can come to an informed decision.

Rheumatologist

Rheumatology is a subspecialty of internal medicine, comprising the study and treatment of arthritis and many diverse rheumatologic disorders affecting joints and numerous other tissues and organs throughout the body. Rheumatologists treat all forms of arthritis and specialize in the evaluation and diagnosis of the many diffuse inflammatory conditions, such as rheumatoid arthritis, SLE, and psoriatic arthritis. They plan medical treatment, including physiotherapy, occupational therapy, medication, and injection therapy. Apart from a small number performing simple office diagnostic arthroscopy, they do not perform surgery.

Some rheumatologists take a special interest in back pain and can be very helpful, not only in ruling out generalized inflammatory diseases such as rheumatoid arthritis and anky-losing spondylitis, but also in the non-operative management of spinal conditions. This may involve physical therapies, medication, or injections, depending on the cause. In the presence of symptoms or findings that suggest a rheumatologic cause for your back pain, evaluation and testing will help identify the underlying inflammatory process. In some cases the rheumatologist may then suggest a progressive trial of medication to control your symptoms.

Orthopedic Surgeon's Role

- Evaluates complicated or 'Red Flag' back problems.
- Evaluates back pain after significant trauma.
- Uses examination and investigations to determine diagnosis in persistent, recurrent, or chronic low back pain.
- Suggests invasive treatments such as injection therapy.
- Evaluates for surgically treatable pathology.

Rheumatologic Symptoms

- Known pre-existing rheumatologic condition.
- Family history of inflammatory disease.
- Pain, swelling, and stiffness in other joints.
- Fever, skin rash, bowel upset, visual disturbance.
- Associated heel or foot pain.
- Back pain for over 3 months *improved* with exercise.
- History of sexually transmitted disease or other infection.

Physiotherapist

Physiotherapy provided by a registered therapist has a number of important roles to play in the management of low back pain. Physiotherapists provide a valuable interface between the patient and the low back condition, one that offers a human aspect with understanding, compassion, and encouragement. True, many treatments and programs can be instituted by the patients themselves without formal referral; however, this might be likened to the difference between an automated customer service telephone line and one where you actually get to speak to a real person. For many, the interaction with a trained professional instills confidence through a greater understanding of the problem while allaying fears. At a time when doctors, in particular, are often unable to offer sufficient time with a patient to explain the condition and answer the many questions it arouses, the role of the physiotherapist is of increasing importance.

Physiotherapy involves a number of processes all aimed at recovery and prevention of further injury. The first of these is education. Reinforcement of the reassurance provided by other medical practitioners is supported by a more in-depth explanation of the anatomy and biomechanics of the low back pain. Even in the many cases where a specific diagnosis is elusive, an understanding of the way the back works and the mechanisms behind pain development will help the patient rationalize the problem. This will reduce fear and encourage participation in a program to recover.

Physiotherapist's Role

- Provides patient education and instruction.
- Develops and monitors treatment program.
- Employs formal modalities and manipulation.
- Modifies activity and technique.
- Develops strategies for preventing re-injury or recurrence.

 BACK FACTS

Many patients with back pain have probably never even attempted a sit-up, let alone been involved in a comprehensive gym-based exercise program. For these individuals, instruction is vital for establishing a routine and for checking technique to prevent injury. Once established, many routines can be performed independently with periodic review, modification, and encouragement.

The physiotherapist can help improve function by instruction on correct posture, gait, bending and lifting as well as positions for rest and relief of pain. Activity modification and ergonomic evaluation will further help progress an individual on their return to normal daily life.

Manipulation involves the mobilization of joints and soft tissues to improve range of motion and reduce pain and clearly involves a direct 'hands-on' approach. Use of diagnostic tests to categorize low back pain (for example, the McKenzie technique) improves the specificity of treatment and becomes more important as back pain persists beyond the acute phase or shows little response to standard treatment.

Here the physiotherapist will assess and monitor the program and modify it according to clinical parameters.

Use of modalities such as ice, heat, and ultrasound offer additional therapeutic options to enhance a rehabilitation program. Ultrasound or diathermy require monitoring and are performed largely in the physiotherapy setting. Modalities such as heat and ice can be harmful if used inappropriately, so instruction is important before progressing to independent use.

Educating a patient in the prevention of re-injury is a vital role for the physiotherapist. Technique modification, posture, ergonomics, combined with an ongoing independent exercise and conditioning program, offer the back pain sufferers an opportunity to take self-responsibility for their condition and avoid recurrence.

Occupational Therapist

Occupational therapy, like physiotherapy, can play a pivotal role in the treatment and management of low back pain. A physiotherapist may work closely with an occupational therapist with respect to posture and ergonomics (teaching correct and safe techniques for tasks at home and in the workplace). Occupational therapy is also involved with splinting and the provision or adaptation of devices that enable easy functioning.

Occupational therapists are involved in patient education, particularly with reference to daily activity. Activity modification involves pacing and postural retraining to minimize discomfort and maximize function. Recommending and providing of mechanical aids is an aspect of the OT's work that is extremely varied. It extends from provision of a simple cane through devices for home or the workplace, such as a foot-stool, improved seating, or lumbar supports. A full assessment of a work-station can often offer tremendous ergonomic improvements to prevent recurrence of low back pain.

Occupational Therapist's Role

- Provides patient education.
- Modifies activity and offers ergonomic training.
- Advises on activity aids for home and work.

Chiropractor

The term chiropractic comes from the ancient Greek word 'cheiro', meaning 'hand', and 'praktikos', meaning 'doing'. Chiropractors use their hands to diagnose and treat disorders of the spine, joints, and muscles. Chiropractors use two types of manual spinal movements, 'mobilizations' and 'manipulations', to correct 'malalignment' within the lumbar spine thought to be responsible for pain in a number of low back conditions.

Chiropractic care was originally developed by Canadian osteopath Daniel David Palmer. In 1895, Palmer manipulated the spine of his office janitor, who had been suffering from back pain for 17 years. The janitor heard a 'click' noise, and

- Assesses presence of 'Red Flag' causes of low back pain.

- Manages acute low back pain episodes.

- Prescribes exercises to prevent further episodes of low back pain.

- Organizes other aspects of a preventive program.

his back pain was said to be completely resolved. Although this is a very dramatic result from a single chiropractic treatment, this type of care continues to provide a popular form of relief for back pain sufferers.

Chiropractic treatment remains extremely popular in North America despite the fact that its efficacy remains largely unproven, mainly due to lack of adequate clinical trials. A review of 36 randomized trials published in the journal *Spine* concluded that although there appeared to be indications that spinal manipulation was beneficial in some groups, further research efforts were recommended. The most significant benefit from chiropractic care appears to be for individuals with uncomplicated *acute* low back pain, a conclusion supported by a number of studies. In addition, patient satisfaction is found to be higher with chiropractors than with other medical practitioners. As yet, there is no evidence that long-term chiropractic care in the absence of symptoms prevents back pain or other spinal pathology such as arthritis.

Osteopath

Doctors of Osteopathy (DOs) have widespread acceptance in the United States and the United Kingdom, where their professions are recognized on par with regular medical doctors. DOs, like MDs, are fully licensed and authorized to prescribe medication and perform surgery. While the majority of manipulative spinal care in the United States is carried out by chiropractors, Doctors of Osteopathy (DOs) have become increasingly popular and respected. In the United Kingdom, where chiropractic has yet to make a significant impact, osteopathy is an integral part of the medical system for back care. In Canada, the Ministry of Colleges and Universities has not yet recognized the only college of osteopathy in Montreal and the profession remains without official government designation.

Osteopaths employ a method termed Osteopathic Manual Medicine (OMM) to increase flow of body fluids, combining body positioning with gentle pressure to predominantly soft tissue areas rather than bones or joints. In addition, a DO may use manual therapy in combination with traditional treatments such as medication or surgery. Osteopaths treat all forms of medical and musculoskeletal illness, much like a family doctor, using a combination of treatments aimed at enhancing the body's own unique ability to heal itself.

Research supports a role for osteopathy predominantly in the sub-acute phase of uncomplicated low back pain, after about 10 to 14 days. Overall the treatment appears to reduce discomfort and promote a more rapid return to function. There is no research to support long-term treatment as a preventive measure.

Osteopath's Role

- Assesses for presence of 'Red Flag' causes of low back pain.

- Manages sub-acute low back pain episodes (2 to 10 weeks).

- Advises on exercises to prevent further episodes of low back pain.

- Offers comprehensive and holistic medical management.

Massage Therapist

Massage has long been used as a technique for controlling pain. Defined as the treatment of disease or injury through the manual manipulation of body tissues, massage is employed to relieve pain and spasm, to induce relaxation, to stretch and break down scarring and adhesions, and to increase circulation and metabolism. Massage promotes the resorption and metabolism of toxins and the residua of inflammation.

On the basis of a number of clinical studies, massage therapy is shown to be beneficial in the treatment of low back pain. No matter what type of massage therapy is administered, most people experience both pain relief and a sense of relaxation and well-being after a treatment. It can help relieve the muscular spasm associated with back pain and known to increase pain and sensitivity.

However, we would not generally recommend massage during the acute phase (first 48 to 72 hours) of low back pain secondary to a lumbar muscle strain or a disc herniation with sciatica.

Acupuncturist

Acupuncture is a therapeutic method for promoting natural healing of the body through the insertion of needles. It is most widely employed in the treatment of musculoskeletal pain and has specific application to the management of low back disorders where the National Institutes for Health in the USA has approved its role. We have found it particularly efficacious in the treatment of radicular or radiating 'nerve pain', such as sciatica, and for the relief of muscle spasm.

Chronic Pain Specialist

Only a small number of back pain sufferers will need a specialist of this type. Treatment in this field is reserved for those with 'chronic back pain syndrome', a complex of symptoms involving significant mental and emotional involvement. A chronic pain specialist will often not work alone, drawing on a number of medical and counseling professionals, including psychiatrists and social workers, to best manage all aspects of your low back pain and their effect on your lifestyle.

Massage Therapist's Role

- Begins treatment of lumbar strain after first 48 hours.
- Manages recurrent or persistent low back pain.
- Works to relieve muscle spasm.
- Plays part in a stress management program to reduce back pain recurrence.

Acupuncturist's Role

- Treats acute and persistent low back pain.
- Treats radiating 'nerve pain' such as sciatica.
- Manages recurrent or persistent low back pain.
- Helps in back pain secondary to arthritis.

Chronic Pain Specialist's Role

- Determines if your symptom complex fits the 'chronic back pain syndrome' picture.
- Educates you as to the numerous facets of care vital to your recovery.
- Assesses your status to produce a multi-dimensional diagnosis.
- Coordinates specialist care to address all issues, including your back.

How Is Back Pain Diagnosed?

The experience you have when seeing a medical professional about your back pain will depend on a number of factors. A consultation in a busy emergency department is going to be very different from a visit to the family doctor you have known for 30 years. Family doctors and specialists may have a different approach to your problem and, depending on the circumstances of your visit, will likely have different amounts of time available.

Although varying in approach taken and time given, the pattern of assessment is much the same whomever you see. Investigations aimed at securing a diagnosis may increase anxiety in the patient and even confusion in the physician. There are, however, categories and diagnoses that, when identified and used correctly, will be of benefit.

✔ BACK FACTS

The role of diagnosis varies according to the circumstances and timing of low back pain. Recent onset back pain requires that serious 'Red Flag' pathology be ruled out, but beyond that, a specific diagnosis is not required. Remember that 90% of cases will settle within 4 to 6 weeks with standard treatment, making identification of individual causes irrelevant. Reassurance and an active treatment plan can be instituted with arrangement for follow up.

Benefits of Diagnosis

From the patient's point of view, a diagnosis is a marvelous thing to have. It gives you a reason for your pain, making it easier to rationalize and justify. When friends or colleagues or employers ask you why you are not at work or are unable to play golf, telling them you have 'back pain' rarely arouses much sympathy. The subject of low back pain is so rife with preconceptions and the symptoms so variable that it is hard for someone not suffering to understand your situation. However, tell them you have "facet pain" or a "degenerate disc at L5-S1 with possible nerve compression" and suddenly you have a bona fide problem that sounds serious. A basket of fruit is likely to replace cynical telephone commiserations.

A diagnosis gives the patient hope that the condition is treatable and curable. 'Back pain of an unknown origin' seems such a nebulous term that it is unlikely to respond to any specific therapy and probably will never go away. A diagnosis of 'facet pain', however, offers potential for cause-directed treatment and cure — fix the facet and the pain will be gone.

From the doctor's point of view, a clear diagnosis increases credibility with patients. Low back pain sufferers feel they are in good hands with a knowledgeable professional. A diagnosis also enables doctors to better understand their patients. Pain is notoriously difficult to explain, the experience so individual that a medical professional may have trouble relating to your symptoms. With a diagnosis comes a sense of physical appreciation for the problem, an awareness that 'yes, that must hurt'. With that understanding comes the ability to explain the cause of the pain and thus to give reassurance to the patient.

Once the physician has a possible cause, the investigations can begin. This again will comfort the patient, who, like the doctor, is anxious to confirm any diagnostic suspicions. If nothing else, this process will buy some time, which, as we have seen, is often all that is needed for the pain to resolve.

However, if an acute episode does not resolve within the expected time and pain becomes prolonged, there needs to be more effort expended in searching for a diagnosis or category. Ruling out serious 'Red Flags' remains a priority, but defining a cause for the pain will help improve the specificity of treatment and promote recovery.

If surgery is contemplated, then a highly specific diagnosis is required. Clinical findings and investigations should correlate and the surgery should be tailored to treat the identified cause of the pain. Only when these conditions are satisfied is the outcome likely to be successful.

Benefits of Diagnosis

- Reassures the patient.
- Guides type and timing of investigations to be performed.
- Improves understanding and interpretation of tests.
- Directs treatment protocols.
- Allows discussion of prognosis and outcome.

History

Perhaps the most important part of the diagnosis of back pain is evaluating your medical history. Here you will be asked to describe your symptoms, when they started, how long have they been present, and if you have had them before. It is important at this stage to indicate if you have had previous investigations, treatments, or surgery on your back. The nature of the pain will be elucidated, the location, temporal pattern, radiation and referral, and severity, along with associated symptoms. The predominance of back or leg pain is a valuable piece of information. Factors that make the pain better or worse are important, as are limitations the pain incurs.

Past medical history is important, especially as it relates to infections, osteoporosis, or cancer. Pre-existing osteoporosis, post-menopausal symptoms, or an association with steroid medication would raise the suspicion of vertebral compression fracture. A history of osteoarthritis or rheumatoid arthritis may indicate involvement of the spine if back pain develops. Arthritis in the hips can result in back pain; it is distinguished by associated groin pain, a limp, and trouble reaching the toes. Past history of cancer with recent onset of back pain should be evaluated to rule out spread to the bones of the spine.

General health will also be assessed, including systemic symptoms such as fever, weight loss, and fatigue. Family history is useful, particularly as it relates to arthritic conditions. Any medications, including herbs or supplements, should be discussed and any allergies noted.

Information regarding your lifestyle, family situation, sports involvement, and employment duties will help better determine your abilities, degree of incapacity, and most appropriate treatment regimen.

Finally, it is often helpful to find out if there is one particular concern about the back pain. For example, some individuals are convinced they have a malignant tumor, others a serious fracture, still others are fearful that they will need immediate surgery. Patients may have had a bad experience with a friend or relative and have often received misguided and often frightening advice from friends, co-workers, or even other physicians. Knowing this allows the physician to tailor explanations and discussion to reduce anxiety.

Health History Workup

Pain Characteristics	pain onset and duration, recurrence and persistence, intensity previous investigations, treatment, surgery
General Health	presence of infections, osteoporosis, cancer
Family History	other conditions or diseases, especially arthritis
Medications	current use of drugs, herbs, vitamins, etc.
Lifestyle	family, work, and sports demands and limitations
Anxiety	fear of fractures, tumors, surgery

Examination

Having formulated a provisional diagnosis from the history, the physician will proceed to a physical examination, which will either confirm suspicions or lead to alternative possibilities and further questioning.

Examination of the spine requires it to be visible and free to move. Taking a pair of shorts to the examination is a good idea. This allows access to the spine and legs without getting undressed down to underwear. A gown should be available for warmth and modesty.

 BACK FACTS

Try to cooperate with the exam as much as possible, and let the doctor know if there are any particularly tender areas or movements before the exam begins. As doctors we want to know what hurts but we do not want to hurt you. Remember, the more we can test and examine, the more we are likely to be able to help with a diagnosis and treatment.

The examination involves both observation and testing. The physician will be able to evaluate posture and gait, abnormal rhythm and alignment, spinal curvature and motion through watching you move during the evaluation. Tests of mobility include flexing or extending in different directions — again, try to do these within your range of comfort and let the doctor know when it hurts and where the pain is. Remember, exaggerating your pain is not helpful. Your physician is less likely to make objective interpretations of your pain if you grimace and scream with every tiny movement or slightest touch. The physician will be less likely to perform a complete examination for fear of hurting you and may therefore miss important diagnostic information.

Many of the tests carried out during the examination are specifically designed to assess the status of your nerves. Maneuvers such as the straight leg raise and thigh extension (femoral stretch) aim to discover the presence of nerve root irritation and referred or radicular pain. Tests of reflexes, strength, and sensation look for nerve dysfunction, a sign of damage by compression or traction. If there is cause for concern, a more detailed assessment of sensation including pin-prick, cotton wool touch, and vibration will be made. A rectal exam may be requested if there is concern about cauda equina syndrome as it provides extremely important information about this emergency condition.

Evaluation of the hips will help rule out arthritis at this joint as a cause of your back pain. Assessment of leg lengths both lying and standing is valuable to look for potential postural factors. Checking the pulses in the groins and remainder of the legs can reveal evidence of arterial blood flow insufficiency, which produces pain in the legs on walking. The differences between this 'vascular claudication' and the 'neurogenic claudication' of spinal stenosis (narrowing due to arthritis or disc herniation) include location, character, and aggravating or relieving factors.

Vascular vs. Neurogenic Claudication

An important diagnostic distinction to make is between spinal stenosis (also called neurogenic claudication) and vascular claudication (resulting from narrow arteries and inadequate blood flow to the muscles of the legs). Careful examination and measurement of blood flow using Doppler ultrasound will enable the correct diagnosis to be made.

Vascular claudication pain results from inadequate blood supply to exercising muscles. Any exercise can bring symptoms on, and pain is only eased by resting those muscles. The clothing shopper who has walked for hours has to stand and look through store windows for a while.

Neurogenic claudication results from compression of nerve root within the spine and is brought on by having the spine in an extended position. Thus, walking uphill or cycling in which the spine is flexed may not induce symptoms. Rest has to be with the spine flexed forward. The grocery shopper has to sit down or bend over the supermarket trolley to keep moving around the store.

Symptom	Vascular Claudication	Neurogenic Claudication
Pain location	Most frequently in the calf, can be one side	Lower legs, feet, sometimes thighs, usually both sides
Pain type	Deep, cramping pain	Burning, heaviness, numbness
Inducing factor	Any walking, particularly uphill, cycling	Walking upright or downhill, standing for long periods
Relieving factors	Rest, standing or sitting	Rest in flexed position, walking or sitting

Classifications of Symptoms

There are numerous ways to categorize back pain symptoms: the timing and severity of symptoms; the pattern of pain, including site and aggravating or relieving factors; and specific anatomic or pathologic diagnosis. Each has advantages and limitations in diagnosis, depending on the individual and the circumstances. Employing a combination of the various systems provides the best individual approach. For example, an individual with back pain following a lifting injury might usefully be diagnosed with 'disc strain', but treatment will be based on a combination of symptom chronology and pattern. A patient with severe leg pain and numbness will be best served with a diagnosis combining chronology along with 'disc herniation'. If surgery was planned for this patient, then the specific anatomic level and side of the disc herniation would be essential.

Temporal Classifications

The language you learned for describing your pain in terms of onset, duration, recurrence, and persistence can now be used to assist in diagnosis. Categorizing low back pain according to these timeframes and patterns is relatively easy because it does not rely on the vagaries of symptoms, rather on the more precise parameter of chronology.

The value of this system of categorizing low back pain is in planning treatment and initiating further investigations. While not specifically providing a diagnosis, it helps guide the physician in timing of tests, such as X-rays, CT or MRI, making referrals to specialists, and gauging the progress of therapy.

Medical Protocol Based on Temporal Classifications

Healthcare professionals follow this kind of protocol based on temporal classifications when diagnosing back conditions.

Acute
- Rule out serious 'Red Flag' pathology.
- Reassure patient.
- Institute initial phase of treatment.

Sub-Acute
- Order investigations appropriate to age, presentation, clinical findings.
- Consider specialist referral.
- Modify treatment to target clinically suspected cause of pain.

Recurrent and Persistent (Chronic)
- Review investigations and treatment to date.
- Re-evaluate possible causes of pain.
- Expand scope of investigations as indicated.
- Refer to specialist.
- Consider injection tests (discogram, facet blocks, nerve blocks) to aid diagnosis.
- Plan therapy to address diagnosis, including therapeutic injections and surgery if indicated.

The Clinical Practice Guideline for Categorizing Pain

- Potentially Serious Spinal Conditions.
- Sciatica.
- Non-specific Low Back Pain.

The Clinical Practice Guideline (Seriousness)

Low back pain can be categorized into degrees of 'seriousness', using The Clinical Practice Guideline. This guideline is designed for acute, uncomplicated back pain of less than 3 months duration, primarily in the 18 to 45 year old working population, and excludes chronic low back pain.

Three degrees of seriousness are defined: potentially serious spinal conditions; sciatica; and non-specific low back pain. The 'potentially serious' category is designed to include those conditions suspected by 'Red Flags' in the presentation (trauma, cauda equina, infection, cancer and osteoporosis) as well as non-spinal causes of back pain such as kidney disease or ulcer. The non-serious conditions are either 'sciatica' due to nerve compression or 'non-specific', a category that includes almost everything else and by far the majority of people with back pain. The division into 'sciatica' and 'non-specific' is of benefit in predicting outcome and longevity of symptoms as recovery is usually longer in the presence of leg pain.

Quebec Task Force Classification

The recognition that doctors were particularly poor at identifying the specific anatomic origin of pain encouraged development of a system of diagnosis based on patterns of symptoms. The results of the 1987 Quebec Task Force study produced a classification aimed at identifying subgroups of 'non-specific' back pain patients. Individuals in each subgroup would have similar symptoms, pain patterns, and clinical findings. These characteristics would have predictive value in

Quebec Task Force Classification

The first four categories incorporate the majority of back pain sufferers in the acute phase. Evaluation of these has shown groups 3 and 4 to have predictive value in identifying individuals with poorer prognosis and longer recovery time.

Category	Definition
1	Pain without radiation
2	Pain with proximal radiation (above the knee)
3	Pain with proximal radiation (blow the knee)
4	Pain with distal radiation and neurologic signs
5	Presumed spinal nerve root compression

appropriate treatment and likely outcome. The classification system also incorporated the results of X-ray investigations and the response to treatment

The McKenzie Classification

The McKenzie method involves assessment, treatment, and prevention of common problems of the spine and extremities. This non-invasive method uses simple movements and positions to examine and treat structures that may be a source of pain. Robin McKenzie, a physical therapist from New Zealand, is the founder of Mechanical Diagnosis and Therapy (MDT). McKenzie introduced his techniques in mid 1950s, which gradually attracted many clinicians and researchers. He established the McKenzie International Institute in 1982.

McKenzie believes the majority of disabilities of the lumbar spine to be mechanical, and thus can be treated in a mechanical manner. Mechanical evaluation uses repeated end-range movements and sustained positions in multiple directions in both upright and lying positions. Physical therapists using the McKenzie system classify a patient's condition into one of the three syndromes: postural, dysfunction, and derangement.

Postural Syndrome: This has been attributed to mechanical deformation of soft tissues and is seen commonly in individuals with poor postural habits. Maintenance of certain postures and positions places specific soft tissues under prolonged stress. Over time, poor posture can lead to premature aging and advanced wear and tear of the spinal joints.

This section written by Helen Razmjou, BSc (PT), MSc, Cred. MDT, Physical Therapist, Orthopaedic and Arthritic Institute, Sunnybrook & Women's College Health Sciences Centre, Toronto, Ontario.

Category	Definition
6	Confirmed spinal nerve root compression (on CT or MRI)
7	Spinal stenosis
8	Post-surgical pain 1–6 months after procedure
9	Post-surgical pain beyond 6 months after procedure
10	Chronic pain syndrome
11	Non-spinal causes of back pain
Category	**Duration of Pain**
a	Less than 7 days
b	7 days to 7 weeks
c	Greater than 7 weeks

Dysfunction Syndrome: The pain of dysfunction syndrome results from the stretching of structures that have become sensitive and shortened. The shortening can be caused by either prolonged, poor postural habits or incomplete recovery from an injury to the spine. Adaptive shortening leads to the loss of spinal movement in certain directions and causes pain to be produced before normal full range of movement is achieved. Thus, the dysfunction syndrome is characterized by intermittent pain and a partial loss of movement.

Derangement Syndrome: This is the most commonly seen syndrome in the lower back area. McKenzie describes this syndrome as a mechanical deformation of soft tissues as a result of internal derangement. Alteration of the position of the fluid within the disc causes a disturbance in the normal resting position of the two vertebrae. Although the derangement syndrome is usually characterized by constant pain, intermittent pain may be seen depending on the size and location of the derangement. In acute stages of derangement, certain types of 'deformities' (for example, a sudden shift of the trunk or inability to straighten the spine) may also be seen. Treating such deformity requires a skilled, McKenzie-trained practitioner, but fortunately the incidence of these acute spinal deformities is very low.

The concept of 'centralization' that was introduced by McKenzie in the mid '50s is the key to treating derangement syndrome. Centralization phenomenon describes a change in the location of pain from the foot or leg toward the midline of the spine. Centralization of pain is thought to result from a reduction in the degree of deformation or compression of the soft tissues that cause referred pain, including discs and nerve roots. Movements and positions that cause centralization are therefore desirable as they reduce the size of the derangement. It makes sense to choose an exercise that moves the pain from foot to the knee, followed by a reduction in thigh pain.

Usually in the early phase of centralization, pain in the lower back area becomes a bit more intense. However, it is permissible for pain to increase centrally, provided there is a reduction in the leg or foot pain. Movement of the pain or other symptoms, such as numbness, further away from the midline into the periphery should be avoided because it indicates that the disc or nerve root is being further irritated or compressed.

Recent studies have shown that the centralization phenomenon is a reliable predictor of final outcome. Inability to centralize pain is thought to suggest the probability that surgical intervention may be necessary.

Basic McKenzie Classification

Using the McKenzie system, patient's symptoms can be classified as 'non-mechanical' or 'mechanical'. Symptoms associated with inflammatory arthritis such as rheumatoid or ankylosing spondylitis are considered 'non-mechanical', whereas those influenced by movement and position are termed 'mechanical'. Individuals with mechanical symptoms can be divided further according to aggravating and relieving factors, movement characteristics, and clinical tests into one of the three syndromes: postural, derangement, or dysfunction.

	Symptoms	Syndrome
1.	Not produced by test movements Produced by prolonged postures	Postural Syndrome
2.	Pain on movement Rapid changes in pain location Symptoms change with repeated motion Possible spine deformity/curve Range of motion improves as pain relieved	Derangement Syndrome
3.	Pain only at end range of motion Symptoms unchanged with repeated motion Little change in range of motion as pain relieved	Dysfunction Syndrome
4.	Symptoms not reproduced with test movement Pain source outside spine	'Other'

Hamilton Hall's Pain Patterns

Toronto-based orthopedic surgeon Hamilton Hall developed one of the most patient-friendly classifications of low back pain, popularized in his book *The Back Doctor*. As with the McKenzie system, while spinal pathology may be inferred by placing a patient into one of the four 'patterns', Hamilton Hall is clear to point out that "knowing the precise physiological source of the symptoms is not relevant to recognizing the pain pattern or choosing the initial treatment."

Hall emphasizes the importance of making a distinction between 'back dominant' and 'leg dominant' pain but notes the not infrequent co-existence of both. Back dominant pain includes all pain as far as the lower extent of the buttock; below that it is considered leg pain.

The next vital step is to elicit whether the pain is constant, invariant with time of day or activity, or intermittent, allowing times or positions of pain-free comfort. Constant pain constitutes a 'red flag' and indicates a need to exclude possible systemic or non-spinal causes. Intermittent pain generally points to a mechanical cause, which can then be categorized into one of the four 'pain patterns' through further careful history and physical examination.

The four pain patterns are not exclusive; an individual may have symptoms and findings suggestive of two or more patterns at one time or sequentially. However, overall, the pattern system of categorization achieves two of the primary goals of back pain management at this stage, reassurance with explanation and direction for treatment. This latter goal provides the basis for Hall's Canadian Back Institute regimen, a three-stage program to eliminate pain, restore movement, and promote physical conditioning. The first stage in particular uses the 'pattern' diagnosis to guide postural education and exercises, although symptoms remain the most important indicator of success. They are used to modify the program according to response.

Hamilton Hall's Pain Patterns

Hall's four pain patterns can be used as an indicator of the anatomic location of the underlying spinal problem and its pathologic basis.

Spinal Pathology in Patterns 1–4

Pattern 1	Disc injury, degeneration, disruption
Pattern 2	Facet joint injury, strain or degeneration
Pattern 3	Disc herniation with nerve compression
Pattern 4	Spinal stenosis (narrowing of the spinal canal usually due to arthritis

Anatomic or Pathologic Classification

Traditional medical management of a condition or disease involves establishing a clear diagnosis combining both anatomic (where the disease is occurring) and pathologic (what is causing the disease) descriptors, achieved through a clinical history and examination, along with a battery of other investigations. Once this process is complete, a specific treatment plan is invoked aiming to cure the condition.

Unfortunately, low back pain rarely offers a clear causative diagnosis initially, and one may even remain elusive after prolonged and intensive investigation. As such, the process becomes frustrating to the doctor, who yearns for a concrete diagnosis, and to the patient, who wishes only some relief and reassurance.

In most cases of acute low back pain, the diagnosis is less important than the treatment, which can be generalized and guided by symptoms and response. In the absence of clinical findings to the contrary, the patient can be reassured that the condition is benign and likely to resolve quickly. There are, however, times when an accurate diagnosis becomes more important; indeed, in the event of surgery, it becomes essential. A diagnosis might be helpful in back pain lasting longer than 6 weeks without improvement or response to treatment. A more specific treatment regimen may improve outcome and therefore investigations are carried out, not only to exclude serious pathology, but to try and elucidate a cause. The same applies to chronic and recurrent back pain. In cases where there are 'Red Flags', a diagnosis is essential and should be sought aggressively. It is also essential in cases of persistent or progressive leg pain indicating nerve compression. With planned surgery, an accurate diagnosis of both the cause of the pain and its specific location is essential to ensure a successful result.

Sample Classifications

In cases where a diagnosis is sought, the spinal causes of back pain can be grouped according to anatomic locations and disease process. Examples include an L5-S1 disc herniation, L4-5 degenerative arthritis with spinal stenosis, or an L3-4 disc infection. With certain diagnoses, the specific location may be less specific, such as with a lumbar muscle strain or inflammatory arthritis, and occasionally the location may be clearer than the disease process — L5-S1 disc disruption, for example. Certain diagnoses may fit into more than one category. For example, disc infection could be placed in both the anatomic classification of 'disc problems' and the pathologic classification of 'infection'.

A simplified anatomic classification is to divide problems into *anterior* (front) or *posterior* (back). The anterior structures include the intervertebral disc, bony vertebral bodies, and longitudinal ligaments. The posterior structures would include the facet joints with associated capsule, bony arch, and attached ligaments. Working along similar lines to the Hamilton Hall system, it implies anterior injury is aggravated by flexion, and treatment is therefore predominantly extension, while posterior injury causes extension pain and is best managed with a flexion program.

Kirkaldy-Willis Degenerative Cascade

W.H. Kirkaldy-Willis and colleagues describe a 'degenerative cascade' involving progressive injury and deterioration in the spinal motion complex comprising two adjacent vertebrae, the disc between, and the two posterior facet joints. This classification correlates pathologic changes within the disc and facets to clinical symptoms and hence directs treatment options. This cascade has some useful applications in both

Anatomic or Pathologic Classification

Diagnosis Essential:
- Acute back pain with 'Red Flags' indicating a serious underlying cause.
- Persistent radicular (leg) pain or nerve dysfunction (numbness, weakness).
- Progressive nerve dysfunction.
- Surgical procedure planned.

Diagnosis Helpful:
- Persistent back pain beyond 6 weeks not responding to treatment.
- Chronic low back pain.
- Recurrent low back pain.

understanding and managing certain low back problems but implies a natural and inevitable progression of degeneration, which is misleading and likely to increase fear in the patient. In addition, as noted above, symptoms rarely predict pathologic changes in a reliable manner.

Besides being confusing, the anatomic-pathologic classification often requires significant medical knowledge, and as such is of limited benefit in the majority of cases of low back pain. More importantly, it does not help the patient get better except in certain, less common circumstances.

Kirkaldy-Willis Degenerative Cascade

Phase	Disc Disorder	Facet Disorder	Clinical Correlate
Phase I			
Dysfunction	Circumferential tear	Inflammation Reduced mobility	• 'Lumbar strain' • Acute back pain, tenderness • Stiffness • Flexion or extension pain
Phase II			
Herniation	Radial tear	Degeneration	• 'Discogenic' pain • Flexion pain, leg pain
Instability	Internal disruption	Joint laxity	• Chronic or recurrent back pain • 'Catching' pain on motion • Intolerance to rotation
Lateral nerve Entrapment	Disc resorption	Joint subluxation	• Narrowing of intervertebral disc • Back + leg pain with activity
Phase III			
Stenosis Spondylosis	Arthritic changes in vertebrae	Arthritic changes in facets	• Chronic back pain • Arthritis symptoms • Spinal stenosis symptoms

Diagnostic Tests

While the history and physical examination are the most important part of the physician's assessment of your back pain, most patients are convinced they need further tests and can be a little put out if nothing is ordered immediately. In response, doctors may order X-rays or other tests to comfort patients and make them feel some thing is being done to help their pain. Unfortunately, this often backfires as the tests may show up some pre-existing, inconsequential variation of 'normal' that has no bearing on the back pain in question. The patient, rather than just getting better, then becomes increasingly anxious and follows a long, blinkered path through numerous consultations and tests with progressively more complex and contradictory findings.

A classic example is the patient experiencing acute back pain after digging the garden. After a brief assessment, the doctor orders X-rays that show 'mild degenerative change'. The doctor calls this 'arthritis' and the patient assumes this is the cause of the pain. Arthritis cannot be cured, the patient reasons, so 'obviously' the patient is always going to have back pain. The truth of the matter is that this 'mild degenerative change' has been there for many years, completely harmless and painless, certainly not the cause of the acute onset pain. The gardening has resulted in a lumbar muscle strain, a common, easily treated and rapidly resolving condition with nothing to do with arthritis. In this case, the X-ray test led to more problems, with increased patient anxiety, than it solved.

With this cautionary case in mind, the following section will examine the various tests available, what they involve, what they show (both 'normal' and 'abnormal'), and when they are appropriate.

'Red Flags'

- Significant injury
- Symptoms of cauda equina syndrome
- Severe, unremitting night pain
- Fever
- History of cancer
- Rapid and unexplained weight loss
- History of osteoporosis or steroid medication

 BACK FACTS

Tests are mostly used to confirm a diagnosis based on the medical history and physical examination. Tests may also be used to rule out certain conditions or pathologies in suspicious cases or as part of a pre-operative work-up. Tests can also be misinterpreted.

Plain X-rays (Radiographs)

Plain X-rays remain the best initial imaging modality for the spine. Besides showing the entire lumbar spine on one film, these X-rays also allow visualization of the sacrum and sacro-iliac joints (where the sacrum attaches to the pelvis). They provide the highest quality resolution of bone, so are useful in the assessment of bone quality. They are also better at

Spina bifida occulta Childhood Symptoms

- Low back pain.
- Progressive scoliosis (curvature of the spine).
- Muscle weakness or wasting.
- Diffuse back pain.
- Loss of pain and temperature sensation in the legs.
- Absent knee and/or ankle reflexes.
- Foot deformities or claw toes.
- Overflow bladder incontinence.

demonstrating some of the subtle abnormalities of such conditions as inflammatory arthritis. Plain X-rays also allow evaluation of alignment, although it is often impossible to tell whether this is structural and fixed or postural and actively correctable.

The number of vertebrae may be counted best on plain X-rays. The number of lumbar plus sacral vertebrae always adds up to 10. Most people have 5-lumbar and 5-sacral. However, about 5% of people will have the 5th lumbar vertebra fully or partly fused to the sacrum (sacralization of L5) and thus 4-lumbar and 6-sacral vertebrae. A similar number will have the 1st sacral vertebra separated from the rest of the sacrum (lumbarization of S1) leading to 6-lumbar and 4-sacral vertebrae. Although it was originally thought that these variations on 'normal' imposed added instability to the spine and increased risk of arthritis, current evidence indicates that this is not the case. They pose no increased risk of back pain or spinal disorders.

For uncomplicated, recent onset low back pain there is no need for this investigation during the first 4 to 6 weeks. Although the radiation exposure is minimal, the dose is unjustified. Between 4 and 6 weeks if the pain is not subsiding, or in the presence of pain after 6 weeks, lumbar spine radiographs are indicated. This should include oblique views, radiographs taken at 45 degrees to the front-back axis as they have been shown to reveal abnormalities sometimes missed on the standard antero-posterior (front to back) and lateral (from the side) views.

Recurrent episodes of low back pain also warrant investigation, which would include plain X-rays. Acute exacerbation of low back pain or a significant change in symptoms occurring in someone with chronic low back pain should be treated like any initial attack. Clearly the history may be more complex and the presence of recent or remote surgery will have to be considered in the equation. However, the same 'Red Flags' can be used to help in the decision-making process.

Spina Bifida Occulta

About 10% to 20% of the population will have incomplete formation of the arch over the spinal canal at L5 or S1, a condition termed 'spina bifida occulta'. Seen well on plain X-rays or CAT scan, there may also be a corresponding tuft of hair on the skin overlying this area on the low back. This condition is associated with spinal cord abnormalities in children where, in the presence of symptoms, it should be further investigated. In the adult with back pain, spina bifida occulta should be considered an incidental finding; there is no evidence that it is associated with an increased risk of low back pain. In one study looking at X-rays of a large population of normal, pain-free subjects, 20% had spina bifida occulta.

Plain X-rays (Radiographs)

What are they?
- A beam of penetrating rays from a single X-ray source passes through the body and is collected on a photographic X-ray plate. Certain tissues, particularly bone, impair the passage of the X-rays resulting in an image on the plate.

What do they show?
- Primarily bony structures including vertebrae, facet joints, sacrum and pelvis.
- Can show dense soft tissue as a shadow.
- Alignment and number of vertebrae.
- Arthritic changes.
- Narrowing of the disc 'space'.

When are they appropriate?
Within the first 4 weeks:
- In the presence of a 'Red Flag' symptoms.
- Significant injury, impact or fall (or lesser injury with age over 50).
- Patient over 70 years of age.
- History of osteoporosis or steroid medication.
- Associated fever, weight loss, history of cancer.
- Severe, unremitting night pain unrelieved or worse with rest.

After 4 to 6 weeks:
- Persistent back pain after 4 to 6 weeks.
- Recurrent episodes of low back pain.
- Increase or change of pain in chronic low back pain.
- Symptoms suggesting instability (catching).
- Suspicion of arthritis or spondyloarthropathy.

Isotope Bone Scan (Technetium and SPECT)

The isotope bone scan (technetium) test measures 'bone cell activity'. It involves injection of a (non-harmful) radioactive marker into a vein in the hand, followed, two hours later, by a scan of the whole body or a specific area. This test, as with others involving radiation, is not advised during pregnancy. Active areas show up as 'hot spots'.

A bone scan is very sensitive at detecting fractures and can pick up minor bony injuries not seen on X-rays. It can help distinguish between acute and old fractures, although the bone scan may remain 'hot' for 12 to 18 months following a fracture. The bone scan is also a sensitive test for the presence of infection and primary or secondary (metastasized) tumors. Arthritis is a common finding on bone scans of the spine but has poor correlation with symptoms (this is not true for SPECT scanning discussed below). This scan is also helpful in localizing pathology and directing further tests such as CAT scan or MRI.

Care must be taken when interpreting this test. There often is no way of determining whether a hot spot is due to a fracture or the result of infection or tumor. Correlation with the patient's symptoms and X-rays is essential. Due to their poor specificity and high sensitivity, 'hot spots' are remarkably common with regular bone scans. Even completely asymptomatic joints can appear with increased uptake.

This is one test where taking the findings in the context of the patient and the symptoms is of utmost importance. The radiologist interpreting the test results frequently has very little information about the patient and may not have access to other tests or X-rays. The radiologist will report findings in terms of possibilities. Patients will often be sent for assessment of 'arthritis' or 'fracture' on the results of a bone scan without any correlating symptoms or findings. It is often difficult for the patient who has already latched on to the idea that they are suffering from a particularly serious condition to comprehend that in fact the test results represent something of a red herring in their search for a diagnosis.

Isotope Bone Scan

What is it?
- An injected radio-isotope (technetium) labeled phosphonate has particular affinity for areas of high bone turnover or activity and areas with increased blood supply. More sensitive and with less radiation exposure than regular X-rays, these areas show up as 'hot spots' on a special recording camera.

What does it show?
- Fractures of bony elements such as the vertebrae or pars (in spondylolisthesis).
- Occult (not seen on regular X-rays) fractures in osteoporosis.
- Infection of bone or disc (discitis).
- Primary bone tumors or metastases from distant malignancy.
- Arthritis (most useful with SPECT scan).
- Failed bony fusion after back surgery (most useful with SPECT scan).

When is it appropriate in low back pain?
- Within the first 4 weeks if 'Red Flags' present suggesting fracture (not seen on plain X-ray), infection or tumor.
- Significant night-time or rest pain.
- Persistent back pain in children or adolescents.
- Identification of arthritic facet joints prior to injection (SPECT scan only).
- Evaluating failed fusion post spinal surgery.
- Pain over 6 weeks, age over 50.

SPECT scans work in a similar way to a regular bone scan but, like a CT scan, can give 3-dimensional localization. This has proved particularly useful in the identification of arthritic facet joints prior to injection therapy and for the evaluation of failed fusion post surgery.

Computerized Axial Tomography (CAT) Scan

A CAT scan (also called CT scan) uses regular X-rays to provide an image, but, unlike plain X-rays, which give only a two-dimensional projection, CT scanning is able to look inside areas of the body, giving a three-dimensional representation of the anatomy. The CAT scan procedure can be quite rapid, depending on the area to be examined and the detail required. The patient passes through a doughnut-shaped or horseshoe-shaped gantry while lying on a platform. The scanner moves around the body with sensors on the opposite side collecting information about the X-rays transmitted. Once collected, the data is converted into a cross-sectional 'slice' of the body. The thinner the slices, the more the detail. While radiation exposure is higher than plain X-ray, it is still minimal and is only cautioned in pregnant women due to the sensitivity of the fetus. The images collected by the CAT scan can be reformatted to show slices in different planes, and in some cases can be turned into a realistic three-dimensional picture or model. CT can be combined with myelography (see below) to improve imaging of the neural elements.

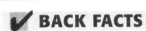 **BACK FACTS**

While providing the best visualization of bony structures, soft tissues can be seen much more clearly with CT than with plain X-rays. Discs, nerves, and ligaments can be seen, allowing identification of disc herniations, spinal stenosis, and nerve compression. Resolution, however, is not nearly as good as with MRI. For evaluation of bony pathology such as fractures, erosions due to infection or tumor, central and lateral recess stenosis (spinal canal narrowing in arthritis), facet joint arthritis, and ligament calcification, CT scanning remains a better imaging modality than MRI.

CAT scanning can be used to assess disc degeneration and herniation but is not considered as good as MRI, increasingly the standard procedure in evaluating these problems. The CAT scan is indicated for assessment of fractures, for example, in post trauma, in osteoporosis, and in bone destruction such as that caused by infection or metastatic tumor spread. Pre-operative evaluation of spinal stenosis due to arthritis is best done with a CT scan. This imaging modality also provides the best pictures of the bony abnormalities seen in spondylolisthesis (slipping of one vertebra upon another). It is particularly useful for the diagnosis of stress fractures of the posterior spinal elements (the pars interarticularis).

With regard to imaging of facet joint arthritis, CAT scanning does provide excellent imaging. However, if an MRI has been performed, the CT adds no further useful information. In addition, CT has not been shown to help identify the symptomatic facet joints in patients with facet joint syndrome back pain, and is unable to predict outcome after injection therapy. Finally, CT is an excellent way of looking at the spine after surgical implantation of screws, plates, and other hardware, for example, after spinal fusion. Screw placement and the success of fusion can be assessed.

Computerized Axial Tomography (CAT) Scan

What is it?
• Regular X-rays are taken from many different angles allowing a 3-dimensional picture of the spine to be compiled by computer from the collected data.

What does it show?
• Fractures of bony elements such as the vertebrae or pars (in spondylolisthesis) — including stress fractures.
• Fractures in osteoporosis.
• Bone destruction due to infection.
• Bone destruction due to metastases from distant malignancy.
• Spinal canal narrowing in arthritis (central and lateral recess stenosis).
• Position of metallic hardware after spinal surgery/status of fusion.

When is it appropriate in low back pain?
• Emergency evaluation of cauda equina syndrome (MRI is better).
• Within the first 4 weeks if 'Red Flags' present suggesting fracture (not seen on plain X-ray), infection, or tumor.
• At 4 to 6 weeks in the presence of radicular (nerve compression) findings.
• At 4 to 6 weeks with symptoms of spinal stenosis.
• Evaluation of degenerative changes in recurrent or persistent (over 6 weeks) back pain.
• Evaluation of spondylolisthesis seen on plain X-ray.
• Evaluating failed spinal surgery.

Magnetic Resonance Imaging (MRI) Scan
Magnetic resonance imaging uses changing magnetic fields rather than X-rays to image the different structures in the body. Different tissues have different 'resonance' properties, and these properties change if the tissue is inflamed or

altered by disease. Different sequences (termed T1-, T2-weighted) can be used to gain different types of information and image different tissue types. Injected gadolinium is sometimes used to enhance visualization of certain tissues, particularly scar tissue.

MRI scanning requires you to lie very still for up to 30 minutes at a time in a very small tube. Recent advances in MRI technology have allowed 'Open' MRIs that are not as claustrophobic. Lying still may a problem for some people, and motion while in the scanner is the major cause of poor imaging. 'Rapid' MRI scanning is a recent development that markedly reduces scan time and will likely solve this problem as it becomes more widely available. Because the MRI machine incorporates huge magnetic fields, the presence of mobile metallic devices within the body can be a contraindication to the procedure. You will be asked to complete a screening form prior to the scan and may require further tests (such as an eye X-ray to check for metal debris) or assessment before proceeding.

MRI provides an almost anatomy-book like picture of the spine with superb detail of soft tissue, such as discs, muscles, and ligaments. Of all imaging modalities currently available to evaluate the spine, MRI provides the most detailed and comprehensive information. MRI scanning is an excellent tool for the evaluation of the intervertebral disc. It is useful in the evaluation of the patient with narrowing of the spinal canal due to arthritis (spinal stenosis). Finally, MRI provides the best imaging of spinal cord damage or neural compression due to infection or tumor, both primary and metastatic (spread from other areas such as prostate or breast). It is the test of choice in progressive nerve deficit or acute compression such as cauda equina syndrome.

Unfortunately, MRI scanning technology and availability exceed the ability of many medical practitioners to understand and interpret the findings. MRI should *not* be used as a

MRI Contraindications and Cautions

Presence of any of the following does not permit MRI scanning:

- Metal clips in the brain (used on vessels during neurosurgery).
- Heart pacemakers.
- Implanted infusion pumps.
- Certain heart valves.
- Certain ear and eye implants.
- Metal fragments/shrapnel in the eye, brain or spine.

Presence of the following indicates caution in proceeding with MRI scan:

- Pregnancy.
- Recent heart or blood vessel surgery.
- Some nerve stimulators (used in chronic pain).
- Severe claustrophobia.

✔ BACK FACTS

Studies show that 50–80% of adults without any symptoms of back pain or sciatica have bulging or protruding discs on MRI. Nearly 30% have disc herniations. Research also shows that herniated discs tend to resorb or shrink over time, so scanning too early may overestimate the pathology. Research is underway to identify MRI features that correlate with pain because a disc bulge or protrusion is not in itself always symptomatic. The more severe the herniation and the more disc material there is in the spinal canal, the more likely there is to be nerve compression or damage, pathology that can also be identified on MRI. However, the MRI findings need to match the patient's symptoms and clinical examination for them to be significant.

'screening tool' for patients with low back pain as it may lead to inappropriate diagnosis and over-treatment in the majority of cases. Before ordering an MRI, physicians should be aware of indications, understand the pathology they are looking for, and rationalize how it will affect patient care. MRI scanning should generally be reserved for evaluation of more specific pathology such as cauda equina syndrome, tumor, or infection, and for pre-operative evaluation in cases of disc herniation and spinal stenosis.

Magnetic Resonance Imaging (MRI) Scan

What is it?
- Magnetic resonance imaging uses changing magnetic fields rather than X-rays to image the different structures in the body.

What does it show?
- Excellent resolution of the disc and disc herniation.
- The best imaging of neural elements such as the spinal cord and nerve roots.
- Abnormalities in ligaments and other soft tissues.
- Bone or tissue damage by infection or tumor.

When is it appropriate in low back pain?
- Emergency evaluation of cauda equina syndrome.
- Progressive neurologic deficit (numbness, weakness).
- Within the first 4 weeks if 'Red Flags' present suggesting infection or tumor.
- At 4 to 6 weeks in the presence of radicular (nerve compression) findings.
- Pre-operative evaluation of disc herniation.
- Pre-operative evaluation of spinal stenosis (combine with CT scan).
- With Gadolinium for persistent pain post disc surgery.
- Evaluation of degenerative changes in recurrent or persistent back pain in cases where it will alter management.

Disc Herniation in Normal Pain-Free Individuals

Percentage of Subjects with No Back or Leg Complaints Showing Disc Herniation on Testing:

Myelography	24%
Discography	37%
CAT scan	20%
MRI scan	28%

Myelogram

This test involves the injection of radio-opaque dye into the sheath containing the spinal cord and nerve roots within the spinal canal. Plain X-rays are then taken. The dye outlines the cord and nerve roots, allowing assessment of neural compression. Besides the invasive nature of the test (a long needle has to be inserted into the back), side effects include nerve root irritation and headache. Sometimes used in association with CAT scanning, myelography has been largely replaced by MRI.

Blood Tests

In the presence of any 'Red Flags', a blood count (CBC) and ESR (erythrocyte sedimentation rate — a test of generalized disease or inflammation) should be ordered. These tests are also appropriate if pain persists longer than 6 to 8 weeks. Other tests may be ordered depending on the clinical situation, for example, a rheumatology screen if inflammatory arthritis is suspected, or calcium, protein, and enzymes for possible malignancy.

Blood Tests

When should blood tests be conducted in the presence of back pain?
- CBC/ESR if 'Red Flags' present or with pain over 6 weeks.
- Possible infection — CBC, ESR, C-reactive protein, TB test, blood cultures.
- Possible malignancy — CBC, ESR, calcium, phosphate, serum protein levels and analysis, liver enzymes, PSA (prostate screen) in men.
- Arthritis — CBC, ESR, rheumatology screen, HLA-B27 (screen for spondyloarthropathy, e.g., Ankylosing spondylitis).

Nerve Tests

Nerve tests are used either for diagnosis or for monitoring during spinal surgery. This latter application is complex, involves a large, highly-trained team, and is used only during major surgical procedures. It will not be discussed here. Diagnostic testing is used to evaluate nerve dysfunction such as might occur with compression or traction from a herniated disc.

Nerve tests require no preparation but relaxation is essential. Discomfort is usually minimal with mild needle insertion pain and tingling from the electrical stimulation.

Electromyography (EMG) and nerve conduction tests involve insertion of fine needles or placement of surface electrodes on the skin. The EMG test records electrical information from muscles at rest and with activity. Compression and damage to a motor nerve in the spine will produce an abnormal pattern of firing within the muscle.

Nerve conduction tests involve the stimulation of a nerve at one point with a small electrical current, and recording of that impulse further down the nerve. Slowing of impulse transmission indicates a damaged or compressed area of the nerve. This test is useful for conditions such as carpal tunnel syndrome but do not give reliable information about nerve compression in the low back.

Diagnostic Nerve Testing

What does diagnostic nerve testing involve?

- Electromyography (EMG), which tests the function of motor nerves, those supplying muscles and making them contract.

- Somatosensory evoked potentials (SSEPs), which tests the integrity of sensory nerves.

- Nerve conduction studies, which examine the speed of transmission of electrical impulses along a nerve.

Somatosensory evoked potentials (SSEPs) are signals detected by electrode sensors placed on the spine or scalp in response to stimulation of sensory nerves in the periphery. For example, stimulation of the peroneal nerve (part of the sciatic nerve) at the knee can be recorded at the level of the spine or brain (through the scalp). A pattern of electrical wave activity is produced as the stimulus activates sequential parts of the sensory pathway.

A combination of EMG and SSEP testing gives the most accurate assessment of nerve root compression. It is used to confirm clinical suspicion of nerve dysfunction and isolate the specific nerve root level or levels.

Injections for Diagnosis

There are many patients in whom, despite careful history and examination, the diagnosis remains elusive. Typically, the individual complains of back pain with referred or radicular pain in the leg but normal neurological findings. Despite tremendous advances in imaging of the lumbar spine, tests still fail to reveal the source of the pain. This surprisingly common scenario leaves the physician somewhat helpless, unable to provide the patient with a diagnosis or treatment plan. It renders the patient frustrated and abandoned, often labeled with the non-specific term 'mechanical low back pain' or 'lumbar spinal pain of unknown origin'. Given the fact that 90% of low back pain resolves within 4 to 6 weeks, such a diagnosis, along with reassurance, is probably sufficient during this period. The same is true for short-duration, recurrent back pain with long pain-free intervals. However, for those with persistent back pain or more regular and longer lasting recurrence where definitive treatment is sought, further diagnostic endeavors are recommended.

 BACK FACTS

The most useful way of localizing a pain source is to isolate it by stimulation (effectively inducing the pain) or by anesthesia (removing the pain). The techniques of needle localization aim to achieve these goals, thereby identifying a specific pain source that can then be treated. The three principle methods are discography (injection of dye and salt water into a disc); facet joint blocks ('freezing' facet joints or their associated nerves); and nerve root blocks ('freezing' a nerve root with local anesthetic).

Discography

Discography involves the placement of a needle using X-ray guidance into an intervertebral disc, followed by injection of radio-opaque dye and saline (salt water) under pressure. Discography is most frequently performed by a trained radiologist and a medical doctor specializing in the interpretation of tests such as X-rays, ultrasound, CT, and MRI. Certain radiologists will be trained in 'interventional' X-ray techniques involving the insertion of needles and injection of dye, anesthetics, or other materials.

The technique of discography is performed under sterile conditions with the guidance of real-time X-ray or CT scanning. A needle is inserted into the disc followed by injection of a small amount of liquid that appears opaque on X-ray. This confirms the position of the needle within the disc and allows an assessment of the disc integrity. Saline is then injected into the disc under pressure and the patient reports any symptoms. Although uncomfortable, the test is generally carried out without sedation or general anesthesia as the patient needs to be alert enough to accurately report what they feel. Local anesthetic can be used for the skin prior to needle insertion.

Discs that are anatomically normal on discography (injection of the dye) have been shown to be painless even after injection of large volumes of saline. Those discs that are very painful and exhibit symptoms comparable to the patient's regular back pain show tears through the annulus on discography. Strict guidelines have been established to improve the accuracy of discograms. Not only must stimulation of a certain disc exactly reproduce the patient's pain, stimulation of adjacent disc at the same session must be painless.

While the value of discography and disc stimulation remains controversial, this procedure remains the only available test to determine whether or not a disc is actually a source of low back pain. MRI scanning is able to identify degrees of disc degeneration and internal disruption but the significance of these findings remains elusive. Changes are often found at numerous levels, making it impossible to determine which one is the source of the patient's symptoms. In addition, MRI has been shown to miss significant disc pathology in up to 20% of cases. Discography provides the potential to localize disc pathology and pain accurately, which, when correlated with MRI, may improve treatment and outcome.

Indications for Discography

- Identifying the intervertebral disc as a cause of low back pain.
- Establishing a diagnosis of internal disc derangement.
- May aid in predicting outcome from minimally invasive disc procedures.
- May aid in planning and predicting outcome from surgery.

Facet (Zygoapophyseal) Joint Blocks

Facet joints can be stimulated by injection of X-ray dye or saline under pressure in a technique similar to discography. This produces low back and leg pain. As a diagnostic test, however, it is unreliable. In contrast, 'freezing' the joint by instillation of local anesthetic into the joint itself or around the nerves supplying it has proven to be a useful investigation.

As with discography, facet blocks are usually performed by a trained radiologist. Sterile conditions and X-ray guidance are essential. Injections carried out without radiologic confirmation of needle position are of no proven benefit. Due to the high placebo effect and large false-positive response (up to 60% in some studies), 'control' blocks need to be performed. These are of two types. Either a series of blocks is carried out on three or more occasions using local anesthetic or saline; or two types of anesthetic are used, one short-acting, one long-acting, on different days. In neither case is the patient told which is which.

In the former test, a positive result would be a clear improvement in pain with local anesthetic but none with saline. In the latter, a positive test would see a longer pain-free period with the long-acting anesthetic. While this protocol is time and resource intensive, it is the only way to ensure that the results are reliable and therefore useful for planning treatment.

The value of facet blocks lies in their potential for direct treatment. Most important in this regard is the use of long term 'freezing' of the joint. By using cortisone within the joint to reduce inflammation or by interrupting the nerve supplying sensation to the joint, a permanent 'block' can be achieved. Recent studies using SPECT (bone-scan CT) to localize symptomatic facets has shown great promise in identifying painful joints likely to respond to a block. While diagnostic facet blocks alone have not conclusively been shown to offer the same valuable information, the combination of both tests may significantly improve specificity and outcome.

Nerve Root Blocks

A nerve root block is the injection of local anesthetic around a specific nerve root as it exits the spinal canal. The aim of this procedure is to isolate a specific root as a cause of referred or radicular back and leg pain.

Compression or traction of a nerve root by a herniated disc will, for example, cause inflammation and damage to that root. This will cause pain and possibly numbness or pins and needles to be felt in the region of the body that nerve supplies. Unfortunately, due to variations in anatomy between individuals and the diffuse distribution of painful sensation in the

Indications for Facet Joint Blocks

- Identifying the facet joint as a cause of low back pain.
- Correlating pain with CT or SPECT findings.
- Combined with steroid injection can be a useful treatment modality.

low back, it can often be hard to isolate the affected nerve on history and clinical examination alone. If, by using a nerve root block, the pain the patient is experiencing can be made to disappear, then the level is identified.

As with other procedures of this type, nerve root blocks are carried out using X-ray guidance and sterile technique. A needle is introduced through anesthetized skin into the intervertebral foramen, the gap in each side of the spinal canal through which the exiting nerve root leaves on its way to the periphery. Long acting local anesthetic is then injected through the needle to 'freeze' the nerve root.

It is important to realize that nerve root blocks do not identify the cause of the pain. They demonstrate that nerve damage, inflammation, or compression exists at a certain level, and that this nerve damage is responsible for the majority of the patient's pain. They do not specify what exactly is causing the compression or damage. However, a positive test can help guide treatment and plan surgical intervention if required.

Nerve root blocks can be used to identify patients that are likely to benefit from therapeutic injection of steroid to reduce inflammation and pain. However, the role of this treatment is largely pain relief and does not address the underlying cause. It may enable sufficient increase in function to allow the patient to resume a more normal lifestyle until the problem resolves spontaneously, or by permitting the patient to participate in a therapy program such as physiotherapy, promote recovery.

Indications for Nerve Root Blocks

- Unusual or diffuse leg pain.
- If CT and MRI findings and clinical presentation do not correlate.
- If EMG studies and MRI or CT do not corroborate.
- In cases of irregular nerve root or vertebral anatomy.
- Failed back surgery syndrome with atypical extremity pain.

What Causes Back Pain?

Now that we have been able to diagnose and classify your back pain, let's step back and discuss its causes by looking at the anatomy of the back and the pathology of pain. Understanding how the spine is constructed, the way it moves and functions, its weaknesses and limitations can help us know why we get back pain and why that pain hurts so much. The more we know, the less it hurts, we would like to think. While back pain seems to resist one-to-one cause and effect anatomical and pathological analysis, much can be gained from a knowledge of back bones and muscles for developing successful treatments.

 BACK FACTS

Understanding the sources of back pain, the complexities of its transmission and the paradoxes of its interpretation, allows individuals with back pain to begin to rationalize their discomfort. They can then begin to explore the numerous treatments and modalities available while incorporating a more confident, less fearful mental attitude. They will be able to tune in to their symptoms and differentiate pain from varying sources.

Back Anatomy and Pain Pathology Illustrations

As you read the following information, you may want to bookmark the 'Back Anatomy and Pain Pathology Illustrations' at the front of the book for quick reference. In this case, a picture may be worth a thousand words.

Spine Anatomy

Try to imagine 24 children's building blocks stacked one on top of the other. At its most simple this represents the bony components or so called vertebra of the spine. Now imagine that this structure has to remain balanced throughout an endless array of movements, bends and lifts, twists and turns, to accommodate positions as diverse as gymnastic moves or yoga — and tolerate tremendous loads estimated at 300 lbs per square inch. No wonder that occasionally things go wrong.

Understanding the way the spine works is an important step in comprehending what happens in back pain when it stops functioning as an efficient, coordinated, and symptom-free structure. Being familiar with the so-called 'biomechanics' of the spine allows you to appreciate how the spine can be injured and what steps you can take to prevent injury.

It permits comprehension of factors such as posture, ergonomic motion, exercise, and flexibility. Finally, it is important when interpreting patterns of pain and following a treatment plan for recovery.

Functions of the Spine

- Resists extreme motion to protect the spinal cord and roots.
- Provides adequate motion to position head and trunk for activities of daily living.
- Offers sufficient balance to maintain erect posture without undue effort.
- Provides strength to resist extreme forces associated with activities such as strenuous lifting.
- Provides a strong central core to support the head and limbs.

Numbers

There are five areas of the spine: the cervical, the thoracic, the lumbar, the sacral, and the coccyx. The cervical spine (C), at the level of the neck, has 7 vertebrae. The thoracic spine (T), at the level of the chest, has 12 vertebrae. The lumbar spine (L) is at the level of the low back, with 5 vertebrae normally. The sacral spine (S) or sacrum, at the level of the pelvis, has 5 fused vertebrae; and the coccyx, the tailbone, has 4 or 5 fused vertebrae.

At each level the vertebrae are numbered sequentially. In the cervical spine, the top most vertebrae is 'cervical-one' or C1, the one below that is C2 and so on as far as C7. The next vertebra within the thoracic region is called 'thoracic-one' or T1. There are normally five lumbar vertebrae numbered L1 to L5, with L5 typically being the last mobile or individual segment. Below this level in the sacrum and the coccyx, the elements are fused together to form a single mass of bone, although the individual segments are still visible at S1 to S5. The coccyx or tailbone similarly has four or five fused yet recognizable segments.

The disc between adjacent vertebrae is labeled according to the vertebra above and below. For example, the disc between the L2 and L3 lumbar vertebrae is called the L2-3 disc. The disc between the lowest thoracic and first lumbar vertebrae is called the T12-L1 disc. Similarly, the disc between the lowest lumbar and the first sacral vertebrae is called the L5-S1 disc.

Functional Spinal Units (FSUs)

In order to understand the component parts of the spine and their functions, the spine has been divided into 'motion segments' called 'functional spinal units'. Each unit exhibits characteristics similar to the entire spine.

The spine can be thought of functionally as a single unit composed of individual elements. These elements are called motion segments or functional spinal units (FSUs). Functional Spinal Units comprise two adjacent vertebrae, the intervertebral disc between them, and all the associated ligaments. There are three joints or articulations between the two vertebrae: two facet joints at the back and one disc at the front. The two facet joints are true synovial joints, such as the hip or knee, though much smaller. In the lumbar spine, for example, they are approximately 1 cm in diameter.

 BACK FACTS

The term 'slipped disc' implies that the disc moves out of place. This is, in fact, not true. The term refers only to displacement of the soft inner core of the disc as it bulges or extrudes from the main body of the disc. The body itself never moves.

The facet joints are fairly flat, allowing the two surfaces to slide across each other. Unlike the hip or the knee, however, range of motion is very limited. The disc between the two vertebrae is not loose or mobile. These discs are very strongly attached to the bony plates at the top and the bottom. Weight is supported through the disc and vertebral body. The vertebral body contains columns of bone that act as struts to achieve this arduous function.

The disc carries the entire compressive load at each level. This can amount to three or four times body weight, depending on position. The structure of the disc includes the main body of the disc ('annulus fibrosis' or AF), a tough outer shell composed of layers of fibrous collagen, and a gel-like core (the 'nucleus pulposus' or NP). The NP takes up about 30% to 50% of the cross sectional area of the disc and is about 70% to 90% water. It acts as a hydrostatic pressure distribution system.

Motion within the FSU is limited by the conformity of the facet joints, the strength of the disc attachment, and the resistance of strong supporting ligaments. The individual FSUs therefore provide protection and strength but limited motion.

While individual FSUs have limited mobility, the association of 24 of them (7 cervical in the neck, 12 thoracic in the chest, and 5 lumbar in the low back) allows sufficient movement to achieve the remaining functions of posture, flexibility for daily function, and support for the head and limbs.

Vertebrae (Bones)

A typical lumbar vertebra has a large barrel-shaped body that sits at the front of the spine with a network or honeycomb of bone surrounded by a more rigid bony casing. The top and bottom of the barrel are called the end plates that attach to the vertebral discs.

Behind the vertebral body is a ring or arch known as the spinal canal, containing elements of the spinal cord, nerve fibers, and some blood vessels. The arch is supported by two columns called pedicles that arise from the upper half of the back of the body. The arch has a roof with two sloping sides called the lamina meeting in the midline at the back of the spine and forming a spinous process. This is quite a substantial structure, particularly in the lumbar spine, the tips being the palpable nodules that can be felt through the skin in the midline of the back. The back of the body, the pedicles, and the arch enclose a triangular canal called the vertebral foramen. From each side of the vertebra extending out horizontally from the lamina are the transverse processes. These, again, are quite substantial in the lumbar spine and represent major attachments for muscles and ligaments. In a thin person, these may also be palpated 1 to 2 centimeters to the side of the central spinous process.

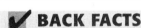 **BACK FACTS**

The individual bony components of the spine are called the vertebrae. There are 7 in the neck, 12 in the thoracic or chest region, and generally 5 in the lumbar or low back region. All vertebrae are basically comprised of the same units, the size and proportion and orientation of each varying throughout the length of the spine.

The structures thus far have provided one important function of the spine, a bony shield or canal to protect the sensitive nerves of the spinal cord. However, they are still no more stable than the pile of building blocks. The added feature of the vertebrae that does improve stability is the facet joints. Looking at the spine from the back, these facet joints form what appear to be butterfly wings extending out from the side of the spine. The lower wings of one vertebra contact the upper wings of the vertebra below. These facet joints are actually synovial joints, the same type of joints as the hip or the knee, with an outer capsule, slippery articular surface coverage, and a synovial membrane that produces lubricating fluid. Like synovial joints elsewhere in the body, these joints are prone to osteoarthritis.

The facet joints in the lumbar spine do add a modicum of stability to the bony elements. While the facet joints do limit the ability of the vertebra to move in certain planes such twisting, they really do not provide anywhere near sufficient resistance to movement to withstand the daily forces across the spine. For this we have to look outside the bony elements and look at the soft tissues that surround the vertebrae. These include the intervertebral discs, the ligaments, and the muscles of the spine.

Intervertebral Discs

My favorite analogy for the intervertebral disc is to a type of fruit candy popular in England that has a sugar-coated, firm outer shell surrounding a sweet and somewhat runny central core. A poorly placed bite through the outer shell leads to a somewhat messy escape of the runny fruit contents. Although not quite as tasty, the intervertebral disc is much the same. Its outer shell or annulus fibrosus (AF) is composed of sheets of dense fibrous collagen tissue alternately angled at approximately 30 degrees to each other. This surrounds a central and slightly posterior soft gelatinous core called the nucleus pulposus (NP). The gelatinous material is rich in molecules called glycosaminoglycans with the ability to attract and hold water molecules, thereby maintaining strength, flexibility, and ability to withstand load. The NP stores energy and acts a cushion, its hydrostatic properties acting to distribute forces evenly throughout the intervertebral discs. Interestingly, as the day progresses, forces of gravity directed through the intervertebral disc lead to loss of water and subsequently loss of height, almost 2 centimeters in an average person, which is regained while in bed at night.

✔ BACK FACTS

Under sustained load the disc undergoes gradual deformation or 'creep'. An example of this property is seen in the substance known as silly putty. A sudden force such as bouncing a lump of this material on the floor will not cause it to change shape. However, a constant pressure with your thumb will cause it to indent. Once your thumb is removed, it will gradually return to its normal shape. This factor may be significant in the spine when considering prolonged postures or repetitive tasks.

Part of the aging process of the intervertebral disc involves deterioration of its component parts. Loss of number and the quality of glycosaminoglycans molecules in the NP results in desiccation and loss of the disc's ability to transmit loads effectively. This has a profound affect on the integrity, function, and motion of the spine. In the aging spine, deterioration of the NP with loss of water and its hydrostatic properties transfers more of the compressive force to the AF periphery and vertebral endplate.

While the facet joints attach the vertebral bodies together at the back of the spine, the discs attach them together at the front.

Ligaments

Together with the unique anatomy and bony structures of the vertebrae, ligaments provide checkreins on the amount of movement occurring between vertebrae. The importance of this is in protection of the spinal cord and associated nerves, which are unable to tolerate extremes of movement at individual levels. Due to the unique characteristic of the bones and the ligaments at different levels throughout the spine, movement at individual segments is somewhat limited, but overall in acting as a unit the spine is able to achieve a fully functional range of motion for the numerous and often obscure activities of the human.

 BACK FACTS

Ligaments are bands or cords of strong fibrous tissue (collagen) that join adjacent bones together. They exist around all joints. Most people are familiar with strains of the ligaments about the ankle or the knee. Ligaments in the spine also form strong stabilizing structures between adjacent bony vertebrae that can be injured.

Ligaments run down the front and the back of the body of the vertebral bodies and along the tips of the spinous processes. They also run between the transverse processes and surround the facet joints. The ligamentum flavum (so called because of its yellow color) runs between the laminae. It is unique in that it contains the highest proportion of elastic fibers of any tissue of the body. Most ligaments are predominantly collagen, which is relatively rigid with only a small proportion of stretchy elastin fibers. The reason for the unique structure of the ligamentum flavum relates to its proximity to the spinal cord. By virtue of its elasticity, in a normal spine it does not buckle during movement, which would be likely to cause undue pressure on the neural elements. Unfortunately, as we shall see later, with aging this property is lost and in combination with other degenerative changes ultimately results in reduced space for the spinal cord and subsequent neurologic symptoms.

Muscles

The muscles of the spine function to maintain balance and alignment, minimizing the effort required to stand erect against the downward force of gravity. This incorporates the principles of posture and balance, crucial to normal pain-free function of the spine and central in both the prevention and treatment of back pain. These same muscles also provide the force to move and hold the spine in the many and varied positions required for work and play. Their strength and endurance is vital to the performance of these functions and this will also prove to be an essential component in the management of back pain.

 BACK FACTS

Surprisingly, despite the stability of the individual FSUs, the spine itself is remarkably weak. Without the benefit of muscular support, the spine buckles under only 90 Newtons of force!

Factors Influencing Muscle Strength and Fatigue

- Overall muscular deconditioning.
- Poor posture and lifting technique.
- Disc herniation.
- Pain and inflammation.
- Vibration.

The importance of the muscles surrounding the spine cannot be over emphasized. Reference to an anatomy book will show what appears to be an overwhelming and incomprehensible mass of muscles surrounding the spine.

The muscles of the back are not just a single mass. There are two anatomic types and three major functional groups. Muscle fibers are generally classified under two types. The Type I (slow twitch or red muscles) have endurance and fatigue slowly. These are the muscles of the marathon runner. Type II muscles (fast twitch or white muscles) are strong, fast acting, and fatigue easily. These are the muscles of the sprinter. The deepest muscles contain the highest percentage of slow-twitch fibers, about 62%, the remaining 48% being fast-twitch.

The spinal muscles are predominantly Type I (slow twitch), responsible for posture. Poor conditioning, fatigue, or inhibition of activity by injury result in weakening of these muscles and substantially increase loads across the vertebrae and the discs. Type II (fast twitch) are most prone to injury. Certain movements, such as asymmetric lifting, put undue strain on these muscles. Injury to these muscles results in pain and inflammation, further decreasing their ability to function as a unit and provide support for the spine. This appears related to their tendency to fatigue more easily.

We need to expend constant energy generating the muscular tone needed to maintain an erect posture. Our position, alignment and balance will significantly affect the amount of energy expended, an important concept when trying to minimize stress and fatigue in the spine.

Functional Muscle Groups

Within the Type I and Type II muscle fiber types found in the back are three functional muscle groups performing the different tasks of posture, stability, and motion:

1. Short muscles running across each FSU.

2. Deep 'multifidus' fibers close to the midline crossing 2–4 segments.

3. Longer, shallower 'erector spinae' fibers on the sides of the spine attaching to the pelvis.

These groups appear to have different nerve supply and different function in posture, stability, and movement of the spine.

Spine and Muscle Dynamics

The feedback between spinal posture and muscular contraction is provided by nerves that sense position and movement through structures such as the ligaments and the disc. Impaired communication can interfere with this system, leading to further imbalance and fatigue. This unfortunately happens in spinal conditions such as disc herniation, muscle inflammation, chronic pain, arthritis, and disc degeneration. It is also affected by adverse external factors such as prolonged posture and vibration — typically 4–6 Hz, the same frequency as most vehicles! This creates a vicious cycle in which one back problem exacerbates another, leading to increased pain and dysfunction. Fortunately this has an 'up-side! While the underlying pathology can often not be remedied, the strength, balance, and feedback can be restored, minimizing the associated pain.

Spine and Muscle Dynamics

The ability of the spinal muscles to provide adequate support balances their strength and endurance against spinal alignment and posture.

Weak Muscle	Strong Muscle	Unbalanced Spine
PAIN	Balanced Spine	PAIN

Planes and Curves

The spine is balanced in two planes, the coronal and the saggital. When viewed from the coronal plane — that is, from the front or the back — the spine is normally straight. Viewed from the saggital plane — that is, from the side, it has natural curves. You can test these by standing with your back against a wall: your head, shoulders, and buttocks will touch the wall with gaps elsewhere due to the saggital spinal curves.

✔ BACK FACTS

When viewed from the side the spine has a definite and normal curvature. Often described as an S-shape, there are actually four curves. Curves with the apex backwards are called 'kyphosis' and those with the apex forward, towards the front of the body, are called 'lordosis'. The cervical spine normally has a lordosis, as does the lumbar spine. The thoracic spine has a kyphosis, as does the sacral spine.

The thoracic kyphosis ends at approximately T10. The region between T10 and L2 is almost straight as seen from the side. The lumbar lordosis then commences, progresses from L2 to S1 with 60% to 70% of it occurring between L4 and S1. Variations in the amount of thoracic kyphosis in the lumbar lordosis occur between individuals within a fairly wide range of normal. Range for the thoracic kyphosis is from 20 to 50 degrees, and for the normal lumbar lordosis from 20 to 70 degrees.

When compared to four-legged animals, humans have developed an erect posture leading to marked alteration and spinal alignment and curvature. Not only has the spine become more stable a result of its reduced role in locomotion, it has developed a lumbar lordosis in order to bring the body's center of gravity posteriorly to maintain balance. Although disc degeneration and arthritis do occur in other mammals, the increased stressors resulting from erect posture and lumbar lordosis, particularly at the L4-S1 levels, is thought to account for the tremendously high incidence of degeneration at this level in man.

When balanced, the shoulders are level and the head positioned directly above the midpoint of the pelvis, the center of the L5-S1 disc. From the side, a line drawn downward from the top of the head, through the seventh cervical (neck) vertebra will pass through the same disc. These lines of balance represent an alignment where muscular force is minimized in the erect posture. Changes in spinal curvature affect this balance, the muscular effort needed to stand, and the forces across the vertebrae.

Minor curves can occasionally be seen as a result of

posture or muscle spasm and are therefore correctable. Other curves in this plane may be due to structural abnormality. The larger and less correctable these curves are the more likely they are to be abnormal. Curves in this plane are termed 'scoliosis' (and often have a rotational element included).

While balanced, little muscular control or effort is required. However, once the spine curves into an unstable position and balance is lost, increasing muscular effort is needed to stop it collapsing. A limbo dancer achieves a seemingly impossible position through balance rather than pure muscular strength! Under increasing load the back muscles tire easily, leading to pain and 'collapse', interpreted not as falling over, but as inability to remain upright without undue discomfort.

Abnormal Spine Curves

Structural   Curves that are essentially unchangeable are called structural. They result from abnormalities in the shape, development, or articulation of the vertebrae.

Functional   Curves that are reversible by movement are called functional. These curves arise as a result of unequal leg length, muscle spasm, or as compensation for other curves or muscle imbalance. Persistence of a functional curve may lead to it becoming fixed and therefore structural.

Spinal Cord and Nerves

The nervous system of the body is divided into three parts: the central nervous system or brain; the brainstem and the spinal cord; and the peripheral nervous system, comprising the nerves that travel from the brain and spinal cord to the rest of the body.

The back is the home of the spinal cord, which starts at the base of the skull and travels within its fibrous membrane covering downward through the bony tunnel in each vertebral body. The spinal cord itself ends at approximately L1 or L2 (the top part of your low back just below your ribcage). From this point on, the vertebral canal is filled with nerve fibers originating from the end of the spinal cord and traveling on their way to the pelvis and legs. This area is called the 'cauda equina', a Latin term for the original anatomic description of this leash of multiple nerve fibers with the appearance of a horse's tail. This arrangement of nerves within the spinal canal is important to understand when interpreting patterns of low back pain and especially sciatica.

Nerve Paths

Let us follow two simple nerve paths: the first involves movement or motor fibers, the second sensation.

When you decide to raise your big toe, an electrical message is initiated in the cortex of the brain. It travels down through pathways in the brainstem, then into the spinal cord. The electrical impulse is transmitted through a single long nerve fiber from the cortex to the bottom of the spinal cord. Here it communicates with another nerve cell, which is part of the peripheral system. The nervous impulse passes out of the spinal canal and into one of the peripheral nerves in the cauda equina. This nerve finally leaves the vertebral canal through a gap between the L5 and S1 vertebrae. It joins other nerves from the spine to form the sciatic nerve, which travels down the back of the leg to reach the muscle that elevates your big toe. The message is complete, the muscle contracts and up goes the toe.

A similar but reversed pathway occurs for sensation. A pinprick to the great toe stimulates a sensory nerve fiber that travels back up through the sciatic nerve into the vertebral canal and upwards to join the spinal cord. From there, further pathways carry the impulse up towards the brain, where the sensation of a pinprick is interpreted.

Now we can understand how pressure by a disc on a motor nerve in the low back can influence muscle function in the foot, and similarly how pressure on a sensory nerve by the same disc will be interpreted as pain in the foot or big toe. Disc herniation, for example, can cause direct nerve root pressure, which not only results in radiating pain into the leg or foot, but can also cause back pain and spasm through stimulation of the posterior nerve roots. Inflammation within the facet joints can cause pain through the sensory fibers coming from these joints.

Autonomic Nervous System

Let's compare the motor system of the central nervous system to the autonomic system. The motor system controls movement. For example, when you want to bend your finger, the cerebral cortex of your brain sends impulses along nerves that travel out through the brain stem into the spinal cord and from there along peripheral nerves that travel through the neck and the arm to the muscles in your forearm, which then contract allowing you to move the finger. You have done this voluntarily and are able to control the amount the finger moves. You are also aware that the finger is moving and can stop it at any time. While other circuits within the brain may modify the speed and smoothness of the movement, it is essentially under your control. Although there are some reflex components to this system (for example, the 'knee jerk' reflex) that can occur involuntarily, you are still aware that they are happening and to a certain extent can exert control over the reflex.

 BACK FACTS

At its most basic the autonomic nervous system may be thought of as that part of the nervous system that is not under conscious or voluntary control. It is responsible for the adjustment of such bodily functions as blood pressure, heart rate, intestinal motility, sweating, body temperature, and metabolic rate.

In contrast to the motor system, the autonomic system works predominantly on an involuntary basis acting in a reflex response to numerous stimuli. Some of these reflexes occur at the level of the spinal cord with few impulses reaching the brain. Others involve complex reflexes coordinated in the limbic system and hypothalamus. These reflexes can occur exceedingly rapidly, causing changes in heart rate, for example, within 3 to 5 seconds and blood pressure within 10 to 15 seconds. When you faint, this is essentially an extremely rapid drop in blood pressure, resulting from stimulation of one part of the autonomic nervous system, effectively slowing the heart and dilating the blood vessels. This happens within 4 to 5 seconds, depriving the brain of sufficient oxygen to cause you to pass out.

Autonomic System

Effects of Sympathetic and Parasympathetic Systems

Organ	Sympathetic Effect	Parasympathetic Effect
Heart	Increased rate Increased contraction	Slowed rate Reduced contraction
Lungs	Opens bronchi (breathing tubes)	Constricts bronchi
Eye	Dilates pupil	Constricts pupil
Skin	Restricts blood flow	No effect
Gut	Reduced activity	Increased activity
Sweat Glands	Increased sweating whole body	Sweating on palms
Muscle	Increased strength Increased glucose production	No effect No effect
Metabolism	Increased metabolic rate Increased blood sugar/fats	No effect
Mental Activity	Increased	No effect

Sympathetic and Parasympathetic Systems

The autonomic nervous system is divided into sympathetic and parasympathetic components. The sympathetic nervous system is primarily responsible for stimulating the individual to a state of heightened awareness as will occur in the initial stages of the stress response. Because this system uses nerves to transmit its impulses, its response is rapid, providing the first line of defense and reaction during the stress response.

Parasympathetic Nerves

Schematic image of the spinal cord and parasympathetic nervous system with the organs that are innervated by each nerve.

Sympathetic Nerves

Schematic image of the components of the sympathetic nervous system with the spinal nerves and organs they innervate.

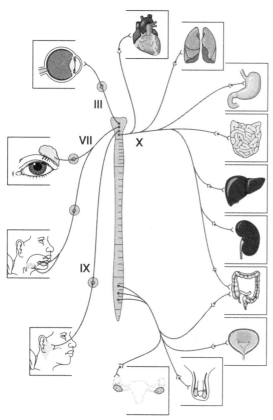

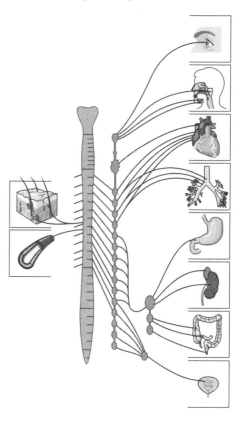

Pain Sensation and Control

The bones, joints, ligaments, discs, and muscles of the spine do not produce pain; rather, the nerves that supply these various structures transmit the sensation of pain. To understand the source and nature of back pain we must discover why the components of the spine sometimes cause these nerves to fire and why these impulses are interpreted as 'painful.'

Pain Receptors

There are two types of pain receptor: nociceptors and sensory receptors. Conscious sensations, including pain, arise from stimulation of these receptors. Messages travel along nerves from the skin, joints, muscles and other structures to reach the spinal cord, where they are relayed up to brain.

Nociceptors

These essentially pure pain sensors are distributed throughout the body with varying concentrations. The cornea (surface of the eye) and the dental pulp of the tooth have a very high density of these receptors such that touch alone is painful.

Sensory Receptors

These receptors carry a multitude of impulses such as light touch and pressure. They become painful when a certain threshold is reached. For example, gradually increasing thumb pressure on your wrist will eventually become painful. The threshold can be lowered by a number of factors such that normal sensations of touch or movement become painful.

Pain Pathways

Let us follow the course of one typical sensation, light touch, for example, by stroking your index finger gently across the underside of your great toe. The sensory receptors in the skin responding to this particular stimulus fire impulses that travel along nerves from the toe, up the leg (within the sciatic nerve), and into the vertebral canal. The nerve root corresponding to this area is the L5 root, but as the spinal cord ends at the level of the L1 or L2 vertebrae, the nerves travel up within the vertebral canal (in the cauda equina) until they reach the appropriate section of the spinal cord. (Note that in this region of the spine the numeric segment of the spinal cord does not line up with the corresponding vertebra.) Once within the spinal cord, they form connections with other nerve cells, then travel upward to the brain within defined pathways specific for this sensation. Most sensory fibers reach the thalamus, a transfer and processing station within the brain. Its name means 'meeting place' in Latin.

From there the messages are passed to the surface of the brain, the cerebral cortex. Most people are familiar with the idea of a representation of the body on the brain, the homunculus, with the size of a body part indicating the density of nervous innervation. The tongue and hands are huge compared to the toes, for example. The interpretation and conscious awareness

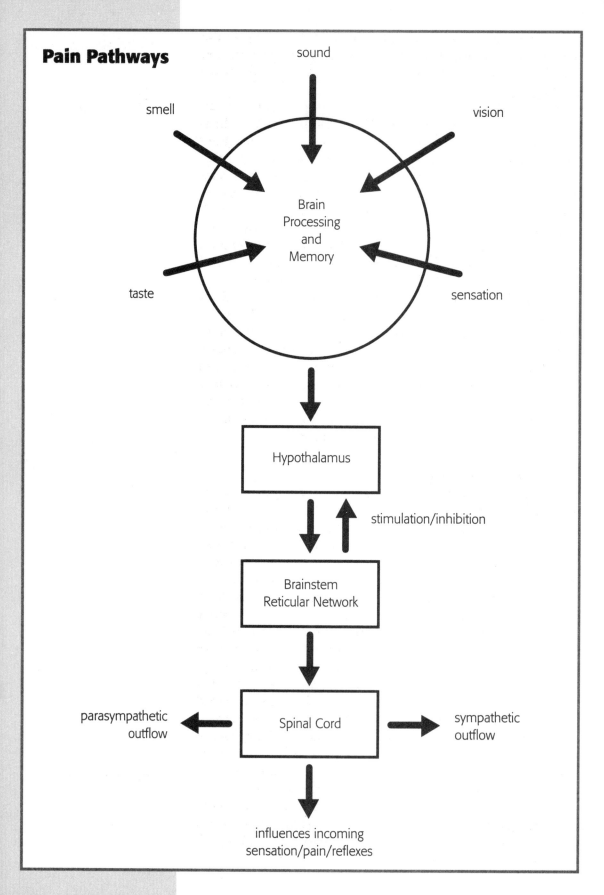

Pain Pathways

sound

smell

vision

Brain
Processing
and
Memory

taste

sensation

Hypothalamus

stimulation/inhibition

Brainstem
Reticular Network

parasympathetic
outflow

Spinal Cord

sympathetic
outflow

influences incoming
sensation/pain/reflexes

of that light touch to the toe is finally made here. Due to the specificity of the pathways and the in-depth representation of body parts in this sensation, the feeling is easily identified and localized.

Pain sensation travels a similar route. Pain sensors or nociceptors exist in all tissues, including the skin, muscles, ligaments and tendons, and the internal organs. Their threshold for stimulation is normally quite high but is strongly influenced by local factors such as inflammation (think how sore the skin is to touch in sunburn), and central factors such as nerve irritation or damage, chronic pain, and emotion. A pinprick to the great toe sends a pain impulse up the same nerves as for light touch to the spinal cord. The fibers enter a different area of the spinal cord, forming local connections, and then travel up toward the brain in specific 'pain tracts'.

Unlike light touch, much of the sensation of pain is dealt with in the thalamus in a 'subconscious' manner. The thalamus coordinates evasive moves to avoid or reduce the pain, such as lifting your foot off the pin! Once the pain reaches a certain threshold, which varies according to the source and location of the pain stimulus, the thalamus allows the cortex to become aware. By this means we are spared much of the pain experienced by the body on a daily basis — and most would agree this is certainly a good arrangement.

Reticular Formation

The reticular formation is an extensive neuronal network located within the brainstem that not only controls basic functions, such as heartbeat and breathing, but also has a profound affect on the overall activity of the brain, level of arousal, behavior, and response to external stimuli. The reticular formation is similar to the hypothalamus in that from an evolutionary perspective it is has been around for a very long time. It is, for example, prominent in the brain stem of reptiles.

Some pain fibers traveling up the spinal cord toward the thalamus connect with the reticular formation. The activity of the reticular formation itself is influenced by both external stimuli, such as pain, and by the overall state of the brain. For example, following a stressful stimulus, the 'fight or flight' response induces a hyper-activity that increases awareness and sensitivity, though may reduce awareness and response to pain. The reticular formation sends messages back down the spinal cord that reinforce 'gate control', thereby exerting unconscious modification of pain sensitivity and reaction. This pathway provides the potential for conscious or voluntary modification of painful sensations and may also have a role in the influence of stress on the development and experience of pain.

Limbic System

Pain messages reaching the thalamus are forwarded to the temporal lobe of the brain, specifically the hippocampus. Through complex neural circuitry, the message is relayed back to the thalamus, the newly created pathway forming the basis of pain 'memory'. This is how we learn that fire is hot or a pin, sharp. When there is emotion, there is memory retention. A child cries from pain because he or she does not try to hide it like and adult. However, adults have the same reaction. The hippocampus also sends messages to the amygdala and hypothalamus, where a 'fight or flight' stress response is initiated, increasing adrenaline and cortisol production, protecting the body from a threatening environment. This response, designed to be beneficial, can have numerous adverse effects when chronically active.

A threatening event such as pain triggers the 'fight or flight' stress response. This is initiated in the amygdala and hippocampus, where external events are interpreted in the light of both innate behavior and life experience. The 'set point' of this process is under the influence of the serotonin system, which also controls mood, hunger, sleep, and aggression. The lower the set point, the more reactive the system and the more likely the stress response is to be triggered. In addition, the emotional memory of the event stored in the amygdala is stronger and carries greater influence when interpreting future events. This is called 'conditioned fear', the basis of the perceived stress.

✔ BACK FACTS

An important aspect to the sensation of pain is its emotional connotations governed by the limbic system, the extensive and complex neuronal circuitry that controls emotional behavior, motivation, and control of the internal and external environment. As such, the limbic system is central to the control of the stress response. Located within the temporal lobe of the brain, it comprises a number of elements, including the hippocampus and the amygdala, centers intricately involved in the stress response, emotion, and memory.

With perceived stress, minor stimulation such as slight pain — even the thought of an event or situation that induces pain — can trigger the 'fight or flight' reaction. As a result, anxiety increases, amplifying both the sensitivity to, and the severity of, pain. This perceived input or thought comes from the medial prefrontal cortex, an area exerting direct influence over the amygdala and hippocampus.

Limbic System

Saggital view of the brain with the structures of the limbic system.

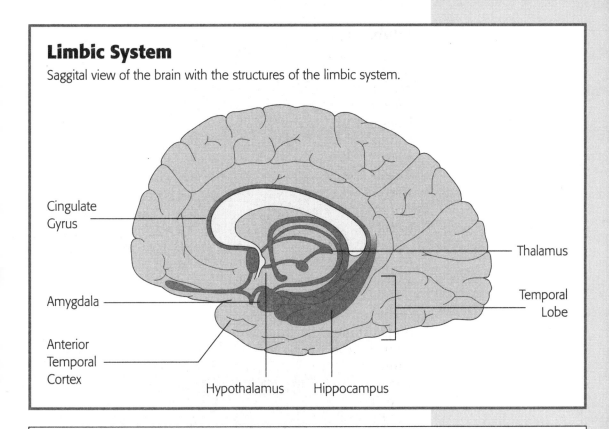

Cingulate Gyrus

Thalamus

Amygdala

Temporal Lobe

Anterior Temporal Cortex

Hypothalamus   Hippocampus

✔ BACK FACTS

Behavioral modification through simple techniques and counseling can significantly affect the influence the cortex has over the limbic system. This will prove to be important in some aspects of pain control in low back pain.

Types of Pain

Pain sensations arise from three types of body tissue: skin and its associated structures; ligaments, muscles, and tendons; and organs such the stomach or kidneys. We have followed a pain pathway for skin and have seen that, due to its dense innervation and detailed representation in the brain, the sensation is well localized. When we get a needle in our foot, we know exactly where it is.

The body has much more difficulty localizing pain when it comes from ligaments, muscles, and bones. Arthritis in the hip, for example, is often felt as thigh or knee pain. A ligament strain in the back can be felt from the shoulder blades to the knees. Organs are even worse. Take, for example, damage to the heart in a heart attack. Pain can be felt anywhere from the chest to the chin to the tips of the fingers.

Organ pain is named visceral pain (the organs are otherwise known as *viscera*). Pure visceral pain is vague, deep-seated, and accompanied by nausea or sweating. Think of the pain associated with a bad stomach flu. This pain likely travels through the autonomic nerves, part of the involuntary nervous system that controls the function of our organs and responses such as 'fight or flight'. This explains the associated symptoms. Once visceral pain reaches a certain intensity, pain is felt in areas supplied by other nerves from the same spinal cord level. This is the chest or arm pain of a heart attack or umbilical pain of appendicitis.

✔ BACK FACTS

Despite the fact that pain 'hurts', most of the time we tolerate it and continue to function. Fortunately, we are not incapacitated with every scratch or bruise. As adults we have learned to accept and control certain levels of pain that seem to be part of daily life. One of the players on our 'experienced' soccer team likes to say, "After 40, the pain never really goes away, it just changes location from time to time!"

The brain is not used to feeling pain from organs. The organs are actually insensitive to cutting or burning. Thus, when sensory input exceeds a certain level, cross-stimulation of other sensory nerves in the spinal cord is interpreted as pain.

A similar situation occurs with sensations from joints, ligaments, and muscles. Even though they possess considerable nerve supply and have a strong representation in the brain, the sensations associated with them are predominantly positional. The receptors feel tension, stretch, movement, and vibration, allowing us to determine body image and joint position. When these nerve fibers begin to feel 'pain', the brain has trouble localizing this sensation, interpreting it as coming from somewhere that normally experiences pain, such as the skin.

Low back pain incorporates elements of all three types of pain. However, the predominance of poorly localized and visceral pain results in back pain being intense, diffuse, deep-seated, and emotionally charged. Just one of the reasons why low back pain hurts so much!

Pain 'Gates'

The gate control theory of pain demonstrates that an increase in incoming messages from sensory fibers, such as light touch and pressure, will inhibit the transmission of pain fibers from sending their message up to the brain. This is why, if we hit our elbow, for example, we rub the area briskly to alleviate the pain. By stimulating the skin sensors to touch, we stop the painful sensation from other tissues reaching the brain. This mechanism may provide some of the basis behind the pain-relieving properties of touch, massage, acupuncture, and certainly TENS machines.

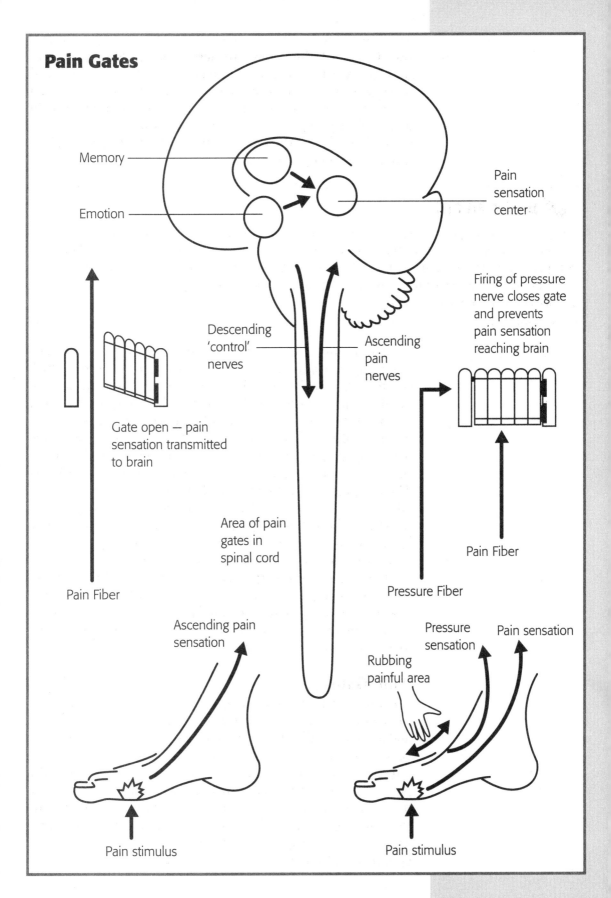

Pain Gates

Memory

Emotion

Pain sensation center

Descending 'control' nerves

Ascending pain nerves

Firing of pressure nerve closes gate and prevents pain sensation reaching brain

Gate open — pain sensation transmitted to brain

Pain Fiber

Area of pain gates in spinal cord

Pain Fiber

Pressure Fiber

Ascending pain sensation

Pressure sensation

Rubbing painful area

Pain sensation

Pain stimulus

Pain stimulus

Sensitization

This is an important and enigmatic feature of low back pain. Through central and peripheral factors, nerves are sensitized such that normally innocuous sensations are felt as pain.

Central Sensitization (when normal sensations feel painful)

Receptors and nerves that normally transmit non-painful sensations, such as light touch and pressure, can cause a feeling of pain if they are stimulated above a certain threshold. Under regular conditions, this threshold is quite high. It takes considerable pressure on the skin to produce a feeling of pain. However, under certain circumstances, this threshold is lowered, a state called 'central sensitization'.

Consider a bad cut on the skin. Even though the surrounding area is not damaged or inflamed, light pressure is painful. This is an example of central sensitization. The persistence of pain messages from the cut itself, transmitted through pain fibers to the spinal cord, causes hyper-excitability at that level. This lowers the threshold at which pressure sensations are interpreted as painful, such that the area surrounding the cut, supplied by that particular area of the spinal cord, is overly sensitive.

Central sensitization is thought to be an important factor in the severity, persistence, and diffuse nature of low back pain. In the presence of one noxious stimulus, an inflamed facet joint, for example, skin pressure, ligament or muscle stretch, and disc movement may be interpreted as painful. Blocking the pathways that promote central sensitization may be a way of decreasing the global pain and dysfunction associated with back pain.

Stress, either acute or chronic, may play a modifying role in central sensitization. Descending messages from the brain, particularly in the limbic system and reticular formation, can alter the level of responsiveness of pain and other sensory fibers, enhancing or reducing perceived discomfort.

Peripheral Sensitization (when pain fibers are extra-sensitive)

The sensitivity of pain receptors to physical (touch, pressure, heat, etc.) or chemical stimuli is influenced by local factors such as inflammation. The chemical transmitters released as a result of tissue damage cause pain receptors to be activated by normally innocuous stimuli such as light touch. In addition, up to one third of pain receptors are 'silent', unable to respond even to strong painful stimulus. In the presence of inflammation, these silent receptors become active, increasing the overall response and sensitivity to pain. The added transmission of pain messages to the spinal cord results in greater central sensitization.

Specific Origins of Back Pain

We have looked at the anatomical structures that make up the spine — the vertebrae, the facet joints, the discs, the innumerable ligaments, and the complex muscle mass. We have also looked at the spinal cord and its emerging nerve roots. Now we can look at these anatomical structures to see how they produce pain. When more than one structure hurts, it may be possible to break the pain down into separate components that may be easier to understand and manage. We shall now look more specifically at where pain arises within the structures of the low back and how that pain is 'felt'.

Understanding the complex pathways and interconnections of sensation and pain allows us not only to begin to comprehend where our back pain is coming from, but also how it is interpreted and why it seems to be so uncomfortable. This understanding is the foundation for developing treatment strategies for overcoming pain.

Pathologic Causes in Low Back Pain

Back pain may be caused by problems in the discs, muscles or ligaments, bones, and facet joints of the spine. More than one structure may be involved.

Disc	Muscle or Ligament	Bone	Facet Joint	More than One Structure
Strain	Strain	Fracture	Strain	Arthritis (with spinal stenosis)
Herniation	Major Tear	Infection	Arthritis	Instability (between vertebrae)
Degeneration/ Disruption		Malignancy	Osteoporosis	Inflammatory Arthritis (rheumatoid, ankylosing spondylitis Infection

Non-Spinal Causes of Low Back Pain

Back pain may also result from other parts of the anatomy.
* Kidney or Bladder Infection, Kidney Stone (associated fever, blood in the urine).
* Stomach/Duodenal Ulcer (associated heartburn, nausea, indigestion).
* Gynaecologic Problems: endometriosis, ectopic pregnancy, fibroids, infection (associated irregular bleeding, pain with periods, vaginal discharge).
* Pancreatic Inflammation or Pancreatitis (associated history of bile stones, alcohol abuse, recent infection).
* Enlarged Abdominal Aorta (severe, unremitting, rapidly worsening low back pain).

Causes of Back Pain

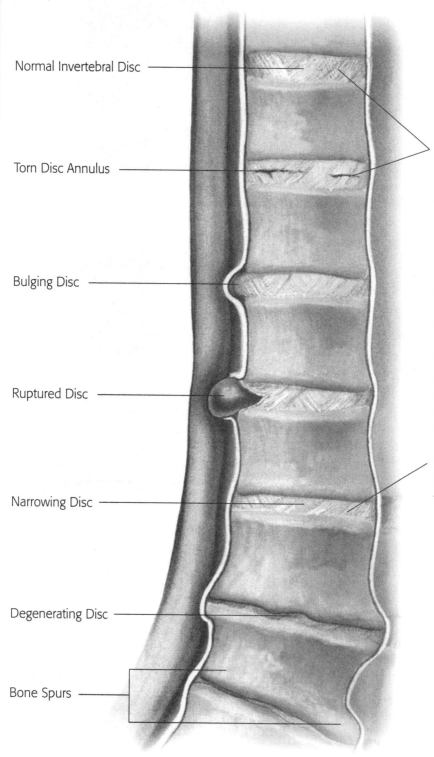

Normal Invertebral Disc

Torn Disc Annulus

Bulging Disc

Ruptured Disc

Narrowing Disc

Degenerating Disc

Bone Spurs

Invertebral Discs commonly wear and may tear, weakening their outer fibrous structure.

Increasing pressure in the spine may bulge and even rupture the disc, causing back or leg pain.

In normal aging, discs lose water and decrease their ability to function as 'shock absorbers.'

Narrowing discs increase stress to the facet joints.

Osteoarthritis may result in narrowing of the disc spaces and development of bone spurs in the vertebral bodies.

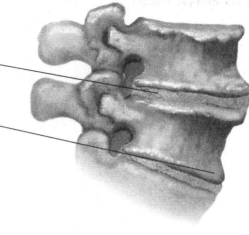

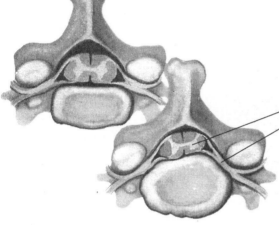

Spinal Stenosis or narrowing of the spinal canal may be the result of arthritis, putting pressure on the nerves and spinal cord.

Instability or abnormal motion may occur in the advanced stages of arthritis or from trauma.

Narrowing discs increase stress to the facet joints.

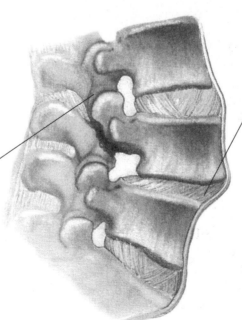

Spondylolisthesis is a forward 'slipping' of one vertebra over another and may be the result of severe instability.

Ankylosing Spondylitis, an inherited form of arthritis, causes swelling, stiffness, and loss of motion in the back.

Intervertebral Disc Pain

The disc is a major source of pain within the low back. Compared to other structures in the area, the disc is relatively richly innervated, although the nerve fibers are confined mainly to the superficial layers. Sensors for both pain and pressure are present with higher accumulations toward the posterior surface. In addition, the anterior and posterior ligaments that adhere closely to the front and back surfaces of the discs contain numerous nerve fibers, predominantly of the pain category. Interestingly, discs showing degeneration appear to have increased nerve supply.

Stimulation of the disc surface in awake patients undergoing surgery (local anaesthetic is used for the incision and dissection) recreates the sensation of back pain in many cases. Even if the sensation is one of 'pressure', under circumstances of central sensitization, these feelings will be interpreted as pain. Injection of salt water into the disc of human test subjects recreates the intense, poorly localized, deep aching discomfort of discogenic low back pain. In these studies, pain was only experienced when the outer shell of the disc was breached. The threshold for this was far lower in degenerate discs. This is thought to be due to a combination of reduced resilience and heightened nerve fiber sensitivity due to chemical changes within the disc — a type of peripheral sensitization.

 BACK FACTS

The dual nerve supply to the disc, involving both regular sensory nerves and those of the sympathetic system, results in a more profound, diffuse, and complex pain.

Disc Degeneration and Herniation

Common Characteristics:

- Repetitive bending with twisting and heavy lifting (over 25 lbs).
- Vibration associated with prolonged driving.
- Male aged 30–50.
- Cigarette smoking.

Disc Herniation

'Slipped disc', 'herniated disc', 'sciatica', 'nerve damage' — these terms are used interchangeably and often inappropriately when dealing with low back and leg pain. Of all aspects of this nebulous subject, the 'disc' is perhaps the most confusing and the one with the most preconceptions. It is frequently considered the principal cause of back pain, demonstrating how poorly understood the pathology and incidence is.

The most important concept to grasp is that the disc comprises a tough outer shell (annulus fibrosus, AF) and a soft inner core (nucleus pulposus, NP). A weakness in the AF may allow the NP to bulge outward, while a tear or split permits the NP to actually extrude from the disc. One further stage involves the NP material separating to form a sequestered mass of tissue lying free within the spinal canal.

Changes in structure and consistency of both the AF and NP that occur with age likely contribute to the development of disc herniation. The hydration and collagen content of the AF falls and small cracks and tears appear. The NP dries out, making it less able to withstand compression, forcing it to flow toward areas of weakness. Typically, the weakest part of the disc is at the back, just to either side of the strong posterior longitudinal ligament. Herniation may occur gradually as part of the degenerative process or as an acute event.

Due to the close proximity of the spinal nerve roots to the posterior aspect of the disc, herniated NP material can compress or stretch these structures. This may result in pain, typically 'sciatica' or nerve dysfunction with numbness or weakness in the leg. In certain cases, cauda equina syndrome may result from a large central disc compressing a number of nerve roots, causing variable sensory loss, weakness, and loss of bladder and bowel control. This presentation requires emergency assessment and surgical treatment.

Disc Herniation and Sciatica

- Almost 90% of individuals will experience at least one episode of low back pain during their lifetime.
- The lifetime incidence of a symptomatic lumbar disc herniation is only 2%.
- 'Sciatica' does not always result from disc herniation.
- MRI scans of individuals with no back or leg pain reveal 28% to have disc herniations.
- 70% of patients with sciatica recover in 6 to 12 weeks.
- Only 1% to 2% of patients with 'sciatica' require surgery.

Sciatica and Nerve Damage

Sciatica refers to pain in the leg below the level of the buttock fold. It relates to the sciatic nerve, a large nerve supplying most of the leg with power and sensation that arises from numerous roots in the lumbar spine. If the pain of sciatica is specific, relating clearly to one nerve root, then it is called radicular pain. Often accompanied by numbness or tingling, the pain radiates down the leg to a specific area such as the great toe or the outside of the foot. The nerve roots from each

Sciatica Causes

- Disc herniation.
- Narrowing due to arthritis.
- Inflammation.
- Facet joint calcification.
- Cyst or tumor within the spinal canal (rare).
- Pressure on the nerve in the pelvis or leg.

level of the lumbar spine supply a fairly specific area of skin in the leg. If the pain of sciatica is more dull, radiating downward but to a more diffuse area, it is called referred pain. Typically this pain radiates through the buttocks and thighs, sometimes into the calf.

Nerve root compression and damage can also cause the nerve to malfunction. In this case, there may be loss of skin sensation in the area supplied by the nerve, loss of power in the muscles it supplies, and loss of reflexes as tested by an examiner. Nerve root dysfunction may or may not be associated with pain. Sciatica does not imply damage, just irritation of the nerve. Even when there is evidence of dysfunction, the nerve is usually able to recover.

Sciatica results from nerve compression or irritation combined with local and central factors producing sensitization. It is not always due to a disc herniation. Anything that stretches or compresses the sciatic nerve roots can produce similar symptoms.

Disc Degeneration

A distinction should be made between disc *aging* and disc *degeneration*. All intervertebral discs go through a number of normal changes during growth, development, and aging. However, not all of them degenerate.

With age, discs naturally lose some height and start to bulge. Proteoglycan (the large matrix molecules) and water content diminish. Flexibility of the structure is lost and fissures and cracks appear. Blood supply to the disk becomes limited and the number of cells living within it, falls. All discs show these changes but to varying degrees and at varying speeds.

Disc degeneration refers to such rapid or extreme progression of the aging process that the disc loses structural integrity and its ability to distribute load. The balance between synthesis of disc tissue and its breakdown shifts toward degradation and the nucleus starts to disappear, resorbed by cells and enzymes. Increased force across the vertebrae and facet joints leads to arthritic change, stiffness, instability, and stenosis.

So at what point does all this become painful? The brief answer is, 'we just don't know'. Why some discs with early changes of 'aging' are extremely painful, while others with advanced degeneration are barely bothersome is an enigma of this condition. Aging does not automatically mean degeneration. Aging and degeneration of a disc are asymptomatic most of the time. The relationship between disc damage and pain is influenced by a combination of factors in the spine along with less tenable elements such as health, happiness, stress, and psychological makeup.

Disc Degeneration Pain Sources

Mechanical
- Increased force transmitted to the vertebrae.
- Loss of height alters biomechanical behavior and increases load through facet joints, ligaments, and muscles.

Nervous
- Tears or fissures stimulate nerves supplying the outer annulus of the disc.
- Altered forces stimulate the autonomic nerves (sinu-vertebral nerves).
- Abnormal loads across the facet joints, inflammation, and arthritis stimulate the dorsal sensory nerves.

Chemical
- Leaking disc tissue induces inflammation and an immune response.
- Cytokines, Nitric Oxide, ProstaglandinE2 produced by degeneration and free radicals induce inflammation.

Sensitization
- A combination of above factors all contribute to peripheral sensitization, which results in even normally benign sensations, such as stretch, being felt as pain.

Types of Disc Herniation

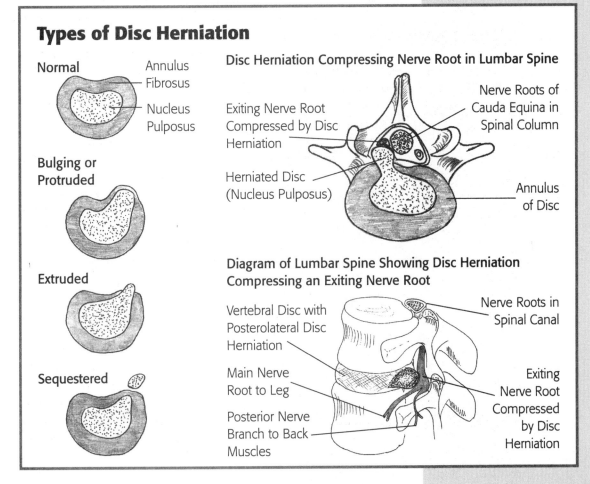

Normal

Annulus Fibrosus

Nucleus Pulposus

Bulging or Protruded

Extruded

Sequestered

Disc Herniation Compressing Nerve Root in Lumbar Spine

Exiting Nerve Root Compressed by Disc Herniation

Herniated Disc (Nucleus Pulposus)

Nerve Roots of Cauda Equina in Spinal Column

Annulus of Disc

Diagram of Lumbar Spine Showing Disc Herniation Compressing an Exiting Nerve Root

Vertebral Disc with Posterolateral Disc Herniation

Main Nerve Root to Leg

Posterior Nerve Branch to Back Muscles

Nerve Roots in Spinal Canal

Exiting Nerve Root Compressed by Disc Herniation

Disc Injury

The intervertebral disc is a complex structure designed to withstand tremendous compressive loads. Values of up to 4000N can be generated during heavy lifting, but due to the way the disc redistributes load to the bony vertebrae, the vertebral body is likely to fracture before the disc ruptures. In contrast, the disc tolerates torsional (rotational) stress very poorly. At between 3 and 12 degrees of rotation, small tears appear in the annulus (outer layer of the disc) and beyond that complete disc failure. Fortunately, the facet joints resist this unwanted rotation, but minor degrees of injury can occur, especially when combined with other movements. The combination of compression with a forward and sideways bending with a twist puts the disc at highest risk of injury. This will result at the least in a 'strain' or minor annulus tear, and may result in frank disc failure with herniation.

✔ BACK FACTS

Disc injury is thought to be an uncommon cause of acute low back pain and is certainly almost never a factor in individuals under the age of 30 in whom disc degeneration has not established a foothold. By the age of 50, however, over 90% of lumbar discs show evidence of deterioration and development of acute annular tears is certainly a consideration.

Fortunately, the vast majority of tears are asymptomatic and concluding evidence of acute disc injury is therefore difficult. Unless there is rapid development of radicular leg pain (sciatica) with associated nerve dysfunction and findings to indicate a frank disc herniation, diagnosis of annular 'strain' remains conjectural.

Injury to the anterior structures, which may include the intervertebral disc, may be implied by symptoms characterized by pain on flexing forward and relief by extending or arching backward. This 'symptomatic' classification is valuable as it helps direct treatment at a time when specific diagnosis is less important than pain relief and functional recovery.

Facet Joint Pain

The lumbar facet joints (zygoapophyseal joints) are the paired synovial joints at the back of each vertebra supplied by branches of the dorsal sensory nerve, the main trunk through which peripheral sensation reaches the spinal cord. Each facet is supplied by two nerves, one from its own level, one from the level above. The capsule of the joint is densely supplied with sensory endings that respond to pressure and stretch. It also contains specific pain fibers. Mechanical stimulation by chronic or acute strain of the joint capsule can give rise to painful sensation, particularly in the presence of sensitization by local factors such as inflammation or by central mechanisms.

Injection of saline into the facet joints of test subjects recreates low back pain with radiation into the buttock and posterior thigh. Studies using local anaesthetic to block the nerves supplying the facets indicate that approximately 15% of low back pain patients have an element of facet pain.

The presence of nerve endings within the synovial tissue lining the facet joint provides an additional source of painful stimuli. This would likely play an important role in arthritic conditions affecting the spine, such as rheumatoid arthritis, ankylosing spondylitis, or osteoarthritis.

Facet Injury

The facets are joints just like the knee or the shoulder and are therefore prone to injury. The surrounding capsule and ligaments can be stretched by movement or force beyond their tolerance, and the joint itself can become inflamed and swollen. The facet joint is a significant pain generator, often resulting in both local and referred pain, muscle spasm, reduced flexibility and tenderness. Next to muscle injury, facet strain is probably the second most common cause of acute low back pain.

As with disc injury, the specific diagnosis is less important than the symptoms in acute low back pain. Injury to the posterior elements of the spine including the facet joints will generally cause pain worse on extension of the spine and relieved by flexion. Again, this is a valuable modifier of treatment.

 BACK FACTS

Facet joint damage or inflammation resulting in chronic pain with peripheral and central sensitization sets up a cycle of pain that is hard to break. The reflex protective muscle spasm associated with pain will increase forces across the facet joints, further contributing to damage and discomfort. Prolonged spasm, leading to damage, and inflammation within the muscle will cause further sensitization as well as inducing pain sensation from the muscle itself.

Muscle and Ligament Pain

Despite the observation that the muscles of the back are richly supplied with nerve fibers, the evidence for a muscular origin for low back pain is limited. Their nerve supply includes receptors for stretch, pressure, and pain, yet muscle fiber damage itself does not appear to be painful. When a sample of muscle is taken for analysis in a surgical biopsy procedure, only the skin and overlying tissues need to be anaesthetized. Cutting the muscle itself is not painful. For pain to arise from this source, other factors have to be in play.

Stretch and Pressure Thresholds

Muscle pain can arise from stretch and pressure inputs if they exceed a certain threshold. This threshold can be lowered by central sensitization within the spinal cord, as occurs in situations of prolonged painful input from other sites. This would explain the muscular pain associated with disc or facet injury or deterioration. Pain can also arise from the pain receptors, although the majority of these appear to be 'silent', requiring a degree of peripheral sensitization to become active. This peripheral sensitization is induced predominantly by local inflammation such as occurs following tissue damage, a mechanism responsible for pain in lumbar strain injury. Inadequate blood flow and oxygen supply, otherwise known as 'ischaemia', also greatly increases sensitivity and may play a role in chronic pain.

Reflex muscle spasm may also play a role in the pain complex that pervades low back pain. It has been shown that facet joint irritation induces spontaneous contraction of muscles on the same side of the spine. This would have a number of effects. Not only would it increase pressure on the already injured facet, it would reduce the threshold for muscle pain by increasing sensory inputs and would promote peripheral sensitization through ischaemia.

Sensory Field Widening

A second factor relates to the way increasing stimulation of sensory fibers within muscle leads to widening of the 'sensory field', the area over which the sensation is perceived as arising. Thus, intense feelings of pain from a muscular source are felt in remote muscles such as the buttocks or thighs, joints such as the hips, and ligaments in the back and pelvis.

Cross Innervation

Cross-innervation of muscles by the sympathetic nervous system, similar to that described above for the discs, leads to deep, burning, diffuse pain, often called 'visceral pain', which has both physiologic effects, such as nausea and sweating, and a strong central emotional component.

Muscle Tear

Muscle injury predominantly occurs through eccentric loading. This is the forcible stretching of a muscle while it is contracting that might occur, for example, during a lifting maneuver in which a load suddenly falls. The back muscles that are contracting to lift the load are stretched by the unexpected increase in weight.

Muscle injury alone is not painful. However, one of the critical events is the bleeding and inflammation that follows muscle injury. While the original damage may be painless or felt as a simple 'pull', the subsequent chemical and cellular changes result in significant discomfort. This takes hours to develop and is the reason why the real pain from a lumbar strain injury is felt later on. Associated with this pain and inflammation is a decrease in the ability of the muscle to contract, resulting in weakness, increased fatigue, and risk of further injury.

A lumbar strain due to a muscle injury is similar to a hamstring tear or calf 'pull'. The mechanism is the same and the muscle injury process identical. The reasons why the back injury seems so much more severe and incapacitating include the inability to rest the affected muscle, patterns of nerve supply, sensitization of pain receptors, and reactive spasm. This seems to create a 'vicious cycle' that exacerbates the effects of the injury far more than might be expected.

Distinguishing features of a lumbar strain due to a muscle tear include localized swelling, tenderness, and bruising, usually only on one side of the spine.

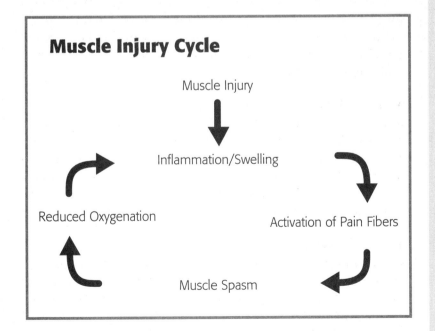

Muscle Injury Cycle

Muscle Injury

Inflammation/Swelling

Reduced Oxygenation

Activation of Pain Fibers

Muscle Spasm

Nerve Pain

While all pain from the back must arise from nerves, it is important to distinguish between pain arising from the end of the nerve (the receptor) and pain arising from stimulation along the course of a sensory nerve. This latter form of input is called 'ectopic' input and provides the basis of radicular or nerve pain in low back disorders, particularly disc herniations, where it is termed 'sciatica'.

Mechanical Abnormalities

Pressure on a nerve does not automatically cause pain. Try, for example, pressing on the ulnar nerve just inside the point of your elbow (the area known as the 'funny bone'). Simple pressure in this soft spot gives only the sensation of touch and pressure locally. Even firm pressure, while painful, is still felt at the point of pressure rather than in the area the nerve supplies, the little finger side of the hand. Although it is not recommended that you try it, tapping on the nerve will cause ectopic firing and a feeling of pain or a sensation of pins and needles in the hand. This is what you experience when you inadvertently hit your 'funny bone'.

Compression or 'traction' on a nerve root such as might occur following a disc herniation does not in itself trigger impulses in normal nerves. However, after a period of prolonged compression (hours to days), the properties of the nerve change such that the mid-portion of the nerve begins to generate electrical signals. These ectopic messages are transmitted to the spinal cord and then to the brain where they are interpreted as if they were true sensations arising from the receptor at the end of the nerve.

Damage due to compression or traction can lead to disruption or loss of the protective insulation that covers a nerve, a process called 'demyelination'. This covering is responsible for nutrition, metabolism, and the electrical properties of the nerve.

✔ BACK FACTS

Why is nerve pain due to pressure such a tremendous problem in some low back conditions? The answer, as with so many other causes of pain we have discussed, lies in the co-existence of other factors, both local and central, that can influence the sensitivity of a nerve, reducing its threshold to ectopic firing.

Chemical Abnormalities

At least part of the alteration in nerve properties is due to the interruption of the blood supply. Nerves, like any other tissue, require blood flow to provide oxygen and other nutrients. When this is impaired, the nerve will begin to malfunction.

Nerves also require nutrient flow of the cerebrospinal fluid (CSF), which bathes the brain, spinal cord, and nerve roots. This flow can also interrupted by compression, further contributing to the metabolic insult. The rapidity of onset of this compression influences the degree of damage sustained by the nerve. More rapid onset is less well tolerated and tends to cause greater impairment of nerve function, whereas slower onset trauma allows the nerve to function but produces more pain. In addition, when multiple roots are involved, the effect is cumulative, greatly increasing pain and dysfunction.

Destructive enzymes can alter the nerve sheath (demyelination) and weaken other supporting structures. Inflammation within the membranes that surround the spinal cord and nerve roots can induce firing in local pain receptors, further adding to sensory input and central sensitization.

 BACK FACTS

Local inflammation resulting from numerous factors, including trauma, arthritis, mechanical irritation, and disc herniation, can lead to the release of chemicals that act directly and indirectly to influence nerve function. As with inflammation elsewhere, locally acting mediators released by involved cells cause swelling or 'edema' that will exacerbate any nerve root compression.

Recent studies have shown that the material released from the disc as a result of herniation of the nucleus pulposus has a significant chemical effect on the nerve in addition to its mechanical action of compression or traction. It appears that the glycoprotein component of the nucleus pulposus, along with enzymes produced by the cells of this structure, are able to damage the nerve root quite significantly. In addition, they induce an immune reaction with inflammation, which further compounds the problem.

Electrical Abnormalities

Besides the mechanical and chemical abnormalities, electrical irregularities within the nerves and spinal cord also contribute to the development of nerve pain. The role of sympathetic nerve fibers in the characteristic deep burning pain of low back disorders is significant. These fibers further influence ectopic pain from sensory nerves. Firing within sympathetic sensory nerves is associated with release of the excitatory chemical noradrenaline (similar to adrenaline), which acts on receptors involved in incoming regular sensory nerves. This stimulation , called 'sympathetic-sensory coupling', lowers their threshold for firing and, in particular, ectopic discharge.

Increased Nerve Sensitivity Causes

• Prolonged Compression/Traction
• Demyelination
• Local Inflammation
• Chemical Stimulation
• Sympathetic-sensory Coupling
• Excitatory Crosstalk

Similar to sympathetic-sensory coupling, 'excitatory crosstalk' occurs between adjacent sensory nerves. This non-neural communication results in heightened sensitivity in sensory nerve roots adjacent to ones that are already stimulated and firing. This is different from central sensitization, which occurs within the spinal cord. A sudden surge in incoming sensory information, as might occur from a sudden movement, would sensitize the entire nerve root at the dorsal root ganglion. The reduced threshold would allow firing in other nerves, which in turn would further add to the excitation. A wave of sensory pulses would then converge on the spinal cord, causing a 'shock-like' spasm of pain, something typically described by low back pain sufferers.

Sciatica (Radicular and Referred) Pain

Sciatica is generally referred to as pain radiating from the back, through the buttock and back of the thigh, often traveling down to the ankle and foot. It may be associated with numbness or pins-and-needles.

Damage, compression, or traction on a nerve root under certain conditions will cause ectopic firing of that nerve. Impulses will be generated at the point of damage rather than at the end of the nerve, where the receptors are located in the skin, a muscle, or a ligament, for example. However, the brain is unable to distinguish ectopic from regular impulses, so the ectopic messages are interpreted as arising from the end of the nerve. Thus, if the damaged nerve supplies the skin of the big toe, that is where the sensation will be felt. This is the basis for radicular and referred pain.

✔ BACK FACTS

The term 'sciatica' and back pain occur together so frequently as to become almost synonymous. However, as we have seen, the sources of low back pain are legion, while sciatica arises purely from ectopic stimulation of the lumbar nerve roots.

If the pain of sciatica is specific, relating clearly to one nerve root, then it is called 'radicular pain'. Often accompanied by numbness or tingling, the pain radiates down the leg to a specific area such as the great toe or the outside of the foot. The nerve roots from each level of the lumbar spine supply a fairly specific area of skin in the leg.

If the pain of sciatica is more dull, radiating downward but to a more diffuse area, it is called 'referred pain'. Typically, this pain radiates through the buttocks and thighs, sometimes into the calf.

Nerve root compression and damage can also cause the nerve to malfunction. In this case, there may be loss of skin sensation in the area supplied by the nerve, loss of power in the muscles it supplies, and loss of reflexes as tested by an examiner. Nerve root dysfunction may or may not be associated with pain.

Pain from Compression of the Bony Vertebra

The bony vertebrae have an identifiable nerve supply and are so closely associated with the discs and the ligaments that bony damage will generally affect sensors in these structures also. Having said that, bone pain is not thought to play a significant role in the majority of low back problems. The exceptions are pain due to fracture, either traumatic or resulting from osteoporosis (thinning of the bones), and invasive diseases such as infection or tumor. These latter two are, however, extremely rare.

BACK FACTS

A compression fracture occurs when the force compressing the front part of the vertebral body is greater than the strength of the bone. This can occur in one of two scenarios:
1. Normal bone strength and excessive force; or
2. Normal force but weakened bone.

Compression Fracture

Lateral view of the vertebral column, showing compression fractures of a vertebra.

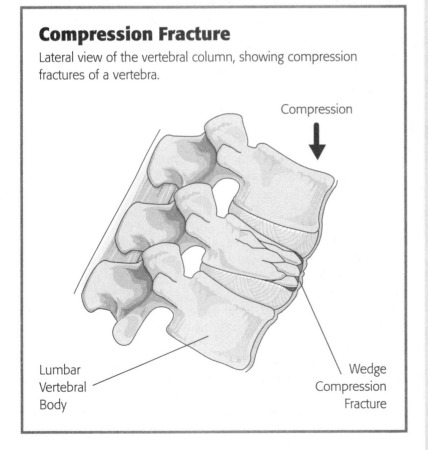

Compression

Lumbar Vertebral Body

Wedge Compression Fracture

Normal Bone Strength and Excessive Force

In a younger individual with normal bone quality, a significant fall or flexion injury can produce sufficient force to overcome the inherent strength of the vertebral bone. This can occur from an injury as innocuous as falling onto the buttocks having missed the chair or from more profound trauma such as a fall in the workplace. Pain from such an injury is normally instantaneous and intense, in contrast to a lumbar strain where initial pain is often minor or goes unnoticed and develops after a number of hours. An injury that results in a fracture is not normally ignored unless there are other factors involved, such as alcohol or drugs. In general, this is a problem that presents to the emergency room.

Normal Force but Weakened Bone

Compression fractures can occur with minor injury or even day-to-day activity if the quality of the vertebral body bone is compromised. Causes include osteoporosis, osteopenia (weakened bone due to illness, immobility, or medications such as steroids), infection, and malignancy.

The most common presentation of a compression fracture in weakened bone is an elderly person presenting with sudden onset of back pain. This may be spontaneous or following a simple fall or lifting injury. The individual may already have recognized osteoporosis and may be undergoing treatment. The pain is usually well localized, although there is likely some associated protective muscle spasm. There is rarely any leg pain or neurologic symptoms. Workup for the elderly individual or the patient with risk factors for weak bone includes a thorough history and physical examination followed by blood tests and plain X-rays.

Arthritis Pain

For some individuals, arthritis is a major cause of their low back pain. Their pain is likely to persist, progress, or recur with great frequency. Pain tends to be back-dominant, associated with stiffness, and likely to follow the pattern of arthritis in other areas, with pain-free periods and gradual step-wise deterioration. There may be evidence of arthritis in joints or tissues remote from the spine. Apart from ankylosing spondylitis in some rheumatoid patients, this is generally an affliction of the older individual (over 60 years).

✔ BACK FACTS

Unlike degenerative disc disease, lumbar spine arthritis (also called lumbar 'spondylosis') tends to affect multiple levels rather than one or two and involves all anatomic components of the spine, including discs, facets, and ligaments.

Defining Arthritis

The word 'arthritis' literally means inflammation of a joint. Arthritis is perhaps best considered as a symptom of an inflamed, stiff, swollen joint that is the end result of a number of disease processes. While inflammation may be the principal underlying process that has resulted in the symptoms of pain and swelling, its cause may be quite varied. In addition, the disease causing the arthritis may affect other tissues in close proximity, or in some cases at some distance from the joint.

By attaching other descriptors to the word 'arthritis' (for example, osteoarthritis or rheumatoid arthritis), we can more closely identify and distinguish the different disease processes and patterns. However, this classic division between 'wear-and-tear' non-inflammatory osteoarthritis and immunological inflammatory rheumatoid arthritis has become blurred recently as more and more inflammatory chemicals, such interleukin-1 (IL-1) and tumor necrosis factor (TNF), are discovered as playing an important part in the development and progression of all forms of arthritis. No longer does it appear that osteoarthritis is purely the result of wear-and-tear, or that rheumatoid arthritis is purely the result of immuno-logical over-activity.

The classification of different types of arthritis nevertheless does help to distinguish different patterns of disease by contrasting presentation of symptoms, clinical findings, and the results of X-rays and blood tests. Such classification is also helpful in organizing thought processes — and in creating guidelines for prognosis and treatment. Not everyone can be slotted conveniently into a particular category or diagnostic group, which underscores the role of the healthcare practitioner plays in establishing a suitable treatment regime for arthritis.

Osteoarthritis vs Rheumatoid Arthritis

Characteristic	Osteoarthritis	Rheumatoid Arthritis
Age	over 65	women 30–50 men 50–70
Common Joints Affected	knees/hips/spine	hands/feet
Number Joints Affected	1 or 2, usually 1 side first	multiple joints, both sides
Systemic symptoms (fatigue, fever, etc.)	absent	can occur
Non-joint involvement (lungs, skin, heart, etc.)	absent	common
Blood tests	normal	rheumatoid factor

Osteoarthritis (Degenerative Joint Disease)

Osteoarthritis is also known as degenerative joint disease (DJD), osteoarthrosis, hypertrophic arthritis, and non-inflammatory arthritis. It is the most common form of arthritis and likely exists to some degree in all individuals by age 65. Over 20 million North Americans over the age of 45 are affected by the disease. Women are affected more than men. Osteoarthritis is not a new disease. It has been identified in the bones of dinosaurs and in the skeletons of pre-historic man and Egyptian pharaohs. It is seen in almost all vertebrates, including those that live in water.

Osteoarthritis is primarily a disease that affects the smooth articular cartilage that covers the ends of our bones within the joint. Articular cartilage is a highly specialized composite of cells, fibers, and matrix 'glue'. It holds water to provide cushioning, yet has the structural integrity to withstand impact and shear force. Its interaction with the synovial fluid that circulates within the joint results in almost frictionless motion. In osteoarthritis, this structure breaks down, resulting in loss of its ability to provide support, resistance, and unhindered movement. The matrix 'glue' becomes weak and the fibers disorganized, leading to over-hydration and softening. Fissures appear and layers of cartilage are lost. Attempts by the few cells to restore order are futile and hindered by the increased production of enzymes that accelerate destruction (collagenases and metalloproteinases). The damaged proteins that are released induce an immune reaction, further increasing inflammation and breakdown.

✔ BACK FACTS

Osteoarthritis in the lower spine, commonly called lumbar spondylosis, is the most common type of arthritis to affect the lumbar spine. Lumbar spondylosis is widespread after the age of 55 and ubiquitous in the elderly.

Osteoarthritis also affects the bone underlying the cartilage (subchondral bone), causing thickening and rigidity along with minute fractures that may be the cause of some of the pain associated with arthritis. The stiffer bone results in more force being transferred to the cartilage, also accelerating breakdown. The lining of the joint (synovium) becomes inflamed by irritation from the debris of cartilage destruction and the associated immune inflammatory response. It becomes thickened, painful, and produces excess fluid, causing the joint to swell.

Tissues surrounding the joint, such as the capsule, bursa, ligaments, and tendons, are also affected, with thickening causing stiffness, inflammation causing pain, and fluid causing swelling.

Lumbar Spondylosis (Osteoarthritis)

Despite its prevalence, arthritis in the lumbar spine remains surprisingly asymptomatic. Arthritis in the hips and knees causes far more pain and disability and results in many more physician visits than arthritis in the low back. As is often the case with arthritis, even the most disastrous looking X-rays are often seen as an incidental finding in patients with complaints in other areas.

Disc degeneration in the spine leads to progressively increased stresses and damage to the posterior facets, with osteoarthritis developing in these small synovial joints. The degenerative "cascade" described by Kirkaldy-Willis shows a graduated deterioration with progressive involvement of all components of the spine. Mild stiffness and intermittent pain may result. Progressive thickening and calcification of ligaments, bone spurs, instability, and loss of disc height contribute to narrowing of the space available for the neural elements, a condition called 'spinal stenosis'.

Rheumatoid Arthritis

Rheumatoid arthritis is one of a number of inflammatory diseases that diffusely affect tissues throughout the body. These diseases include psoriatic arthritis, ankylosing spondylitis, Reiter's syndrome, SLE (systemic lupus erythematosus), dermatomyositis, and vasculitis. The distinguishing feature of rheumatoid arthritis is it predilection for affecting primarily synovial joints. Other conditions in this group of diseases can also affect the joints, but the arthritis tends to be a less prominent symptom as other tissues are more frequently involved (for example, the skin in psoriatic arthritis).

✔ BACK FACTS

Rheumatoid arthritis (RA) predominantly affects the hands and the feet, with the third most commonly affected site being the cervical spine (neck), where significant involvement can lead to instability and spinal cord compression requiring surgery. RA can also affect the low back, where it causes disc space narrowing, facet joint destruction (with typical synovial joint erosions), ligamentous damage, and subsequent instability. In addition, both the disease and the subsequent treatment with steroid medication may lead to osteoporosis, with risk of compression fracture. Fortunately, in most individuals, it causes little or no discomfort.

Rheumatoid arthritis is the most common type of inflammatory arthritis and affects about 1% of the population. Women tend to develop rheumatoid arthritis in their thirties and forties, with men developing it in their fifties and sixties. By age 65, it is estimated that approximately 0.75% of women and 0.2% of men suffer from rheumatoid arthritis.

Arthritis is a systemic disease, and although its focus appears to be primarily in the joints, other tissues can be affected. These include the skin, where nodules can develop, usually in the forearm just below the elbow. Muscles and nerves may be affected causing weakness. The eyes can become inflamed, as can numerous other tissues, including the lung, heart, and arteries. The involvement of these other tissues is fortunately rare and associated with the more severe forms of rheumatoid arthritis.

Patients with RA may experience low back pain but the degree of pain and dysfunction is normally overshadowed by involvement of the hands, feet, neck, hips and knees. A program similar to that employed for osteoarthritis can be used if low back pain is a problem.

Ankylosing Spondylitis

Ankylosing spondylitis is one of a group of diseases called the spondyloarthropathies. These include ankylosing spondylitis, reactive arthritis, Reiter's syndrome, arthropathy (associated with bowel inflammatory disease), and psoriatic arthritis. These diseases are considered a separate entity from rheumatoid arthritis and osteoarthritis, although presentation and involvement of certain joints may be similar. The incidence of ankylosing spondylitis in the general population is about 0.2%. However, in individuals possessing the genetic marker HLA-B27, the incidence is approximately 1% to 2%.

The etiology or cause of ankylosing spondylitis remains elusive. Strong association with the HLA-B27 genetic marker indicates a possible combination of genetic predisposition and environmental stimulus. Infective agents, such as the Klebsiella organism, have been indicated, and there is definite link between another of the spondylo arthropathies, Reiter's syndrome, as well as Chlamydia, Shigella, Salmonella, and Yersina.

By far the most common presentation of ankylosing spondylitis is low back pain. The back pain is usually felt in the upper buttock and comes on gradually. The pain may move from side to side and is associated with stiffness that is worse in the morning. The pain typically is worse at rest and is eased as the individual begins to mobilize. The pain can spread throughout the back and between the shoulder blades. Occasionally chest pain can be felt either at the back of the chest or in the region of the breastbone.

The hips and shoulders are the most common large joint targets for ankylosing spondylitis and are affected in about 20% of sufferers. In some cases, the pain or stiffness in one of these joints may spark the initial diagnosis. One feature that

Ankylosing Spondylitis Symptoms

- Onset before age 40 years.
- More common in males.
- Insidious onset.
- Low back pain for at least 3 months duration.
- Pain in low back and buttocks.
- Pain eased by exercise

ankylosing spondylitis and indeed the other spondyloarthropathis have in common with rheumatoid arthritis and not with osteoarthritis is the involvement of other tissues besides the bones and joints. Ankylosing spondylitis can affect the eyes, heart, lung, and kidneys. Involvement of the feet with tendonitis or plantar fasciitis ('heel spurs') is a common associated symptom.

Psoriatic Arthritis

Psoriatic arthritis is a type of inflammatory arthritis associated with the skin condition psoriasis. Psoriasis is a skin condition characterized by well-demarcated, red lesions covered with silvery scales. It typically involves the scalp and behind the ears, the back of the elbows, the front of the knees, the back, and the buttocks. Involvement of the finger and toenails may resemble a fungal infection with pitting, splitting, discoloration, and debris under the nails. Its association with low back pain groups it with ankylosing spondylitis as one of the spondylo-arthropathies.

 BACK FACTS

Psoriasis occurs in about 1% to 2% of the general population and psoriatic arthritis develops in about 10% of people with psoriasis. Psoriatic arthritis does not occur without psoriasis, although areas of skin involvement may be minor and may require careful searching for by the physician or patient. Men and woman are equally affected with psoriatic arthritis.

Psoriatic arthritis has been identified as distinct from rheumatoid arthritis. The incidence of positive blood test for rheumatoid factor is low. Psoriatic arthritis differs from osteoarthritis in the fact that it is predominately inflammatory and involves tissues other than the joints, most notably the skin and nails. It is different from rheumatoid arthritis in that it tends to involve the joints at the ends of the fingers rather than at the knuckles. It is similar to ankylosing spondylitis in its association with HLA-B27.

As with many of the inflammatory arthritides, the exact cause of psoriatic arthritis is unknown. There is certainly a strong genetic component and involvement of the HLA-B27 gene as well as other HLA genes. There is suggestion that there may be a specific psoriasis gene. There is evidence of auto-immunity (where the body's immune system attacks its own tissues), and relationships have been found between viral and bacteria infections and the onset or progression of the disease. There is also indirect evidence that an episode of trauma in a patient with psoriasis may precipitate the development of arthritis.

Spinal Stenosis

It is estimated that as many as 400,000 Americans, most of them over 60, may presently be experiencing symptoms of spinal stenosis. Most are unaware of their diagnosis and have simply have changed their lifestyles, reducing physical activity in order to control their pain. Many just assume their symptoms are part of getting old.

✔ BACK FACTS

Spinal stenosis is a clinical condition defined by a certain group of symptoms typically caused by any spinal pathology that results in inadequate space for the neural elements (spinal cord, cauda equina, nerve roots). The condition is likely far more prevalent than is currently recognized and is only going to become more so as the population ages.

The classic symptoms of spinal stenosis are pain and numbness in the legs, absent at rest but getting progressively worse with activity, particularly walking or standing in the erect position. The range of symptoms experienced by individuals with spinal stenosis is far more varied. In addition to low back pain, which may accompany all presentations, heaviness, hot and cold, pins-and-needles, 'walking on cotton wool' and burning sensations in the legs and feet are reported. In addition, changes to gait, including 'foot slap' (the heel hits the ground followed rapidly by the front of the foot slapping down), 'foot drop' (an inability to lift up the toes), and frank clumsiness, lack of control or balance, and weakness with falls, can also occur.

Neurogenic Claudication vs Vascular Claudication

Note: See page 38 for a comparison of vascular and neurogenic claudication symptoms.

An important diagnostic distinction to make is between spinal stenosis (also called neurogenic claudication) and vascular claudication (resulting from narrow arteries and inadequate blood flow to the muscles of the legs). In this condition, discomfort is most common in the calves, although all leg muscles may be affected. Pain and cramping are common, whereas numbness is rare. Resting the leg muscles in any position eases discomfort. Thus someone with spinal stenosis will have to sit and the vascular patient will have to stand until the pain subsides. Careful examination and measurement of blood flow using Doppler ultrasound will enable the correct diagnosis to be made.

Spinal Stenosis Causes

There are a number of causes for spinal stenosis, classified as developmental and acquired. Some people with arthritis will have a greater tendency to develop spinal stenosis due to a degree of pre-existing developmental narrowing. Spinal stenosis can be acquired from arthritis and spondylolisthesis, the slipping of one vertebra on another, surgical and traumatic causes, and metabolic bone disease.

A number of anatomic features contribute to the development of spinal stenosis in lumbar spine arthritis. Degenerative narrowing of the disc brings adjacent vertebrae closer together. Not only does this reduce the available space in the neural foraminae (tunnel through which the nerve roots leave the spine), instability with tilting, slip, and rotation further compromise these and the spinal canal itself. Bony excrescences form at the edges of the vertebra and facet joints in a vain attempt by the body to stabilize the spine. These further compromise available space. The ligamentum flavum thickens and buckles as do other ligaments. These can compress nerve roots and blood vessels. Arthritis within the facet joints leads to swelling, more bone formation, and stiffness, adding to the overall picture and narrowing the neural spaces further.

How narrowing within the spinal canal and neural foraminae produce symptoms of spinal stenosis is not fully understood. It is thought to be a combination of direct, posture-related, nerve pressure, compression of the dural tissue covering the nerves, and compromise of the local blood supply.

Spinal Stenosis Due to Instability (Spondylolisthesis)

Spondylolisthesis refers to the slippage of one vertebra upon the other, from the Greek 'spondylos', which refers to the vertebra, and 'olisthanein', the verb 'to slip'. Most of the time the upper vertebra slips forward on the one below, while occasionally it can slip backwards (termed 'retrolisthesis').

There are a number of causes for this instability, including degeneration and arthritis. In this type of spondylolisthesis, the neural arch remains intact, the instability being caused by bony deformity, facet destruction, and ligamentous laxity. The slip may be static, as seen on plain X-rays, or dynamic, occurring only with flexion of the spine and therefore imaged only with X-rays taken in this position.

The most common type is called 'spondylolytic' spondylolisthesis and refers to the defect in that part of the bony arch called the pars. This defect can be genetic (it is present in nearly 50% of the Inuit population), or acquired, typically through sports such as weightlifting or gymnastics. While it may develop at age 5 or 6, it does not generally become symptomatic until the teenage years. Most individuals remain asymptomatic, the abnormality only showing up as in incidental finding later in life. This type of spondylolisthesis is most common over the age of 50 and occurs typically between the L4 and L5 vertebrae. Among adults, estimates put its prevalence at 5% to 6% in males and 2% to 3% in females in the United States.

Spinal Stenosis Causes

Developmental (genetically acquired)
- Hereditary
- Achondroplastic (abnormal bone development)

Acquired
- Degenerative (arthritis)
- Spondylolisthesis (vertebral slipping)
- Post-Surgical
- Post-Fracture
- Bone disease (e.g., Paget's Disease)

Spondylolysis and Spondylolisthesis

Saggital section, showing 'slip' of the L5 vertebra on the sacrum (S1) in spondylolisthesis.

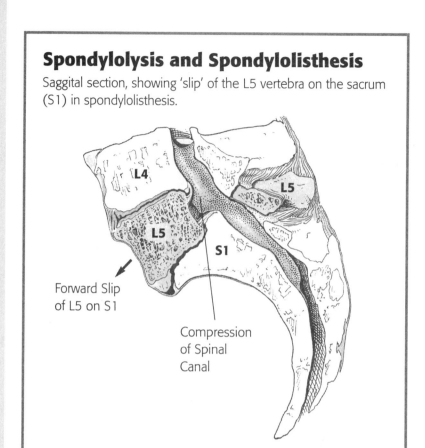

L4

L5

L5

S1

Forward Slip
of L5 on S1

Compression
of Spinal
Canal

Spondylolisthesis Grades

The grade is determined by the percentage of slip measured as a percentage:

Grade 1   25% of vertebral body has slipped forward

Grade 2   50%

Grade 3   75%

Grade 4   100%

Grade 5   Vertebral body completely fallen off
           (i.e., spondyloptosis)

Adolescent Spondylolisthesis

Spondylolisthesis can also occur in younger individuals, including children, not due to degeneration but due to a defect in the bony architecture of the arch at the back of the vertebra. Called 'dysplastic' spondylolisthesis, this adolescent type accounts for about 15% of all cases. Flat joint alignment or incongruous shape fails to provide adequate resistance to the normal pull of gravity and there is a resultant slip. These patients often develop symptoms quite rapidly, with pain, numbness or weakness, and occasionally cauda equina syndrome.

Non-Specific Sources of Pain

The diffuse, burning pain often described by back patients as a band stretching across the low back has more in common with the spreading chest pain of a heart attack than with the sharp local pain of a muscle or ligament injury. It has similar associated general physical and emotional symptoms and is consequently harder to rationalize, understand, and cope with than more basic 'sensory' pain. The reason for this unpleasant characteristic of low back pain is due to involvement of the autonomic nervous system, specifically the sympathetic system. Known as ortho-sympathetic or sympathetic-sensory coupling, it describes the influence of anatomical anomalies at the level of the lower lumbar spine on sensory interpretation.

✔ BACK FACTS

One of the complicating factors in the presentation, interpretation, and localization of back pain is the fact that sensory fibers from a large area and numerous different tissue types often travel within the same sensory nerve. Thus, sensation of touch from the skin, stretch from the muscles, and movement from a joint may all reach the spinal cord at the same time.

The sinu-vertebral nerve supplies the intervertebral disc, nerve coverings, and longitudinal ligament at each level of the spine. The fibers of this nerve contain a strong sympathetic component, and because of this, are unable to travel directly to the corresponding level of the spinal cord. Sensory input from L3, L4, and L5 first travels to the L2 level where they congregate at a spinal ganglion (a confluence of communicating nerve fibers). There is thus a 'hole' in the sensory innervation between L3 and L5 because the dorsal nerves do not reach the skin at these levels. Not only does this result in poor localization, but the pain routes through the sympathetic system impart the diffuse, burning quality so typical of low back pain. The presence of damage or inflammation of these sympathetic sensory nerves may also promote spontaneous firing of adjacent regular sensory nerves further increasing pain input.

The value of understanding this pathway is emphasized by recent work evaluating the use of nerve blocks at the L2 level in chronic low back disorders to treat chronic diffuse pain.

Psychic Pain

More often than not, individuals with exactly the same pathologic process, the same size disc pressing on the same nerve, will have completely different experiences and outcomes. One person may be back at work in a week, while another remains disabled for years, unable to recover, plagued by the accompaniments of chronic pain such as depression, anxiety, and fatigue.

In 1992, a study from California looked at the influence of childhood emotional trauma (sexual abuse, emotional neglect, parental loss, for example) on the outcome of simple disc surgery. Those with no risk factors showed 95% recovery, those with one or two risk factors, 75%, and with more than two risk factors only 15% had a good result. Furthermore, in a follow-up study, pre-operative psychotherapy vastly improved outcome in the at-risk groups.

 BACK FACTS

While we all have the same nerve receptors, nerve fibers, and pain pathways, some of us 'feel' pain more than others and some of us seem better able to cope with it. While there are undoubtedly innumerable factors at play, the role of the psyche has become increasingly recognized as a contributing factor in pain.

Psychic Pain Triggers

The experience of pain relates to two areas of the brain, the sensory cortex and the frontal lobe. The sensory cortex is where pain is identified, its location on the body mapped, and its nature determined. The frontal lobe is where the emotional component of pain is registered. Through connections with the limbic system, the more primitive areas of the brain, the emotional component interacts with memory and the fear/stress response. Patients lacking frontal lobes can identify pain but do not 'suffer'.

The influence of the psyche on perception of pain may be determined not only by the pre-emptive programming of the frontal cortex and limbic system but also by the overall status of these pathways at the time the pain is experienced. Developmental factors are most likely to have an influence on the way in which the system is 'wired'. Genetic factors combined with developmental emotional trauma have been shown to have a significant influence on the development of both psychological and chronic pain conditions such as fibromyalgia. Post-traumatic stress disorder, for example, is thought to arise from an inadequate cortisol response to a stressful event in a genetically susceptible individual. It is likely that a similar susceptibility exists for back pain, causing some individuals to develop chronic symptoms and experience more profound disability.

Recent studies examining brain activity with MRI scanning revealed that individuals with chronic pain such as fibromyalgia or low back pain showed a marked increase in activity in the frontal cortex and cingulate gyrus (the initial communication point with the limbic system) compared to normal subjects. The cingulate gyrus is also responsible for switching attention; it is thought that an abnormality here leads to individuals 'focusing' on their pain.

The influence of pain on the hippocampus, that part of the limbic system responsible for coordinating the 'fight or flight' stress response, has also been evaluated. Chronic pain is associated with altered responsiveness of the stress pathway, reduced cortisol, and impaired secretion of CRH (corticotropin releasing hormone) from the hypothalamus. This is thought to be partially due to cell death and shrinkage of the hippocampus, a finding also seen in chronic stress. Not only does this affect the way the individual handles new stress, it also has a profound influence on all tissues and systems of the body, leading to the development and progression of illness, both physical and mental.

The brain also appears able to influence the degree of central sensitization within the spinal cord. This is a heightened state in which even normally pleasant sensations are interpreted as pain. A reduced level of the calming neurotransmitter serotonin in stress and chronic pain allows increased activity of the excitatory transmitter, glutamate. Serotonin acts to inhibit pain message transmission within the brain, so there is less control over the incoming pain messages. In addition, a high concentration of the pain transmitter Substance-P has been found in the spinal cord of chronic pain sufferers. This will increase pain fiber firing and induce sensitization within the cord.

Back Pain Syndrome

The causes of back pain are complex. The individual suffering low back pain is not only at the mercy of simple pain fibers. Through sensitization, even pressure, stretch, and touch can begin to be interpreted as 'painful'. The organization of these sensory fibers prevents specific localization of these unpleasant sensations. This results in diffuse, radiating pain throughout a large area, which not only increases overall sensory input, it impairs our ability to rationalize it. Add to this involvement of autonomic nerves with their element of 'visceral' pain, that deep-seated, burning discomfort with a strong emotional component, and we begin to understand how back pain is so unpleasantly unique. Involvement of the brain, specifically the areas associated with emotion and memory, introduce a further dimension to back pain, particularly when it becomes chronic.

Fortunately, a wide variety of effective treatments have been developed to address the causes of back pain and alleviate this suffering.

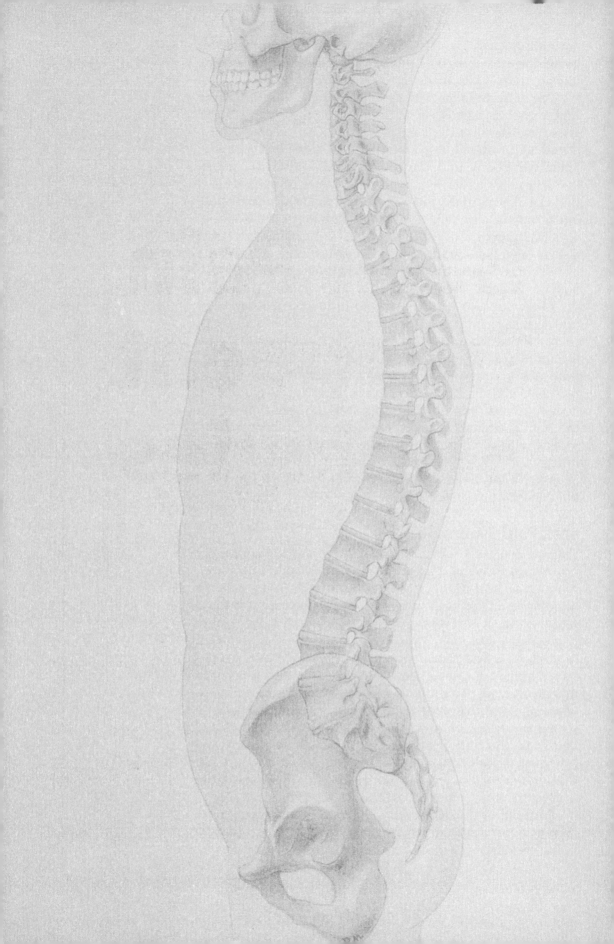

Back Pain Treatment Strategies

Physical Treatments for Back Care

Physical treatments for back pain include non-invasive strategies and 'hands-on' therapies. They provide an important first line of treatment for many low back conditions and are often all that is required to relieve pain, improve mobility, and restore function.

Non-Invasive Treatments

Bed Rest

Working on the assumption that patients with back pain often felt better lying down and that disc pressures are lower in this position, bed rest was viewed as the standard treatment for back pain as recently as the 1980s. I remember admitting patients to hospital for 'bed rest and analgesia'. Of course, lying in bed, being fed and washed to the accompaniment of large doses of pain-killers, was likely to make even the most debilitated patient feel better. This management protocol continued until researchers found out that 4 or even 7 days of bed rest was no more effective long term than just 2 days, the only difference being hospital stay and the delay in return to work.

Having established that early mobilization was not harmful, studies found that patients who returned most quickly to daily activities and work recovered faster, experienced less chronic pain, and encountered less recurrence than those who waited for the pain to resolve completely. While heavier jobs may not have been possible, early return to lighter modified duties improved outcome.

Bed Rest Facts

- Patients with acute low back pain actually do better returning to daily activity than they do by resting or enrolling in an exercise program.
- Chronic sufferers do best with a combination of normal activity plus exercise.

✔ BACK FACTS

Physical therapies are an integral part of all back pain management — for treatment of an acute attack, for prevention of re-injury, or for recovery from surgery. They are often used together, providing complementary and often synergistic benefit. You can carry out some treatments independently; others require input or interaction with a trained therapist.

Ice and Heat Treatments

Ice

Ice treatment, cooling, or cryotherapy is a widely used modality for the treatment of pain and inflammation, particularly following injury. Ice application to the skin has been shown to decrease skin, intra-muscular, and joint temperature. Cooling of nerves reduces muscle spasm and pain. There is a direct effect on the local inflammatory response. The local metabolic rate is reduced and the permeability of blood vessels decreased. The effects last after removal of the ice, and there is no evidence that it causes a reactive increase in blood flow later on.

The most effective form of ice therapy is wet ice. Crushed ice in a plastic bag wrapped in a wet towel applied to the skin for approximately 20 minutes is the most efficient way of reducing tissue temperature. The most convenient form is probably a re-useable 'gel' cold pack. These last about 15 to 20 minutes. Caution is recommended when applying these packs directly to skin. Normally, they should be wrapped within a light towel.

Cold packs can usually be applied for 10 to 20 minutes — it is unusual for applications under 30 minutes to cause injury. The risk increases if ice or gel packs are applied directly to skin. In general, it is safest to have them wrapped in a thin towel. This minimizes the possibility of frostbite. Any numbness or tingling is an indication to remove the pack immediately. Upon removal of the pack, an interval of 40 minutes to one hour should be allowed before reapplication.

Superficial Heat

Besides the psychological effect of comfort, heat has a number of beneficial effects on joints and tissues. It induces muscle relaxation and reduces spasm. It increases the flexibility of tissues with a direct effect on the properties of collagen. Heat also increases the metabolism of tissues, improves blood supply, and relieves pain. Superficial heat also allows penetration through the skin, superficial tissues, and upper layers of muscle, though deeper tissues and joints are reached by heat from ultrasound and diathermy.

Superficial heat is generally applied through heat packs or heating blankets. Superficial heat should not be used during the acute stages of inflammation, for example, in an acute lumbar strain. This should initially be treated with ice for 48 to 72 hours before progressing to heat.

Contrast Treatment

Contrast treatment involves the combination of heat and cold. Besides the effects of heat and cold noted above, contrast

Cold Pack Facts

- Apply in the first 48 to 72 hours of acute episodes of low back pain or lumbar strain.
- Apply post exercise.

Superficial Heat Facts

- Apply after the first 48 to 72 hours of acute low back pain.
- Use in chronic back pain to ease pain and spasm.
- Use *prior* to exercise.

baths are particularly effective at reducing tissue swelling. Generally, a combination of 3 to 4 minutes warm, followed by 1 minute cold over three cycles is recommended.

Ultrasound

Deep heat is probably the most important effect of ultrasound. Ultrasound treatment involves the application of high frequency sound waves to the tissues using a hand-held probe attached to an ultrasound machine. Frequency and penetration can be adjusted as well as length of treatment. This modality requires a trained practitioner.

Ultrasound is mechanical energy in the form of high frequency vibrations, which is transmitted to the tissues. It is applied to the skin through a hand-held device and conductive gel. It has mechanical properties that may alter nerve receptor sensitivity, reducing spasm in muscle and decreasing pain. It may also promote a healing response in cells by improving protein synthesis. Ultrasound is particularly useful in the treatment of muscle and tendon injuries.

Although such benefits as increased extensibility, blood flow, decreased joint stiffness, muscle spasm, and pain are reported from ultrasound treatment, it may be contraindicated in some arthritic conditions where deep tissue heating can accelerate joint destruction. However, ultrasound in the lower, non-thermal energy levels (30 mW/cm^2) has been shown to promote fracture healing and promote cartilage repair.

Short-Wave Diathermy

Diathermy involves passage of a high frequency current with no nerve stimulation creating a rapid vibration that induces deep heat in the tissues. The effect is similar to that of ultrasound. Diathermy should not be used near metal implants or in the presence of heart pacemakers. It is generally contraindicated, as with other deep heating modalities, in the acute phase of low back pain.

Interferential Bio Electrical Stimulation

This treatment involves the application of two 'interfering', medium-frequency, alternating currents. The interference results in the production of variable intensity current within the tissues. This is applied through pads or suction cups and results in bioelectric stimulation without significant heating. Beneficial effects include pain relief, control of swelling, reduced muscle wasting, improved flexibility, and muscle strength.

Ultrasound Facts

- In persistent or chronic low back pain, as part of a comprehensive rehabilitation program, ultrasound may offer benefit similar to heat (reduction of pain, muscle spasm) and promote soft tissue healing.
- May be used in acute injury rehabilitation once initial inflammation has settled.

Thermal Effects:
- Increased metabolic rate and enzyme activity.
- Increased blood flow.
- Increased flexibility of collagen and muscle.
- Decreased sensitivity of neuro-receptors.

Non-Thermal Effects:
- Tissue regeneration.
- Soft tissue repair.
- Increased protein synthesis.
- Reduced swelling.
- Decreased pain and spasm.

Back Pain Treatment Strategies

TENS (Transcutaneous Electrical Nerve Stimulation)

TENS and TMS (transcutaneous muscle stimulation) involve the application of electrical stimulation to nerves and muscles via adhesive pads placed on the skin. Costing between $250 and $700, these units are about the size of a personal stereo and run on batteries or through an adapter. The user can adjust the intensity of the stimulation. Some units allow selection of high (60–100Hz) or low (less than 10Hz) frequency application.

High frequency stimulation is the conventional form of TENS. Although tolerated well for a number of hours, this high frequency stimulation provides only short-term pain relief. Low-frequency stimulation has been likened to acupuncture and provides longer pain relief. It can only usually be tolerated, however, for 20 to 30 minutes at a time. TENS may work in a similar manner to acupuncture and massage. Although not clinically proven, it is thought that a combination of pain-gating (via additional sensory input) and endorphin release is responsible for its beneficial effects in some individuals.

When using a TENS machine, users should try different electrode placements, including directly over the painful area, adjacent to it, or distant along the path of a supplying nerve. Variations of times and frequencies can also be tried. Using the unit for at least a week in various combinations is recommended before concluding it is ineffective.

Side effects of TENS are rare, but include allergic skin irritation under the adhesive pads and transient pain from the electrical charge.

Effectiveness

The efficacy of TENS and TMS is controversial. Some research has found significant benefit to the modality. One study compared the effects of TENS in chronic back pain to placebo-TENS, a unit identical to the regular TENS unit but with no electrical transmission to the skin or muscle. While both groups saw a reduction in pain intensity and unpleasantness, the true TENS group experienced a far more substantial reduction in intensity and its effects were additive over time. Other investigators in a number of randomized clinical studies have not confirmed the superiority of TENS over a placebo treatment. Although predominantly used for chronic pain, a recent study from Montreal suggests a role for TENS in acute low back pain, a role it has played for many years in the field of sports injuries. By gating pain and acting as a physical analgesic, it can promote faster rehabilitation.

TENS Facts

- Generally recommended for chronic and recurrent low back pain with recent studies and sports medicine indicating a role in acute pain.
- May be a useful adjunct to other pain-relieving methods in order to restore function and improve ability to participate in an active exercise program.
- Should not be used as sole treatment as it is likely to induce dependency and detract from other, more useful forms of long-term treatment.

Contraindications to TENS (and other electrical modalities)

- Heart arrhythmias or a pacemaker.
- Pregnancy.
- Do not place on or near the throat.
- Do not place over or near areas of infection or malignancy.

Hydrotherapy

Hydrotherapy is the external use of water-based modalities for treatment. One of the most obvious and frequently used benefits of water for the patient with low back pain is the ability to exercise without significant strain on the spine. Water-based activity does not involve any impact loading and subsequently allows exercise without causing pain or further injury. Water provides variable resistance to movement depending on speed and is therefore ideal for allowing individuals to pace themselves.

Whirlpool baths can be used, depending on their temperature, to provide heat, cryotherapy, or contrast bath treatments. Whirlpools should be avoided for the first 2 weeks following surgery due to the slight increase in risk of infection.

Magnets

The use of magnets or magnetotherapy can be traced back to Cleopatra's time. It is said that she used to sleep with a magnet under her to prevent or slow the aging process. Since then magnets have been used in various ways. The first recorded therapeutic magnet came from material called magnetite, a substance found in the earth with a weak magnetic charge. The substance was then crushed and made into a paste and applied as a poultice to an injured area.

There are several theories as to how magnets may work to alleviate pain and inflammation. One theory employs the nature of the pain signal itself. It is believed that a pain signal when transmitted across a cell depolarizes that cell. Magnets are thought to raise the threshold for depolarization on a cellular level. This would then prevent the cell from depolarizing easily, and therefore prevent the transmission of pain across it.

It is also believed that injured tissue produces a positive charge. If the negative end of a magnet is placed over the tissue, a natural balance of charge is re-established. This is thought to improve circulation allowing blood vessels to dilate and provide more nutrients to the area.

Effectiveness

Several studies have been conducted to determine the efficacy of magnets as a form of treatment for musculoskeletal injuries or diseases. One double-blind, placebo-controlled study took a look at the effect of magnets on arthritis. This study published in the *Journal of Rheumatology* has confirmed the relief of arthritic pain through the use of magnets without any adverse side effects. Another double-blind, placebo-controlled study evaluated pulsed magnet fields on 37 patients with osteoarthritis in either the knee or the hip. The treatments lasted 30 minutes each and were performed on average four times a week. At the end of the study, the patients receiving the real magnet therapy reported a 39% reduction in pain. Only 8% of the placebo group reported a drop in pain. Although more extensive studies need to be performed into the exact mechanism and efficacy of magnets as a therapy for arthritis or other musculoskeletal problems, there appears to be some value to the this treatment modality.

There have been no adverse reactions reported, but there are some situations where magnets should not be used. Magnetotherapy or magnets themselves should not be used in pregnant women. Although it is unclear if there is any effect on the fetus, and until it is known for certain that it is safe during pregnancy, it is best to avoid it all together. In addition, individuals with pacemakers or any other electrical device inside the body should avoid all types of magnet therapy. The change in polarization from the magnet may alter the function of the device.

Orthotics

Orthotics, in their simplest form, are inserts within footwear designed to aid the foot during walking. Behind this simple statement lies a great deal of conflicting opinion within the medical community, and podiatry in particular, as to their role in the treatment of musculoskeletal conditions and back pain.

Orthotics act on the foot directly, but can have influence on the biomechanics of the entire leg, with potentially beneficial effect on the ankle, knee, hip, and spine. However, the orthotic represents only part of an overall treatment plan. It does not in itself represent a sole form of treatment and should be undertaken in conjunction with other treatment modalities, including those from other medical specialists, in order to achieve optimal effect.

Due to the very nature of the disease process, the orthotic should be adjustable to allow for changes as they occur and to ensure that a 'flexible prescription' is achieved. By this it is meant that the orthotic is not acting on the foot too aggressively, leading to trauma (both to soft tissue and joint) that aggravates inflammation and thereby increases discomfort. Effective, ongoing, and timely communication with the prescribing foot specialist is important. The need for adjustments to the orthotic is common in arthritic cases.

Effectiveness

There is no good evidence that orthotics 'cure' back pain. They may be appropriate in cases where there is a difference in leg length or where there is a need to provide extra cushioning to reduce impact — in work boots, for example. They may be tried as part of the comprehensive management of chronic or recurrent low back pain.

Posture Improvement Facts

- Basic improvements to posture — pulling the shoulders back, not slouching, sitting properly — often help to resolve back pain. 'Hands on' techniques such as Yoga, Tai Chi, and the Alexander method also work extensively through correct movement and posture.

- While standing, use a foot-stool intermittently under one or other of your feet to take strain off your lower back. The stool only needs to be about 6 inches high to be effective. A similar stool can be put under your desk while seated.

- Pulling the shoulders back and tucking the chin in will help regain balance and posture. Try looking in a full-length mirror to make sure you are not rounding your shoulders or slouching through your low back.

- Balancing a book on your head may seem a little "Miss Jean Brodie" but it works!

Correct Postures

How To Stand Correctly

In correct, fully erect posture, a line dropped from the ear will go through the tip of the shoulder, middle of the hip, back of the kneecap, and front of the ankle bone.

Incorrect Standing Postures

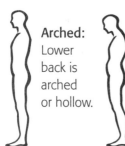

Arched: Lower back is arched or hollow.

Stooped: Upper back is stooped, lower back is arched, abdomen sags.

Corrected Standing Posture

To find the correct standing posture, stand one foot away from a wall, then sit against the wall, bending the knees slightly. Tighten abdominal and buttock muscles. This will tilt the pelvis back and flatten the lower spine. Holding this position, inch up the wall to a standing position by straightening the legs. Now walk around the room maintaining the same posture. Place your back against the wall to see if you have held it.

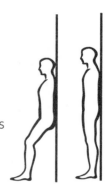

How To Sit Correctly

Incorrect Sitting Postures

Slumping, swayback, forward thrusting, and arching postures cause back strain while sitting.

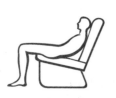

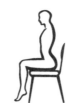

Slumping: "TV" slump strains the neck and shoulders, possibly leading to "dowager's hump."

Swayback: If chair is too high, swayback is increased.

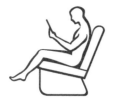

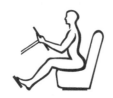

Forward Thrusting: Thrusting the neck forward while reading or doing close work strains the muscles in the neck and head.

Arching: While driving a car, arching of the back can be caused by sitting too far away from the pedals and steering wheel.

Corrected Sitting Posture

To correct sitting posture, throw the head well back, then bend it forward to pull in the chin. This will straighten the back. Now tighten abdominal muscles to raise the chest. Check position frequently.

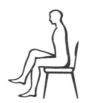

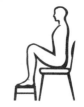

Relieve strain by sitting well forward, flattening back by tightening abdominal muscles and crossing knees.

Use a footrest to relieve swayback. Aim to have the knees higher than the hips.

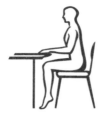

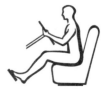

Keep head and neck in as straight a line as possible with the spine. Bend forward from the hips.

While driving, sit close to the floor pedals and steering wheel. Use seat belts and a hard back rest.

How to Work on Your Feet without Back Strain

To prevent strain and pain while standing at work, check your body position regularly, drawing in the abdomen, flattening the back, and bending the knees slightly. Change tasks to avoid fatigue. Lie down periodically, if possible.

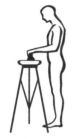

Do not arch back and bend neck.

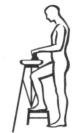

Use a footrest to relieve swayback.

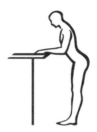

Do not sway your back while standing.

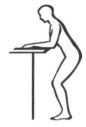

Always flex your knees and keep your back straight while bending.

Stretching

Stretching during the day is an essential component of back pain prevention. The key here is to stretch before it hurts! By performing simple maneuvers, such as pelvic tilts and hamstring stretches, on a regular basis throughout the day, muscle fatigue and tightness can be avoided, reducing your risk of back pain. See the section on stretching exercises in the "Specific Back Exercises" section for many more techniques.

Canes, Braces, and Supports

More often used to reduce pain from the hip or the knee, a cane may actually improve walking tolerance in spinal stenosis by promoting a more forward flexed posture.

Braces for the back come in a wide variety of shapes and sizes, varying in strength and complexity depending on their proposed function. Braces used to treat scoliosis (spinal curvature) in children or fractures are necessarily extremely rigid and conforming, made to measure for individual patients. Braces for low back pain are generally 'lumbar supports' or 'corsets' composed of an elastic band with or without rigid reinforcement and lacing. They are widely available for purchase off-the-shelf.

Lumbar supports, such as the popular 'Obus Forme', are used and recommended extensively. They comprise, at their most simple, a semi-rigid back rest contoured to fit the curvature of the spine that provides support to maintain the lumbar lordosis (forward curve). More complex supports include additions for the car or office, complete chairs, and beds.

Back Brace and Support Facts

- Back braces should be used as an adjunct to other treatment modalities and only then on a temporary basis. Prolonged use leads to physical dependency and contributes to a sense of disability.

- Back supports may offer benefit both in the short term and for prevention of back pain recurrence. There seem to be no drawbacks to their use, and they are less likely than braces to induce dependency.

There is certainly good evidence for the therapeutic benefit of braces, though not for injury prevention. Abdominal obesity significantly limits the effectiveness of a lumbar support and an extension-type device appears to offer most benefit.

Evidence for the effectiveness of support devices is largely anecdotal but their concept of improving posture appears sound. As with lumbar supports, the majority of back pain sufferers seem to gain relief by maintaining the lumbar lordosis, symptoms increasing with its reversal and a slouched position. By providing feedback through pressure, the individual recognizes this position and corrects it. This is particularly important during prolonged sitting, such as at a desk or in the car. Voluntary correction of posture will help strengthen back muscles, adding further benefit.

Mattresses

We have all spent a night on an uncomfortable bed and have woken up the following day with a 'stiff' back. While there is no clinical evidence as to the benefit of one mattress over another in the prevention or treatment of low back pain, experience dictates that a poor bed can have an impact, though a good night's sleep on any mattress will likely make you feel better and more relaxed.

Pillows can also provide a useful addition to the bed. On your back, a pillow under the knees will significantly reduce pressure across the intervertebral discs. Lying on your side with hips and knees flexed will reduce pain caused by extension of the spine, facet strain or arthritis for example. A pillow may be used between the knees. Tilted up 45 degrees to one side with a long pillow beneath your back and pelvis is also a helpful maneuver.

Ergonomic Improvements

There may be a number of work or sport-specific ergonomic improvements that can reduce forces across your low back. General recommendations include concentrating on the task at hand, controlling your breathing, and pacing yourself. Do not perform tasks you know to be beyond your limits — if it's likely to be too heavy, ask for help!

If your work involves standing for a prolonged period, a footstool can reduce the strain on your back. Alternatively, putting one or other foot up on the stool will reduce hamstring tightness and extension stress on the low back. This also applies at home, for example, when tending to the baby in a crib or changing diapers. Adjusting your workstation or desk and incorporating a comfortable chair with a lumbar support is valuable. Avoid low, soft chairs. Stretch often.

Mattress Facts

- **Provide Adequate Space:** A small bed for one or two people can lead to cramped and awkward sleep positions, which may aggravate back pain.

- **Ensure Adequate Support:** Old or thin mattresses with failed springs will reduce spinal support and contour.

- **Use Two Single Beds Instead of One Double:** Tying two single beds together so they do not slide apart, covered with a single large mattress cover and sheets, is an excellent way to prevent the central sag of a larger mattress. In addition, movement from the other side is not transmitted.

With regard to sports, persistent or recurrent pain may be an indicator of poor technique. Spending a few sessions with a trainer or a teaching professional can result in tremendous rewards for both your back and your handicap.

Lifting Ergonomics

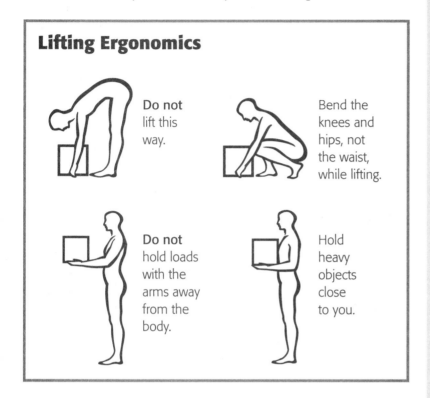

Do not lift this way.

Bend the knees and hips, not the waist, while lifting.

Do not hold loads with the arms away from the body.

Hold heavy objects close to you.

Traction

Traction is a mechanical treatment modality whereby a longitudinal distraction force is applied along the length of the spine. Applied manually or through a pelvic sling, weights, and pulleys, this form of therapy has been used in low back pain for over two thousand years.

'Auto-traction' involves a device in which the lower limbs are anchored and the patient can pull on handles to increase the amount of traction. To achieve any sort of effect on the vertebral bodies, a force equivalent to 25% of body weight must be applied, and even then there appears to be only a slight reduction in disc pressure. However, some studies have shown that auto-traction *increases* disc pressure, possibly due to the muscle contraction required to pull on the traction handles.

Gravity traction (hanging upside down) has been demonstrated to distract the vertebral bodies by between 0.3 and 4.0 millimeters, but this form of traction is physically demanding and associated with headache, increased blood pressure, rapid heart rate, stomach reflux, and, rarely, bleeding into the brain. The lack of control over the amount of traction makes accurate assessment of this treatment modality difficult.

Ergonomics and Lifting Facts

- Do not lift awkward or unbalanced loads and avoid sudden movements. When lifting, always face the task.
- Do not twist and lift.
- Keep the object as close to your body as possible, and if that is not possible due to awkward shape or position, then ask for help.
- Bend your knees and keep your back straight while lifting. Looking up rather than at the object will help with this, as will keeping it close.
- To change direction, turn your feet rather than your shoulders. Reverse the process when setting the object down.

Traction Facts

- Traditionally recommended for disc-related back pain including disc herniation.
- Gravity traction cannot be recommended at this time.
- Traction in the presence of acute disc herniation is also not recommended.

Hands-On Physical Treatments

Chiropractic Treatment

There are several theories as to how both manipulations and mobilizations of the spine offer relief from pain and stiffness. For example, movements may help to release 'trapped' synovium or disc between two or more spinal segments. This trapped tissue is said to be the result of subluxed or altered spinal facet positioning. By returning the spinal segments to the 'normal' position, the tissue regains regular blood flow and pressure.

The movement from the manipulation or mobilization may encourage a stretching and even breaking of tissue adhesions. These adhesions can hold a spinal segment in a subluxed position, impair blood flow or nerve transmission between spinal segments, or increase inflammation of the myelin sheath surrounding the nerves.

The relief of pain through these spinal movements may be accomplished by a release of endorphins. Endorphins are the body's natural painkillers. It is thought that following each manipulation, the body releases these pain-dulling endorphins, bringing about sensations of well being and relief.

Chiropractic Spinal Movement

There are two types of manual spinal movements in chiropractic treatment, 'mobilizations' and 'manipulations'.

Mobilization

A chiropractic mobilization is a controlled passive force with low velocity yet variable amplitude. This type of manual treatment takes place within the joint's physiological space; it does not move the spinal segment beyond the joint's normal passive range of motion. A mobilization is used to decrease pain, increase motion of a joint, and decrease restricted areas of the spine.

Manipulation

Chiropractic manipulation is the gentle movement of joints and the surrounding musculature. The movement is often small and may be associated with a 'pop', thought to be a release of carbon dioxide within the joint. The distinguishing feature of a manipulation is that the pressure applied to the spinal segments can occur with either a high or low velocity, but only a low amplitude force. In addition, the manipulation moves the spine into the paraphysiological space, the space between the joint's passive end range and the anatomical end range. The theory behind chiropractic manipulation is that when a joint becomes 'fixated', it can impart neurologic and biomechanical impairment, increasing irritation and inflammation. Chiropractic manipulation of fixated joints or spinal segments aims to improve biomechanical and neurological function by restoring normal motion, relaxing tight muscles, and improving joint coordination. Chiropractic manipulations can increase the mobility of a joint, helping to relieve back pain. This may have some value in reducing the degree of 'sensitization' in the spine that accounts for so much pain amplification.

A final theory proposed is that the active motion of the manipulation or mobilization initiates a reflexive response in the nervous system. Similar to the gating theory or pain control, these 'new' nervous impulses reduce transmission of painful sensation to the brain. The altered input may reduce central sensitization, resulting in an overall decrease in pain.

None of these theories have been clinically or scientifically tested.

Effectiveness

Despite the widespread use and acceptance of chiropractic care from the general public, its efficacy remains largely unproven, mainly due to lack of adequate clinical trials. A study of treatment of acute low back pain published in the *New England Journal of Medicine* in 1995 found similar outcomes regardless of whether the patient saw a family doctor, a chiropractor, or an orthopedic surgeon. Significantly, patient satisfaction was highest with the chiropractor! In a UCLA study, patients were asked to rank their satisfaction of the outcome of their treatment on a scale from 10 to 50, according to relief of pain, explanation of treatment, confidence in practitioner, and self-care advice. All patients in the chiropractic care group reported greater satisfaction and reduction of pain than patients in the group receiving traditional medical treatment.

There is no evidence that long-term chiropractic care in the absence of symptoms prevents back pain or other spinal pathology such as arthritis.

Chiropractic Facts

- The frequency and duration of chiropractic treatment is decided on an individual basis by you and your chiropractor. Individuals have different spinal problems and heal at a different rates. Your chiropractic protocol should be developed and carried out according to your individual needs.

- Failure to improve after four or five sessions would be an indication to revaluate this treatment.

Chiropractic Safety Concerns

- Although chiropractic care is generally very safe, there are certain conditions where it should not be performed. Such cases include radicular nerve pain (sciatica) with numbness or weakness, surgically fused spinal segments, severe osteoporosis or other metabolic pathologies affecting the integrity of the bone, and cancer.
- The side effects that may accompany a chiropractic treatment are nausea, dizziness, local discomfort for a short period of time, and headaches.
- Arterial complications such as recently reported for neck manipulations are not considered an issue in the lumbar spine.

Osteopathy

Osteopathy, as with many forms of 'natural' therapy, aims to enhance, promote, and support the body's innate ability to heal. In contrast to chiropractic treatment, which aims to correct 'blocks' in the flow or transmission through nervous structures, osteopathic manipulation works to restore the flow of fluids, such as blood and lymph. Chiropractors adjust the spinal vertebrae to enhance neural transmission, most frequently through brief, rapid manipulations. Osteopaths employ a method termed Osteopathic Manual Medicine (OMM) to increase flow of body fluids, combining body positioning with gentle pressure to predominantly soft tissue areas rather than bones or joints. Applying exactly the correct amount of force to restore flow and promote healing is essential to the practice. In addition, a DO may use manual therapy in combination with such traditional treatments as medication or surgery.

Treatment with an osteopath will involve a full history and examination. While chiropractic care remains largely focussed on the musculoskeletal system, osteopathy aims to treat all forms of illness, including digestive, respiratory, neurologic, and infective conditions. History and clinical testing establish the site of blocks or abnormalities that interfere with transmission of the bodily 'rhythm'. This rhythm is generated by the brain, spinal cord, and breathing pattern, then communicated to the rest of the body through soft tissue planes or fascia. By manipulating this fascia, obstructions to flow and hence healing can be removed.

Effectiveness

Despite widespread use of osteopathy in the United States and the United Kingdom, clinical research to support its role in the management of low back pain remains scarce. One randomized study published in the *New England Journal of Medicine* in 1999 compared osteopathic manual therapy to standard medical treatment for patients with uncomplicated low back pain of at least 3 weeks duration but present for less than 6 months. Outcomes in both groups were similar with respect to resolution of their pain, but the osteopath-treated group used fewer pain-killers and required less physical therapy. Both groups of patients reported being satisfied with their treatment; other studies have found increased patient satisfaction with osteopaths as opposed to traditional medical practitioners, a factor most likely related to improved verbal interaction.

Further research reported in the journal *Spine* supports a role for osteopathy in the management of acute or sub-acute, uncomplicated low back pain. The Welsh Randomized

Osteopathic Manipulation Study (ROMANS) in 2003 found improved physical and psychological outcome in patients with back pain of 2 to 12 weeks duration without significant increase in cost over more traditional therapy.

As with chiropractic care, further research is needed to elucidate the value of osteopathy in low back pain.

Massage Therapy

Massage has long been used as a technique for controlling pain. Defined as the treatment of disease or injury through the manual manipulation of body tissues, massage is employed to relieve pain and spasm, to induce relaxation, to stretch and break down scarring and adhesions, and to increase circulation and metabolism. Massage promotes the resorption and metabolism of toxins and the residua of inflammation.

There are several ways in which massage is thought to relieve pain. One involves the blocking or 'gating' of painful stimuli. The theory is that massage gently stimulates nerve fibers adjacent to the pain center, sending another set of messages to the brain. This acts almost like an overload on the system and not all of the messages get to the brain. As the massage is 'new' or different from any chronic or constant pain, it lessens the sensation of the true pain, even though the massage is not actually painful.

Massage has also been shown to stimulate the release of enkephalins and endorphins, the body's natural painkillers. These hormones act on the same receptors as powerful drugs, such as morphine, reducing the awareness and intensity of pain.

Massage helps to increase local circulation, improving the flow of nutrients to an area, thereby increasing the amount of available material for healing. An increase in circulation will also help to remove the inflammatory chemicals, which not only contribute to further inflammation but can act as free radical producers that hinder healing. There is good evidence that prolonged muscle spasm leads to increased and prolonged back pain via a number of mechanisms. Massage may have an important role in resolving these.

Effectiveness

Massage therapy has been consistently shown to be beneficial in the treatment of low back pain. One study examined 24 adults, all 39 years of age with low back pain for more than 6 months, and compared the use of massage therapy to relaxation exercises as a form of pain relief and treatment for low back pain. Treatment sessions were 30 minutes long, twice a week for 5 weeks. At the beginning and the end of the study, patients answered a questionnaire, provided urine samples, and were assessed for range of motion and perceived pain. At the end of the study, the group receiving massage reported much less back pain, depression, and anxiety, as well as improved sleep. The examiners found a much larger range of motion in this study group than in the group receiving relaxation exercises. In addition they found elevated serotonin ('happy hormone') and dopamine ('relaxing hormone').

A similar study conducted nationally across the United States on over 2,000 patients with neck and back pain for more than one year concluded the benefits of massage therapy and other alternative forms of treatment: 65% of the patients reported significant relief with massage therapy, the highest percentage of relief reported when compared to chiropractic

Types of Massage Therapy

There are several different types or techniques that fall under the umbrella of massage therapy.

Swedish Massage

Probably best known is 'Swedish' massage involving long strokes along the superficial layers of muscle fiber. Swedish massage uses strokes such as effleurage, which are smooth gliding motions across the soft tissue applied with both hands.

Effleurage

Effleurage is used to gently relax the muscle fibers. Swedish massage is often combined with active and passive movements of the joint to help stretch the muscle, ligaments and tendons.

Deep Tissue Massage

Deep tissue massage is another popular form of therapy used to release chronic patterns of tension in the body with slow, deep finger pressure and strokes on contracted muscles. Unlike Swedish massage, this type focuses on deeper layers of the muscle. You may feel sore or tender during the treatment, but this subsides rapidly after the treatment session.

Friction Massage

Friction massage is a type of stroke that is very effective for pain and inflammation. It involves deep circular movements applied to soft tissues or muscles, often at right angles to their orientation, causing a degree of friction. The result here is to increase the blood flow to the area and help breakdown adhesions and 'muscle knots'.

Petrissage

Petrissage or kneading massage involves squeezing, rolling, and kneading the muscle bed. This is used in most types of massage with varying degrees of depth and strength. It usually follows effleurage as a way to loosen the muscle fibers and prepare the area for deep tissue or trigger point work.

Trigger Point Therapy

Trigger point therapy, also known as myotherapy or neuromuscular therapy, is the application of concentrated finger pressure to irritated and painful areas in the muscle, otherwise known as 'trigger points'. This type of therapy is used to help relieve spasms and localized pain within the muscle.

Tapotement

Tapotement is a technique used where the therapist places the sides of the hand on the patient's tissues and applies short vigorous taps in a repetitive and rhythmic motion.

and relaxation techniques at 61% and 43%, respectively. Yet another study examined the use of massage therapy on 262 patients with chronic back pain. Aged 20 through 70 years old, these patients received massage therapy, acupuncture, or self-help educational information for over 10 weeks. Symptoms of pain, movement, flexibility, and dysfunction or impairment were monitored. The group receiving massage showed superior improvements and reduced their pain medication the most.

Side Effects

No matter what type of massage therapy is administered, most people experience both pain relief and a sense of relaxation and well-being after a treatment. There are very few contraindications to massage. It should not be performed over or close to a cancerous tumor, nor over the surface of an ulcerated lesion. Massage is not recommended over the sacral area during the first 8 months of pregnancy. Aside from these exceptions, massage therapy has few side effects and mostly positive responses. After a treatment, one may feel a little more sore for 24 hours, as the muscles have literally been 'worked, releasing inflammatory bi-products from that area. In addition, some people may feel slightly light-headed or even dizzy when they first stand up off the massage table. This can be easily alleviated by getting up very slowly and simultaneously taking deep breaths.

Acupuncture

Traditional Chinese Medicine teaches that there are a series of 12 energy channels that run through the body, known as meridians. These meridians are somewhat like blood vessels and nerves in that they are the routes through which energy is dispersed and nutrients are delivered throughout the body. Much as a defect in an artery or nerve causes pain, inflammation, swelling and other pathology, so does an obstruction in a meridian. Energy in Traditional Chinese Medicine is called Qi (pronounced "chee"). Qi circulates through the meridians and heals the body.

Massage Therapy at Home

Simple massage techniques can be practiced at home. Massage is of benefit in all cases except the very acute stage of low back pain. It also helps relieve stress, an important factor in the persistence and recurrence of back pain.

- Use a massaging shower-head, which augments the benefits of superficial heat from the water.
- Move a simple wooden roller-type massager back and forth across the low back.
- Use commercial electric massagers with or without heat.
- Have a partner apply slow, gentle, finger, thumb, or hand pressure.

✔ BACK FACTS

Acupuncture is a therapeutic method for promoting natural healing of the body through the insertion of needles that has been used therapeutically in Asia for over 2000 years. Not until the 1970s did physicians from the United States travel to China to observe and learn acupuncture first hand. Subsequently, several studies were performed to discover the mechanism behind pain relief through needle insertion. It was shown that endogenous opioids or endorphins were released upon insertion of a needle. Since these studies, the acceptance and use of acupuncture in Western society has grown immensely.

There are hundreds of specific points along these meridians. Each point acts like a reservoir of potential energy for that meridian. If there is a block or problem in the meridian, by stimulating a certain point or points, the energy can be released and flow restored. This helps to heal the meridian and to re-establish a beneficial flow of energy though the body. The body continually generates small but detectable charges of energy. The flow of this energy influences growth, maturation, and production of hormones and enzymes — in fact, the functioning of the entire body.

Acupuncture points are concentrated in areas of low electrical resistance with a correlation between electromagnetic fields in the body and these energy meridians. One of the ways acupuncture is thought to work is by influencing the electromagnetic field of the body. The Westernized scientific description of acupuncture is a stimulation of the nervous system by inserting a needle into the body. This stimulation causes a release of specific chemical substances that influence the muscles, spine, and brain. These various chemicals then bring about relief of pain, a decrease in inflammation, and a balance back to the body.

Acupuncture may also work by blocking the transmission of painful stimuli through a 'gating' mechanism. Similar to the principal whereby you rub the skin over an injured area to reduce pain, providing an alternative sensory input through acupuncture may block out some of the pain transmission to the brain.

Effectiveness

Musculoskeletal pain is probably the area where acupuncture is used most widely in our society. One study examined the effects of acupuncture with and without traditional anti-inflammatory pain management. The researchers asked the question, "Does a combination of acupuncture and conservative orthopedic treatment improve conservative orthopedic treatment in chronic low back pain (LBP)?" This study followed 186 patients in a low back rehabilitation center with a history of back pain ranging from 6 months to 5 years. This double-blind, controlled, randomized study had patient groups receiving either true or sham acupuncture treatments in addition to standard orthopedic care or standard care alone with no acupuncture. The group receiving true acupuncture plus conservative care had far greater improvement in pain than both other groups, with all results being statistically significant. Similar results emerged from a recent study from England and from Germany. Collectively, this data showed that acupuncture was statistically superior to various other control interventions.

Studies evaluating the efficacy of acupuncture in osteo-arthritis have also revealed encouraging results. An NIH (National Institutes for Health) panel in the United States concluded in 1997 that there was sufficient evidence to support the use of acupuncture in osteoarthritis and low back pain. Acupuncture is effective in relieving pain, reducing muscle spasm, and improving mobility in back pain due to arthritis. We have found it to be particularly useful in the relief of radiating 'nerve pain' that spreads into the arms or legs.

Side Effects

There are usually no side effects with acupuncture, although it is essential that new needles are used for every treatment (rather than sterilized ones) to eliminate risk of disease transmission. There is no problem with receiving acupuncture while on any pharmaceutical or natural medications. The acupuncture treatment will not alter the efficacy of the drug or supplement. The only place to be careful with acupuncture is during pregnancy. Many of the points have been shown to stimulate uterine contractions, so it is best to refrain from acupuncture during pregnancy.

Because acupuncture involves the movement of hormones, steroids, and natural chemicals in the body to promote healing, very few adverse reactions have taken place. However, there can be an initial flare of symptoms before the relief. You should not be alarmed by this reaction because it is considered a sign that things are changing in the body for the better. This reaction should not last past the first few treatments. If pain persists, stop the treatments and consult your therapist.

There is very little pain on the insertion of the needle. A small pin prick sensation may be felt as the needle passes through the top layers of the skin laden with nerve endings. Once past these layers, there are usually no sharp sensations. Some people feel a pressure or a heavy feeling around the needle. This, too, is considered a positive effect, an indicator that the treatment will be effective.

Acupuncture needles are very thin and are solid, unlike hypodermic needles that are hollow in order to take blood or deliver a drug to the body. As they are so small, they rarely leave any trace of their presence. There is usually no blood or other markings after the needle is withdrawn.

Shiatsu

Shiatsu is an ancient form of therapeutic body treatment that literally means 'finger pressure' in Japanese. The art of shiatsu is based on a combined knowledge of Traditional Chinese Medicine and Western physiology and anatomy. As the principles of shiatsu are similar to acupuncture, and the points

- Continual back pain can have a very profound affect on over all well-being, particularly the psyche. It has been demonstrated over and over again that stress and depression are large contributing factors not only to one's perception of pain, but also to their prognosis. Shiatsu has had great success with decreasing the level of stress and anxiety in people, thereby increasing over all health, recovery from injury and reduction in pain.

- Shiatsu treatments usually last one hour and are not usually associated with any adverse effects. Like any form of body treatment, muscle stiffness, fatigue, headaches, or other mild symptoms may occur.

- As clinical research on shiatsu still remains limited, it should not be the only form of treatment used in any therapeutic plan.

treated are the same (without needle insertion), the therapeutic benefit of shiatsu has great potential, with little to no associated adverse reactions.

Similar to reflexology, in which pressure is applied only to points on the feet, shiatsu employs the application of pressure and motion predominantly to specific acupuncture points along various energy meridians in the body. These energy meridians or channels are located all over the body, so shiatsu treatments involve physically treating the entire body, not just the foot.

Shiatsu treatments take place with the patient fully clothed, lying flat on the ground. Most often these treatments are not done on a massage table as the therapist will combine stretches and joint movements or limb rotation while pressing on the acupuncture points. Shiatsu is said to affect all levels of the body — the physical, the emotional, and the spiritual.

Effectiveness

Research is limited but one study took a look at 66 individuals with lower back pain. Patients were monitored for pain and anxiety about their pain before and after the treatments. After only four shiatsu treatments, all participants reported less pain in their lower back, with less anxiety or stress about their physical pain. All participants also reported that they would recommend shiatsu as a beneficial form of therapy for others with back pain.

Another study evaluating the effectiveness of shiatsu on stress involved 25 volunteers who had a 10-minute shiatsu treatment or a similar treatment where the pressure was applied to other areas of the body, not on the acupuncture points. Before and after the treatment each patient was asked to record stress levels, in addition to using the bispectral index (BIS). Pressure applied to these acupuncture points significantly reduced the BIS values and verbal stress scores when compared to the control group receiving pressure on non-acupuncture points.

Active Release Therapy™

Active release therapy (ART) is a soft tissue technique developed and patented by chiropractor P. Michael Leahy. Different from chiropractic manipulation, massage, and shiatsu, ART addresses chronic injuries to muscles and fascia, particularly those related to repetitive trauma. The technique is taught in specialized centers where practitioners can become certified. ART treatments include both examination and assessment to localize areas of 'scarring' or 'adhesions', followed by soft tissue mobilization to release these abnormalities.

Effectiveness

ART is extremely popular in the field of sports and athletic therapy, where success rates of up to 90% are claimed. The technique is certainly supported by testimonials from numerous high-level athletes. As yet, however, there remain no significant clinical research studies to support these reports. ART is more likely appropriate for more chronic cases of back pain and possibly in the management of post-surgical soft tissue pain.

Yoga

Yoga is a type of exercise that employs both the body and the mind to bring a sense of balance to the body, mentally and physically, so that the body may be in the best possible position to heal. Yoga itself does not create health, but instead helps to provide an environment that allows the body to function optimally.

Yoga is best known as a physical practice that utilizes gentle stretching, breathing, and relaxation techniques. Each of these techniques follows a specific pattern or sequence that helps to relax the mind and energize the body. It begins with concentration on breathing. Focusing on the breath helps to quiet the mind. When the mind is quiet, the release of cortisol, our stress hormone, decreases. Next follows a series of gentle movements and poses that help to strengthen and lengthen the muscles. This also helps to increase the circulation through the body, which in turn provides new nutrients to damaged or inflamed areas and helps sweep away metabolic by-products. In doing this, the supportive muscles of the low back and other areas are strengthened and lengthened at the same time, decreasing spasticity and muscle tightness.

It is often hard to exercise with back pain, for every movement irritates the injured or painful area. Yoga offers a unique way of working the muscles, burning fat, and increasing cardiovascular health without adding the extra stress of pressure to injured areas of the back. As it is a form of exercise that helps, in a postural sense, to lengthen the spine, it can be very useful in low back pain secondary to disc disease or arthritis.

Effectiveness

Yoga has been shown to be very beneficial in the treatment of back pain and in the prevention of re-injury. At work we face many stressors both physical and mental every day. Stress has been shown to be one of the leading factors in musculoskeletal problems, particularly in the back. One study showed that short interludes of yoga at work helped to teach

Yoga Facts

- Useful in subacute, recurrent, and chronic low back pain.

- Yoga can have a beneficial effect on low back pain, both physically and emotionally. Through the use of gentle stretching and deep breathing during yoga, a significant reduction in back pain can be achieved, while strengthening the body and preventing further injury to the back.

- In addition, yoga can offer a positive effect with respect to stress, relaxation, and the diseases or disorders associated with it. Whether due to a decrease in the stress hormone cortisol, lowered blood pressure, increased immunity, or simply relaxation, an improved harmony between the body and mind is achieved through yoga. This can be used as a powerful treatment modality without the use of medications or side effects.

important stress management techniques and relieve muscular tension in the back. This led to statistically fewer back injuries and a more rapid recovery from existing back problems with a non-specific origin. Another demonstrated that regular yoga practices helped to strengthen the back while relaxing muscles along the spine. The participants in this study reported a significant reduction in back pain following regular yoga and less recurrence of injury.

Studies have been performed monitoring stress and its response to yoga. In one study, seven yoga instructors were examined for brain wave activity and cortisol levels while they were performing yoga exercises. All participants displayed a marked increase in alpha brain wave activity, indicating increased alertness with enhanced relaxation. Reduction in cortisol levels directly correlated with these changes in brain wave activity.

There are essentially no contraindications to yoga, although certain movements or postures may need to be limited, particularly during the acute phase of low back pain if they cause irritation. They can then be phased in later as the back recovers. Some people may need to limit the range of motion through some of the exercises. Such caution is advised in the presence of a total hip replacement (due to decreased stability in the joint). This should be discussed with your surgeon. Some individuals may need to begin more slowly with the exercises and build up their strength and flexibility. It is important not to push the body too far. Pain on a movement is indicative that you should move through the exercise with care. Otherwise, yoga should be implemented as a regular stress management technique.

Tai Chi

Tai Chi is often referred to as a moving form of yoga combined with meditation. This form of exercise employs both the mind and the body simultaneously in order to bring about both body awareness and strength. Tai Chi is based on the principal of balancing Yin and Yang forces, opposing characteristics of the same detail, for instance, female/male, hot/cold, and dark/light. This balance is achieved by fostering Chi or Qi, the life force or life energy in the body that runs along the same series of meridians described in acupuncture. When there is an obstruction in this Qi, injury, pain, discomfort, and disease result. The balancing of Qi in the body is created through body movement and meditation, each helping to unblock congested Qi and deliver it to areas that are deficient in Qi. This then restores the natural harmony or balance within the system and ultimately relieves the pain or heals the injury.

There are many different forms of Tai Chi, otherwise known as 'sets', each consisting of a different sequence of coordinated movements. Many of the movements stem from various martial arts practices, such as Qi Gong. Tai Chi movements mimic the natural movements in nature seen in animals and birds, but unlike the staccato movements of these animals, Tai Chi is performed in a slow, continuous, even movement. The basic movements in Tai Chi are pushing movements with the hand that work to move all the joints through their full range of motion.

Breathing is a very important component of Tai Chi. In Tai Chi one is taught to breathe fully from the abdomen, not the simple shallow breath from the upper chest or lungs that most of us use. The breath is a representation of the mind. Its purpose is to relax the mind, as in meditation, but to do so with awareness. It is not simply creating a blank space in the mind. Each breath should be processed by the mind in a graceful and active manner.

Tai Chi then teaches students to match their breath to each movement. In doing so the individual is able to bring together both the mind and the body in a simultaneous awareness that allows for better musculoskeletal functioning. The movements of Tai Chi are timed with the breath. As one extends out or forward, the breath is exhaled. The reverse is true as the movement returns to the center of the body, or a neutral position.

Effectiveness

Scientific research from the Medical Academy of Shanghai, the Tangshen Medical Center, and Bellevue Hospital in New York City have shown that Tai Chi stimulates the central nervous system, decreases heart rate and blood pressure, and gently tones the muscles without strain. It also helps improve digestion and promote regular bowel movements. According to Tai Chi practitioners, one can easily reach the American Health Association standards for exercise by practicing Tai Chi 3 times a day.

Tai Chi has been used therapeutically with the elderly and injured for decades. Since then it has grown in popularity, used by all ages as a form of 'warm-up', cross-training, and body awareness. One study performed on the elderly was designed to evaluate flexibility, balance, pain, and mood. It was found that anxiety and pain perception diminished greatly and mood, flexibility, and balance improved significantly. It was also seen that the rate of falls and injuries diminished and quality of life improved.

Another report showed the beneficial effects of Tai Chi with the pain of ankylosing spondilitis. After daily Tai Chi exercises,

Tai Chi Facts

- Tai Chi helps to coordinate the mind and body so that the mind becomes actively aware of its proprioceptive position and movement in space. This helps to strengthen and stimulate muscles, such as those involved in the core support of the back and abdomen. This then aids in proper posture, both while sitting and moving.

- In addition, Tai Chi helps to instruct the body to move 'correctly'. This means helping the muscles 'learn' which fibers should contract first, in a coordinated sequence of stimulation to increase strength, promote range of motion in a joint, and decrease injury.

- The gentle movements of Tai Chi also help to smoothly rotate all the joints and stretch them, freeing up the blocked Qi that can create pain.

pain weakness and general malaise were significantly alleviated. If the Tai Chi was stopped for more than one week, symptoms returned. In addition to relief of pain, much of the flexion
deformity of the spine caused by the ankolosing spondilitis was
minimized and balance and strength improved.

Tai Chi, although not proven to be a clinical form of treatment for back pain, has shown many beneficial therapeutic
effects that are non-invasive and promote a healthy lifestyle.

The Rosen Method

The Rosen Method is a physical therapy based on the theory
that a natural and optimal state of one's physical and mental
health exists. In this state, the body is better balanced, free of
pain, and more resilient to disease. The aim is to regain this
state by helping the patient become aware of blocked patterns,
behaviors, or tensions in the body, then allowing them to be
released.

The Rosen Method treats the mind and the body as an
integrated unit, placing emphasis on the role that emotions
play in physical well-being. The belief is that a body will hold
tension in muscles, referred to as barriers, when an emotion
or expression of that emotion has not taken place. The
emotion may have been suppressed in the past because it may
have been too difficult to handle at that point. The body may
have somatized it into the muscle. With treatment, once
relaxed, the chronic tension from that repressed emotion is
allowed to move out of the body, the muscle relaxes, and the
body's optimal state is restored.

Rosen practitioners believe that changes in the mind-body
connection can be seen in the breath. The breath is said to
represent the intersection between the conscious and the
unconscious mind. The diaphragm plays a central role in the
breathing function. Sitting below the lungs, the diaphragm is
innervated by nerves from two different parts of the nervous
system, allowing the movement of the diaphragm and therefore lungs to be controlled with and without our awareness.
Voluntary movements of the breath are linked to the
conscious mind, while involuntary movements are controlled
by the unconscious.

Chronic muscle tension decreases the movement of the
muscles, joints, and organs, increasing pain. To change the
habits of the body, voluntary motions such as stretching and
strengthening are vital, but for the residual chronic tension,
you also need to change the involuntary processes of the body.
By bringing awareness to the area that is chronically tight,
neurological information is then transmitted up the peripheral nerves to the central nervous system, where it replaces
the old information. This process is termed 'disintegrating/

The Rosen Method Facts

- Particularly useful for chronic pain. We know that there is a great deal of emotion associated with chronic pain, whether or not the pain was brought on by the emotional upset or not. This type of therapy, although not rigorously clinically studied, has reported great benefits where other types of therapies have failed.

- Brings body awareness to the patient, teaches important breathing and relaxation techniques, and is free of adverse side effects.

The Rosen Method is not specific to back pain; it is a very useful tool for any pain pattern, emotional or physical.

reintegrating'. When this process takes place, the muscle softens, there may be a change in circulation, or even a quiver in the muscle. This is viewed positively as an indicator that a shift has taken place.

Muscle tension may be held anywhere in the body, but is most often associated with the neck, back, and torso. There are also said to be emotions associated with different parts of the body. 'Trapped' or suppressed fear manifests itself in the lower abdomen, lower back, and pelvis. Anger and sadness present as chronic tension in the neck, top of the shoulders, and thoracic (chest) region. Muscle tension may also present as decreased range of motion of a joint, pain, stiffness, or other symptoms.

Treatment Protocol

Whatever the symptomatic presentation or associated emotion involved, the treatment process is the same. The assessment begins the minute the patient walks into the room. The practitioner observes all movements, voice patterns, breathing, and expressions, including how the patient speaks about the problem, watching for posture, joint movements, holding patterns, and other nuances. Next, the patient lies on the table, on the stomach, with a pillow beneath the pelvis for comfort. Practitioners begin by placing their hands on the patient's back and feeling for muscle tension. They also watch how patients breath, whether they are completely inhaling or exhaling, and whether the breath is coming from the lower abdomen or is a shallow lung-breath.

Once an area of tension is found, the practitioners focus on it by placing their hands on that area and possibly pressing deeper into the tissue, somewhat like a massage. During this time, the practitioner will often feel emotionally and physically what the patient is experiencing. By focusing in on this area, they can 'awaken' the muscle to the suppressed issue. This often brings out memories or simply emotions for the patient. The experience of the emotion itself is often enough to allow the muscle to release and send that relaxed information into the central nervous system. Other times, it may require a few treatments or discussions about the identified emotional issue.

The belief with the Rosen Method is that once the emotion or memory is released, the muscle memory is resolved and this new information is then reset in the body, allowing dissolution of the chronic muscle tension and relief of pain. Whether or not the patient is aware of the specifics of the memory is irrelevant. There has then been a re-patterning of the body and a return to its homeostatic optimal balance.

The Alexander Technique

The Alexander technique, named after F.M. Alexander, is defined as discovering and achieving one's purpose, based on the belief that only when every muscle and cell in the body knows its specific 'purpose' can the human body function optimally.

Many physical therapies treat dysfunction, whether it is pain, inflammation, or spasm, by applying opposing treatments, such as anti-inflammatories or anti-spasmotics, whereas the Alexander technique teaches people to change dysfunctional patterns, removing harmful tension through re-education of the mind and the body rather than with a series of exercises and medications. This method of rediscovering balance in the body and releasing tension can then be applied to all daily activities such as sitting, walking, running, or working at the computer.

Alexander therapy focuses on changing the way we habitually perform activities such as getting out of a chair or walking. The therapist will instruct the patient to perform a specific task and will carefully observe the coordination of the patient as a whole and the patterns of muscle movements and contractions. The therapist will then instruct the patient to make small changes in specific parts of the activity, such as timing of different joint movements, balance, and posture, gently touching these specific areas or joints. This can be equated to a sports instructor aiding athletes in their tennis swing or golf stance.

Teaching the patient to breathe fully from the abdomen rather than shallow chest breathing is also incorporated in this technique. By increasing the available oxygen to each cell, there is more energy for movement, less chance of injury and therefore less fatigue.

The goal at the end of the training is to teach the body to move in a tension-free, almost effortless way to help encourage maximal muscle firing and contraction with the least amount of stress and work in each muscle. This promotes efficient muscle movement, enables healing, and prevents further injury. The same method is then applied to every movement of the body, so that it becomes ingrained into the individual's physique.

Effectiveness

The Alexander technique is supported by numerous testimonials, including the comments of marathon record-holder Paul Collins, who believes it helps protect the body from injury during intense athletic performance. There are also no available clinical studies.

Exercise Treatments for Back Care

Prepared in cooperation with Sabine Stojanovich, CPTN, ACE, CPTN, AAHFP (Certified Personal Trainer and Rehabilitation Conditioning Consultant).

For any machine to function well, it needs to be switched on and used regularly. You cannot simply blow the dust off, press the 'on' button, and expect it to perform without small noises or glitches. The human body is probably the most complex machine of all. It only makes sense that a well-conditioned body will not only last longer, it will have greater resistance to the wear and tear of everyday living and recover from injury more rapidly.

The basis behind exercise as a treatment for back pain is threefold. First, in recovering from injury, controlled exercise promotes healing of damaged tissue and prevents development of the stiffness and weakness that may follow acute pain. Second, according to biomechanical theory, improved control and stability, along with strength and endurance, will restore the ability of muscular support to protect the spine. If pain is due to repeated mechanical irritation of pain-sensitive structures, then preventing that irritation will reduce pain and improve mobility. Third,, maintaining a strong, flexible spine, appropriate weight, and aerobic fitness with endurance will protect the spine from mechanical insult and further injury.

The key to sticking to an exercise program is finding a variety of exercises that you like. Test the wide variety of stretching, strengthening, and cardiovascular exercises presented in 'Specific Back Exercises' section of this chapter. Some will be more comfortable and effective than others. Pay attention to your posture as well, while standing and sitting, working and playing, to relieve any tension that may cause pain.

Exercise Benefits

- Strengthens the muscles that support the spine (abdominal/para-vertebral).
- Increases circulation and nutrient flow to muscles and other tissues.
- Increases flexibility and range of motion.
- Improves posture and muscle tone.
- Essential component of any weight-management program.
- Improves sleep.
- Increases energy.
- Improves mood and feeling of well-being.
- Reduces stress and anxiety.
- Decreases risk of cardiovascular disease, diabetes, etc.
- Reduces injury risk.

 BACK FACTS

Regular exercise several times a week strengthens not only the heart muscle, but also the skeletal muscles that support the back. Exercise is a basic therapy for preventing and treating back injury. Gone are the days where the prescription for back pain was a television remote and a firm mattress. In fact, bed rest is contra-indicated in most cases of acute or chronic back pain. Exercise should become as commonplace in your lifestyle as brushing your teeth.

Exercise Basics

Prior to starting any exercise program, you should consult your healthcare practitioner. This is true whether you have back pain or not. It is also very important that you perform each exercise properly. If you exercise with an incorrect technique, you may do yourself more harm than good. And do start slowly. If you have exercised in the past, but have been reticent for the past few years, do not expect your body to be capable of returning to the exercises you were doing before at the same intensity. This, too, increases your risk of harm or injury, from both cardiovascular and muscu-loskeletal perspectives. Start slowly, and build from there. Do not get discouraged! You should anticipate a six-month program to return to your previous level.

In order to maximize your benefit from any conditioning regimen, it is important to alternate your exercises. This is true for several reasons. First, when you perform the same exercise over and over again, the muscles become very efficient. Thus, you will reach a point where you are actually burning fewer calories and gaining less strength, despite performing the same actions at the same rate of intensity. By alternating the type of exercise you perform and the level of intensity, you can increase the amount of work performed during the same amount of time.

Second, it is important to alternate the muscle groups that you use. By exercising the same muscles over and over again, you can inflame, irritate, and weaken them, leaving them more susceptible to injury or harm. A muscle group needs 48 hours of rest. You can still exercise every day, just alternate muscle groups. For example, upper body one day, lower body the next. By alternating the type of exercises you do and the muscle groups used, you will strengthen a wider variety of muscles, while giving each muscle group time to recover and rest. There is great truth to the adage that 'It is the rest that makes you strong'.

Whatever type of exercise program you choose, it should involve three main components: stretching, strength training, and cardiovascular exercise. Alternating strength training and cardiovascular exercise from day to day is ideal with stretching performed daily. We will consider the general aspects of these before outlining specific exercises for management of your back pain.

Exercise Terminology

- **Resistance:** the force against which you work during an exercise. This may be just body weight against gravity or it may involve external weights, elastic bands, or pulleys.

- **Rep (short for repetition):** one complete movement of an exercise, for example, one leg-lift, one biceps curl, one sit-up.

- **Set:** any number of reps comprise a set. Strengthening involves sets with a low number of reps (8–10), while endurance is built with low resistance and a higher number of reps (15–20).

Stretching

Tight muscles contribute to many types of injury and muscular ailments, particularly back pain. And it is not just the muscles of the spine that affect back pain. Hamstrings (the muscles on the back of the legs), for example, when tight, greatly affect the movement of the pelvis and back. Jobs that involve standing on your feet all day (bank teller or check-out clerk) or leaning over a table (surgeon or dentist) require near constant activity in the hamstring muscles. Failure to stretch is a common cause of back pain in these individuals. Sitting all day tends to shorten the hip flexors, therefore pulling the pelvis forward and applying pressure on the lower back.

Whatever type of stretch you decide to do, it is important to note that when first beginning, do not try to stretch the injured area. Begin with the muscles that surround the injured area. If you try to stretch the affected area at first, you may actually increase the spasm. Wait until the surrounding areas are lengthened and strengthened, and then begin to work the injured segments of the back. No matter what area of the body you are stretching, in order to increase flexibility and elasticity of the muscles, ligaments and tendons, you need to push the stretch to the furthest possible range of motion.

There should be no pain involved with the stretching process. Take the stretch just to the point before it hurts and hold it for 60 seconds. Ease into it slowly and don't bounce the stretch, just hold. There may be some discomfort (not pain!) involved in this at first, and it may take weeks to months before you can take a stretch to its full range. However, if you keep working at it, each time you stretch, you will move a little bit further.

In order to determine how much discomfort you should endure before causing injury, use correct posture and motion through the stretch as your guide. If you have to bend a nearby joint, like the knee, in order to move that hamstring stretch a little further, then you are compromising the stretch and risking injury. Go as far as you can in the correct position without having to compensate in any other area to push further.

Stretching is often relegated to the last few minutes of a workout. This is probably the biggest mistake you can make. An adequate stretch program should comprise at least 15 to 20 minutes.

Benefits of Stretching

- Reduces risk of injury during exercise or other activity.
- Improves muscle function.
- Prevents muscle 'tightness' with associated postural compromise.
- Increases muscle blood flow and clears metabolic waste products.

Types of Stretching Exercises

There are seven main types of stretching: static stretching, active stretching, dynamic stretching, passive stretching, isometric stretching, proprioceptive neuromuscular facilitation, and ballistic stretching. They vary in their intensity and complexity, some requiring a second individual to assist. In order to determine which type of stretch is best suited for you, seek out advice from a trainer or healthcare worker. If you have exercised and stretched in the past, start slowly on your own. Begin with the easier stretches, such as the static, active, and dynamic stretches, and gradually build up to isometric and PNF (proprioceptive neuromuscular facilitation) stretching to increase both the strength and flexibility in your muscles and joints. This will not only help support the muscles that surround the spine, but will also stabilize your abdominal, pelvic, and leg muscles, creating a very strong core to support your body and prevent further injury. And remember, warm up *before* you stretch!

Static Stretching

Static stretching is the simplest type of stretch. The muscle or joint is taken through a slow and controlled range of movement until the limitations in the muscle or joint are reached. The stretch is held for a minimum of 15 seconds and for up to 30 seconds, if possible. In order to achieve this, the muscle group or joint is not pushed quite as far as it is in active stretching. The stretch is performed slowly, in a controlled manner, with enough support to ensure that no sudden movement occurs.

Active Stretching

Active stretching is probably the most popular and best-known form of stretching. It involves stretching the muscle to the limits of motion and then holding that position for a short period of time, around 10 to 15 seconds. The stretch is held 'actively' by the individual whose muscles are being stretched, rather than having another person hold the limb in position. This active contraction in the opposing muscle groups actually helps relax the muscles being stretched. It is a more aggressive stretch than the static stretch and is used to increase flexibility and to strengthen opposing muscles. This type of stretch is best utilized after exercise as a warm down.

Dynamic Stretching

Dynamic stretching, as the name implies, involves moving the body gradually through a movement. This is done with increasing speed as the stretch progresses.

As opposed to ballistic stretching, where there is bouncing and small, fast movements, dynamic stretching employs long, controlled movements that gently take the muscle or joint to the limits of the range of motion and not beyond.

This type of stretching is very beneficial for increasing flexibility and warming up muscles prior to an aerobic activity but can also be used after exercise.

Passive Stretching

Passive stretching is also called relaxed stretching because most of the work involved in passive stretching is not performed by the person whose muscles are being stretched. In passive stretching, the muscle group that is being stretched is usually held in place by another individual or occasionally by another body part.

Passive stretching is performed in a very slow and controlled manner to help lengthen and relax a muscle group. This type of stretching is particularly useful for muscles that are extremely tight or in spasm. It is difficult to engage the stretch reflex and increase tension through a passive stretch. This type of stretch also helps to clear metabolic waste products in muscle after a workout and is therefore often utilized as a cool-down stretch.

Isometric Stretching

Isometric stretching is a form of stretching that helps to increase the strength and integrity of the muscle being stretched while increasing flexibility. Isometric stretching involves moving the muscle or joint to its full range of motion, and rather than simply holding it there, applying a resistant force in the opposite direction. This forces the stretched muscle fibers to contract. By doing so, the muscle is strengthened in a stretched position. The tension or force is applied for 10 to 15 seconds and then relaxed for 20 seconds before repeating.

This type of stretching is best used after a workout. It is not an ideal for stretch for beginners or when there is damaged tissue. Isometric stretching is best used in a conditioning program to increase strength and flexibility.

Proprioceptive Neuromuscular Facilitation (PNF) Stretching

Proprioceptive neuromuscular facilitation or PNF stretching is a very useful and popular type of stretching among athletes. A combination of isometric stretching and passive stretching, it involves resistance placed upon the muscles while in tension. During this type of stretching, the muscles are put through the fullest range of motion that the muscle bed or joint will allow. However, rather than one continuous movement, the motion is stopped frequently and an opposing resistance force is applied. This then forces the stretched muscles to engage and create tension within them. The resistance is applied for at least 20 seconds before moving the muscle through further range and applying resistance again.

Between each force application in a new position there should be at least a 20 second rest to allow the muscle to recuperate and recover before firing once again. This greatly increases the strength of the muscle being stretched.

This type of stretch, like the isometric stretch, is not suitable for injured areas of the body and is best used with a knowledgeable trainer or healthcare worker who can assist you.

Ballistic Stretching

Ballistic stretching uses the momentum of a body part to create a force that will allow the body to move beyond the normal range for that joint or muscle. This is a type of stretch that helps to increase circulation quickly and warm up the muscles and joints. It is a bouncing type of motion, where the muscles are used like springs, bouncing in and out of a stretched position. This type of stretching has limited use and needs to be performed very carefully in a warmed muscle to prevent injury. It does not allow the muscle to relax in the stretched position, and can in fact tighten the muscle more by engaging the stretch reflex. This is particularly true if you are applying this technique to an injured or inflamed area of the body. It should always be avoided in this situation.

Stretching Exercises

This charts presents the stretches recommended for the treatment of various types of back pain After reading further, you may find it convenient for developing your own exercise program, ideally in cooperation with a medical doctor, physiotherapist, or occupational therapist. Remember to warm up before you stretch.

Type of Back Pain	Static	Active	Dynamic	Passive	Isometric	PNF	Ballistic
Sudden Onset							
Lumbar Strain							
Acute Phase 0–48 hours	X						
Subacute Phase	X	X	X				
Prevention Phase		X	X	X	X	X	X
Disc Herniation							
Acute Phase	X						
Subacute Phase	X	X	X				
Prevention		X	X	X	X		
Recurrent							
Acute episode	X	X					
Prevention	X	X	X	X	X	X	
Persistent							
Degenerative Disc Disease	X	X	X	X			
Arthritis	X	X		X			
Spinal Stenosis + Instability			X				

Strengthening

The second component of exercise involves strength training — muscle force and muscle endurance. Muscle force is the ability to contract against resistance — basically how much you can lift. Muscle endurance is the ability to contract repeatedly — how long can you lift for. With respect to the spine, both of these aspects are important, but given the role of spinal muscles in postural support and the preponderance of slow-twitch nerve fibers, endurance is essential for back health.

Strength training does not mean using heavy weights! Start with a weight that actually feels too easy. Get used to the exercise and get your muscles used to resistance training. Only then can you gradually and carefully increase resistance. In order to reduce the muscle loss that occurs so rapidly with inactivity, strength training should start as soon as acute back pain has begun to subside. Non-involved muscle groups can even be trained during the acute phase as long as there is no

Basics of Strengthening Exercises

- Muscle force is increased by exercising against high resistance with few repetitions.

- Endurance is increased by exercising against lower resistance with a higher number of repetitions.

aggravation of the back or leg pain. In either case, exercises should be started very gently so they seem almost too easy. This will allow you to gauge your tolerance and prevent injury. As pain subsides and tolerance improves, resistance and repetitions can be increased.

Good Pain vs Bad Pain

Strengthening exercises should not be painful. However, it is not uncommon to experience discomfort afterward. This may be after a few hours or even the next day. Individuals who are used to exercise will recognize this as the 'healthy' muscle ache indicative of a hard work-out. However, those not used to such sensations often confuse it with re-injury or aggravation of their back pain. In fact, in those with chronic or recurrent pain, any sensation in the back area will immediately be interpreted as 'my back pain', even though the cause may be completely different.

Learning 'good' from 'bad' pain is essential for making progress. This may have to be taught by a therapist or other practitioner. Adequate warm-up, controlled exercise with slow resistance increments, and sufficient stretching along with modalities such as heat and ice will minimize discomfort from your workout.

Performing exercises correctly is essential in maximizing their benefit and reducing risk of injury. Isolating muscle groups improves exercise specificity, and avoiding excessively heavy resistance will augment this. Individuals at the gym lifting those enormous dumbbells by swinging their arms and arching their back are giving the arms a poor workout and risking back or shoulder injury. By using lighter weights with smooth, controlled movement of the arms, you will build more muscle, increase endurance, and avoid damage. As a rule, think posture first and form second. Once you start to compromise either of these it means the weight you are using is too heavy!

Bad Pain Indications

The following are indicators that you are doing more harm than good with your exercises:

- Sudden sharp pain that occurs during exercise.
- Pain that radiates or spreads beyond the exercised area.
- Pain that fails to subside after resting the muscle for 2 to 3 days.
- Pain that persists and prevents you from making progress in your program.

Cardiovascular Exercise

Cardiovascular exercise is the third crucial component to any preventative or therapeutic musculoskeletal program. As with strengthening, trying to remain active even during the acute phase of low back pain will reduce the deconditioning caused by immobility. Cardiovascular fitness is crucial to the management of recurrent, persistent, and chronic low back pain.

Benefits of Cardiovascular Exercise

- Improved muscle tone, blood supply, endurance and flexibility.
- Reduces spasm and removes toxic metabolic by-products.
- Improves health of the heart, blood vessels, and lungs.
- Releases pain-relieving endorphins.
- Assists weight management.
- Improves mood and energy.
- Helps reduce stress.
- Helps lower blood pressure.

Measuring Your Heart Rate

1. Find your pulse at your wrist or on the front of the elbow.

2. Count beats per minute (bpm) at rest, during exercise, and before the warm-down.

3. Measure your heart rate (bpm):
   - Number of beats in 10 seconds multiplied by 6
   - Number of beats in 15 seconds multiplied by 4

4. Calculate your 'Maximum' heart rate = 220 minus your age = Maximum beats per minute (bpm)

   Cardiovascular Exercise Stages
   - Warm-Up: 5 to 10 minutes
   - Stretch: 5–10 minutes

   Heart Zone Exercises:
   - Healthy heart zone = 50% to 60% of Maximum, 20 to 60 minutes
   - Fitness zone = 60% to 70% of Maximum, 20 to 60 minutes
   - Aerobic zone = 70% to 80% of Maximum, 20 to 60 minutes

   Cool-Down: 50% to 60% of Maximum, 10 to 15 minutes.
   Stretch: 15–20 minutes

5. Some people find the concept of 'perceived exertion' easier to follow. Ask the question, 'on a scale of 1 to 10, how hard am I working?' 1 is rest, 10 is flat-out.
   - Healthy heart zone = 5–6
   - Fitness zone = 6–7
   - Aerobic zone = 7–8
   - Above 8 = working too hard, slow down!

Warm-Up and Stretching

Make sure you warm-up for 5 to 10 minutes by performing your planned activity at low intensity. Then stretch the principal muscles used in the activity for a further 5 to 10 minutes. This will prepare your body and muscles both physiologically and psychologically for exercise and help prevent injury.

Frequency, Duration, Intensity

Frequency, duration, and intensity are the three important components of any cardiovascular program.

To gain cardiovascular benefit, it is recommended that you exercise at least three times per week and ideally three to five times. If you are just starting to train, then you will need a good 24 to 36 hours between sessions to allow adequate recovery and to reduce injury and exhaustion risk. This can be gradually increased as you become fitter.

Exercise duration should be at least 20 minutes and is best varied between 20 and 60 minutes. However, beginners should take things very cautiously and start at low intensity for 5 to 10 minutes, gradually increasing duration over a few weeks. Always increase duration before you increase intensity; walk for longer before you start to walk faster.

The easiest way to monitor the intensity of your workout is to measure your heart rate. This should be done at rest, during, and on completion of your session. Some fitness machines have built-in heart rate monitors and may even have cardiovascular programs you can follow. You can buy a separate heart rate monitor to wear (chest devices are most accurate) if you are exercising outside or on other types of equipment. Or you can take your pulse, preferably at your wrist. Count the number of beats in 10 seconds and multiply by 6 or count for 15 seconds and multiply by 4 to get a value of beats-per-minute (bpm).

Cool-Down

As important as the warm-up, the cool-down should be performed at 50% to 60% max for about 5 to 10 minutes. This is followed by stretching for 15 to 20 minutes to complete your workout.

Cardiovascular Exercise Components

- **Frequency:** To improve fitness and maintain optimum body fat you should perform cardiovascular exercise at least three times per week.
- **Duration:** Cardiovascular exercise should be performed for at least 20 minutes.
- **Intensity:** Percentage of maximum heart rate should be monitored.

Heart Zone Training

Using your heart rate to determine intensity is called 'Heart Zone' training. It uses percentages of your age-adjusted maximum heart rate. This is most simply determined by subtracting your age from 220. So, if you are 40, your age-adjusted maximum is 180 bpm. A more accurate assessment is a Max Heart Rate fitness test but this needs to be performed by a professional.

Healthy Heart Zone

This is exercise performed at 50% to 60% max. This is the lowest level at which benefit is achieved and is generally a good starting point for beginners. It has been shown to reduce blood pressure, cholesterol, and body fat but not to greatly improve fitness.

Fitness Zone

This involves exercise at 60% to 70% max and adds cardiovascular fitness and greater fat burning potential. You should aim to reach at least this level within a few weeks of starting to train. The advantage of this level is that it generally involves less stress on the musculoskeletal system and spine.

Aerobic Zone

This is where you really begin to increase your cardiovascular endurance and efficiency. Performed at 70% to 80% max, it greatly improves heart and lung function. It also burns far more calories and is therefore more effective for weight loss.

More advanced training includes anaerobic and interval training which will not be discussed here. Further information is easily obtained from books, the internet, or a personal trainer.

- **Supine:** lying on your back looking at the ceiling.
- **Prone:** lying on your front looking at the floor.
- **Spine Extension:** curving your spine so it forms an arch toward your tummy.
- **Spine Flexion:** curving your spine so it form an arch toward your back (as in bending to touch your toes.
- **All Fours:** on your hands and knees on the floor with your back parallel to the floor.

Specific Back Exercises

Many exercises have been developed to assist in alleviating back pain, some more effective and some safer than others. Complicating any recommendation that you pursue one or another form of exercise is the wide variation among individuals with respect to their level of fitness, familiarity with exercise, type of back pain, and response to treatment.

In general, exercises in each section are listed in order of increasing difficulty. Always start with the easiest and progress slowly.

Caution

If you are in any doubt about the suitability of an exercise or the way in which it is performed, then you should first seek the assistance of a knowledgeable healthcare professional. If you are new to exercise, then clearance should be obtained from your doctor before proceeding.

Postures and Stretches

Postures are the easiest form of 'exercise'. They involve positions and movements aimed at reducing discomfort, particularly in the acute stage of low back pain. Stretches, as discussed above, should be mostly confined to static, active, and dynamic in the early phase.

Basic Pain-Relieving Postures

These techniques do not constitute 'exercise' but are useful to alleviate pain before or after exercise and during the acute phase.

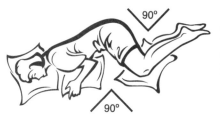

Figure 'Z' Lying: Lie on your side, pillow between your knees, between your arms and under your head, hips and knees flexed to 90 degrees.

Supine 'Z': Lie on your back on the floor, pillow under your head, hips and knees to 90 degrees with your lower legs resting up on a stool or chair

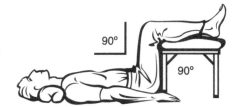

Extension Postures and Stretches (for Back Pain Worse with Flexion)

Standing Extension: Position feet shoulder-width apart, hands on hips or holding a support such as the back of a chair. Look up at the ceiling and try to make an arch in your low back with the top of the arch pointing forward. Perform slowly, do not arch too much!

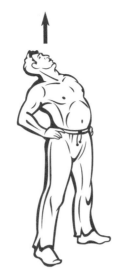

Sitting Extension: Sit up straight and tilt your pelvis forward, pushing out your stomach.

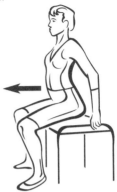

Prone Extension: Lie prone with your chin on your hands as if watching television.

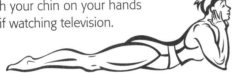

Sloppy Push-Up: From the prone extension position, push your chest away from the floor with your hands.

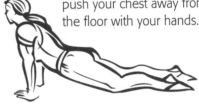

All Fours Arch: From the all-fours position, tilt your pelvis so as to push your tummy to the floor.

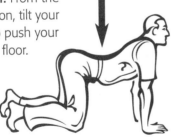

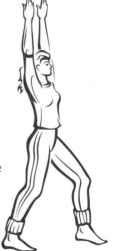

Warrior Pose (yoga position): Place one foot forward in lunge position with arms extended above the head.

Flexion Postures and Stretches (for Back Pain Worse with Extension)

Single Knee to Chest: Lying supine, hug one knee to your chest.

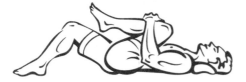

Both Knees to Chest: Lying supine, hug both knees to your chest.

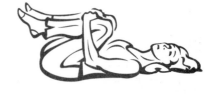

Sitting Flexion: While sitting on a chair, feet on a low stool, curl forward as if to put your head between your knees.

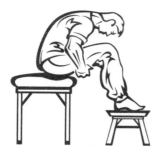

Step Flexion: Stand facing a chair and put one foot on the chair. Then bend forward.

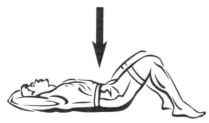

Pelvic Tilt: Lying supine, contract your abdomen to tilt your pelvis backward. Aim to flatten the arch of your low back to the floor.

All Fours Tilt: From the all-fours position, tilt your pelvis so as to push your low back up toward the ceiling (like a cat stretching).

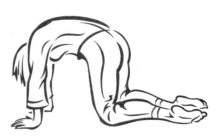

Pelvis and Leg Stretches

Introduce these stretches as acute pain subsides, as part of a preventive program, and incorporate into your conditioning routine.

Hamstring Stretches

(helpful in back pain made worse with extension and for individuals spending a lot of time standing, reaching, bending or lifting):

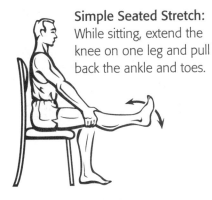

Simple Seated Stretch: While sitting, extend the knee on one leg and pull back the ankle and toes.

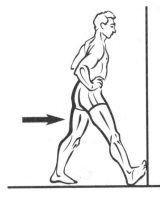

Simple Standing Stretch: Put one leg forward so the sole of the foot is against the wall. Keep looking ahead while flexing your trunk forward until you feel the hamstring stretch.

Sitting Stretch: Sit on the floor, one leg straight out ahead, toes pointed to the ceiling, one bent out to the side. Keep looking up (not at your foot) as you flex your trunk forward along the extended leg. You can wrap a towel around the bottom of the extended foot for leverage to help gently pull you forwards.

Advanced Standing Stretch: Place the foot of the leg to be stretched on a chair or bench in front of you, then flex your trunk forward as in Sitting Stretch. Keep looking forward with your toe pointed at the ceiling.

Quadriceps Stretches

(helpful in back pain made worse with flexion and for individuals spending a lot of time seated):

Simple Standing Stretch: Simple standing stretch — support yourself with one hand with the other grasp the ankle of the leg to be stretched. Pull the foot into your buttock and the thigh backward trying to stretch the quadriceps rather than arching your back.

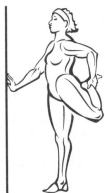

Lying Stretch: Lie prone and pull the foot of the leg to be stretched toward the buttock on the same side. Alternatively try lying on your side, grasping the ankle and pulling your foot towards the buttock while keeping the legs together.

Advanced Lying Stretch: Lie on the edge of a firm bed or bench and support yourself with one arm while allowing the opposite leg to drop off the side. Actively flex the knee or have a trainer assist.

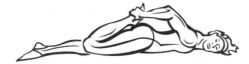

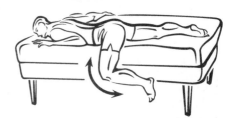

Gluteal Stretches

(helpful for individuals with radiating pain, and for those who spend a lot of time standing):

Easy Gluteal Stretch: Lie supine, flex one knee to 90 degrees, and bring the opposite ankle across to lie on top of the flexed knee. Pushing the knee of the crossed leg away from you will stretch the gluteal on that side..

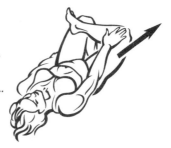

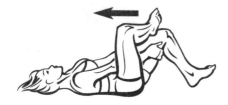

Hard Gluteal Stretch: Start with the easy stretch, then pull the knee of the lower leg up toward your face. If you find this hard, lie facing a wall and put your foot on the wall so your leg is bent at 90 degrees, cross ankle over knee.

TFL Stretch: The TFL (tensor fascia lata) runs down the outer aspect of each leg. Stretch by standing arms length from a wall, hand on the wall and leaning your hips toward the wall.

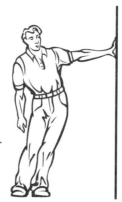

Strengthening Exercises

Core Strengthening (for individual muscle groups)

Abdominal Strengthening:

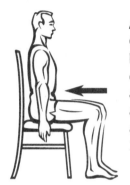

Abdominal Contraction: Either lying on your back or sitting straight in a chair, tighten abdominal muscles and hold for 15 to 20 seconds.

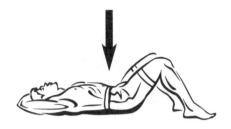

Pelvic Tilt: Lying on your back, knees bent and feet on the floor, contract your abdominal muscles and tilt your pelvis so as to flatten your low back to the floor. Hold for 15–20 seconds.

Wall Sit-up: Lying on your back, put both feet up on the wall so hips are bent at 90 degrees. Then do a partial abdominal curl. By having the feet up, this takes the pressure off the back. An advanced alternative is to have the legs supported over an exercise ball.

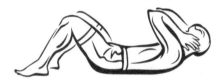

Partial Sit-up: Lying on your back, knees up, feet on the floor and hands beside your ears, lift only your head and shoulders off the floor and hold.

Full Sit-up: Lying on your back, knees up, feet on the floor and hands beside your ears, lift your body until your elbows touch your knees. You may tuck your feet under something to provide stability.

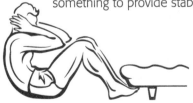

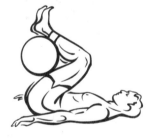

Exercise Ball Lift: Lying on your back, grip your legs over the exercise ball. Lift the ball up to the ceiling by pushing up with your pelvis and abdominals.

Back Muscle Strengthening:

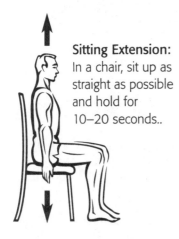

Sitting Extension: In a chair, sit up as straight as possible and hold for 10–20 seconds..

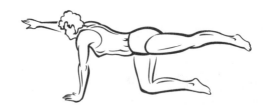

Kneeling Lift: While on all fours, lift the right arm forward and extend the left leg back off the ground. Hold for 5 seconds and then change sides.

Lying Extension: Lying prone, support your body with your elbows and lift your chest off the ground using back muscles and hold for 5–10 seconds.

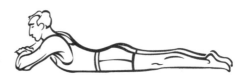

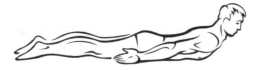

Chest Raise: Lying prone with your arms by your side, lift your chest off the ground and hold for 5–10 seconds.

Oblique Strengthening:

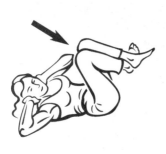

Oblique Sit-up: Lying in the sit-up position, take your elbow up to touch the opposite knee. Repeat on other side. Crossing one leg over the other makes this exercise even easier

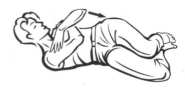

Oblique Crunch: Lying on your side, with your hands across your chest, bring your elbows up towards your hip.

Exercise Ball Oblique: Lying on your back, put your legs up on the ball so your hips are at 90 degrees. Perform the oblique sit-up in this position. An easier option is to place one foot on a wall, say the right, and cross the left ankle over the right knee. Then perform the oblique curl by bringing your right elbow toward your left knee. Then reverse sides.

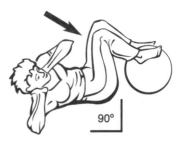

Core Stability (for combining core muscles to provide stability strengthening)

Bridging:

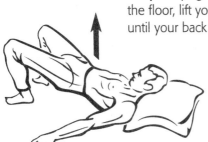

Simple: Lying on your back, knees up and feet on the floor, lift your buttocks and pelvis off the floor until your back is straight. Hold for 20 seconds.

Simple with Leg Raise: Perform the simple bridge with one leg extended out straight off the ground, then repeat with the opposite leg.

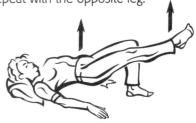

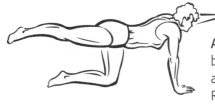

All-Fours Extension: On all fours, keeping the back straight, extend out straight the opposite arm and leg and hold for 10–15 seconds. Repeat on other side.

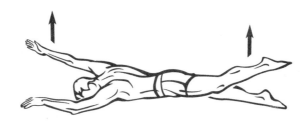

Prone Extensions: While lying prone with your arms extended out past your head, lift opposite arm and leg up and hold for 15 seconds. Repeat on the other side.

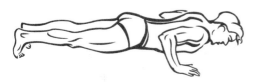

The Plank: While lying prone, lift your body up onto your elbows and toes. Make sure your back is straight, and hold for 30 seconds.

Quadriceps and Hamstring Strengthening

Quadriceps:

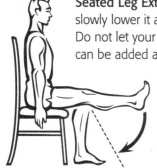

Seated Leg Extension: In a chair, extend your leg out straight, slowly lower it again by 20 to 30 degrees, and then raise it again. Do not let your knee fall all the way back to 90 degrees. A weight can be added around your ankle to increase resistance.

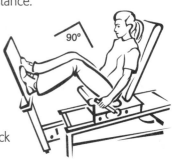

Leg Press: On a leg press machine, place your feet shoulder width apart, with your knees bent to 90 degrees. Slowly straighten your legs out, but do not lock them. Start with a lowest weight, and slowly build up.

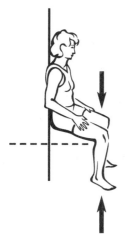

Squat: Standing with your legs slightly wider than shoulder width, tilt your pelvis back, tightening your abdomen, then bend your knees, and lower your body down, keeping your back straight at all times. Make sure that your knees stay over your ankles. Looking down you should be able to see your toes at all times (although ideally you should be looking ahead during the exercise). Do not let your buttocks drop below the level of your knees.

Ball Squat: Face away from a wall and place an exercise ball between you and the wall. Squat, allowing the ball to roll down and up as you move. Hold the squat with the knees at about 80–90 degrees for 5 seconds or longer as your strength improves.

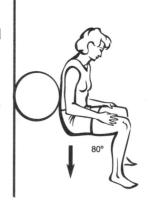

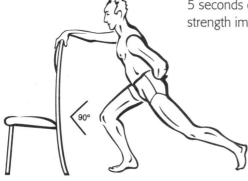

Lunge: With or without support of a chair, step forward with one leg, and bend until your knee is 90 degrees, then return back to standing. Always keep your knee and foot aligned. Do not let your knee go forward.

Hamstrings:

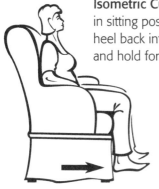

Isometric Curls: On a couch in sitting position, pull your heel back into the couch and hold for 20 seconds.

Regular Curls: Lying prone lift your heel up towards your buttocks. This can be done at home, or on a machine with weight.

Leg Press, Squat, and Lunge: These are described on page 152 and also work the hamstrings.

Hip Extensors (Gluteals):

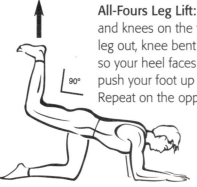

All-Fours Leg Lift: With elbows and knees on the floor, extend one leg out, knee bent to 90 degrees so your heel faces the ceiling, and push your foot up to the ceiling. Repeat on the opposite side.

Dog Lift: On all fours 'cock' your bent leg out to the side.

Prone Leg Lift: Lying prone, lift one leg off the floor while keeping it straight, and hold for 10–15 seconds.

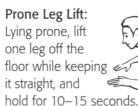

Leg Press, Squat, and Lunge: These are described on page 152.

Upper Back Strengthening:

Seated Row: With your back straight, and elbows bent to 90 degrees, pull the grip bar towards your body, bringing your elbows past your back. Concentrate on trying to get your shoulder blades to touch.

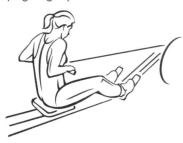

Trapezius Pulldown: On a trapezius pull-down machine at the gym, place your hands slightly further than shoulder width apart on the grip bar, and pull down while keeping the back straight. Pull the bar down in front of your face rather than behind your neck and do not lock out your elbows on the return motion. You can add weight to the machine as you improve.

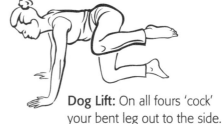

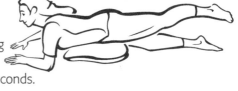

Cardiovascular Fitness Exercises

There are a number of types of cardiovascular exercise all with their own advantages: walking, cycling, swimming, elliptical training, and jogging or running.

Types of Cardiovascular Exercises

Walking
The most simple and easiest to perform, brisk walking requires no equipment besides a good pair of cushioned shoes and appropriate clothing. Duration is increased first by walking for longer periods. Intensity is increased by walking faster and going up hill.

Cycling
The easiest form of cycling is on a stationary bicycle. A reclining bike may be more comfortable but a standard cycle is tolerated well by those with spinal stenosis. Increase duration first and then intensity.

Swimming
Swimming is excellent for exercise without impact. It can be combined with water aerobics, for example, to provide a strengthening component. Back-stroke with or without arms is most comfortable. Using a float and kicking the legs is another alternative. Those with pain on extension may find front-strokes difficult to start with.

Elliptical Trainer
This machine offers a good, non-impact exercise which may include arm movement. Intensity is increased by adding resistance and incline.

Jogging and Running
Jogging and running are probably the most intense aerobic exercises, though running is not tolerated by everyone. It requires good strength, coordination, and body mechanics to feel comfortable and reduce injury risk. Treadmill running provides less stress and impact along with an even surface. Road running is not recommended.

Cardiovascular Exercise Programs

The programs presented here are very basic. To advance your fitness further and with more variety, an experienced and knowledgeable kinesiologist or personal trainer is recommended.

Beginner Program

Never exercise before or during recovery from acute back pain episode. Exercises can be interchanged but try to vary the type of exercise from day to day. Strength training can be carried out Tuesday and Thursday. Take at least one day off per week.

Week 1
Monday	5 minutes brisk walking
Wednesday	10 minutes cycling
Saturday	5 minutes brisk walking

Week 2
Monday	7 minutes brisk walking
Wednesday	12 minutes cycling
Saturday	7 minutes brisk walking

Week 3
Monday	10 minutes brisk walking
Wednesday	15 minutes cycling
Saturday	10 minutes brisk walking

Week 4
Monday	15 minutes brisk walking
Wednesday	15 minutes cycling
Saturday	15 minutes brisk walking

Week 5
Monday	17 minutes brisk walking
Wednesday	20 minutes cycling
Saturday	17 minutes brisk walking

Week 6
Monday	20 minutes brisk walking
Wednesday	25 minutes cycling
Saturday	20 minutes brisk walking

Intermediate Program

This program is recommended for individuals who have exercised in the past 6 months on a regular basis. Exercises can be interchanged but try to vary the type of exercise from day to day. Strength training can be carried out Tuesday and Thursday. Take at least one day off per week.

Week 1
Monday	5 minutes brisk walking
Wednesday	10 minutes cycling
Saturday	5 minutes brisk walking

Week 2
Monday	10 minutes brisk walking
Wednesday	15 minutes cycling
Saturday	10 minutes brisk walking

Week 3
Monday	15 minutes brisk walking
Wednesday	20 minutes cycling
Saturday	15 minutes brisk walking

Week 4
Monday	20 minutes brisk walking
Wednesday	30 minutes cycling
Saturday	20 minutes brisk walking

Week 5
Monday	25 minutes brisk walking
Wednesday	30 minutes cycling
Saturday	25 minutes brisk walking

Week 6
Monday	30 minutes brisk walking
Wednesday	40 minutes cycling
Saturday	30 minutes brisk walking

Sexual Intercourse

Like most aspects of a relationship, communication is the key to concerns about sexual intercourse and back care. It is important to discuss with your partner what positions increase pain and which ones do not. You may also want to talk about what increases arousal more quickly, so the time spent moving around trying to get aroused is reduced, thereby decreasing the risk of aggravating the back pain.

✔ BACK FACTS

Most people shy away from sexual intercourse when enduring back pain. More often than not, this is due to the partner's fear of increasing or creating pain in the sufferer. However, regardless of who has the back pain, no one needs to avoid sexual intercourse. In fact, in many cases it can actually bring you closer together during a difficult period.

Although there are several positions that are less painful than others, there is great individuality, so trial and error are important. Keep changing styles or positions until you find the one that is most comfortable for you. Sex does not have to involve intercourse. Everything from hugging and caressing to mutual masturbation can be incorporated with tremendous success; all you have to do is try it! Consider your back pain an opportunity to explore different aspects of your sexual relationship and make it stronger.

Comfortable Positions

As a guide, the position that seems to aggravate back pain the least is with both partners lying on their sides. This allows the spinal muscles and joints to remains relaxed, without having to contract and hold the abdominal area in a specific position. If you bend the knees slightly, the pressure on the spine is decreased further. This can be performed face-to-face, or in the 'spoon' position, face-to-back.

Another position that is useful in back pain is to have the symptomatic partner lying flat on their back. If this is the female, she can bend the hips and knees so the soles of the feet are flat on the bed. Alternatively, the soles of the feet can be placed on the shoulders of your partner.

If the male has back pain, place a small pillow under the knees while keeping the legs out straight or flex the hips and knees, allowing the woman to sit with her back resting against the man's thighs. Both alterations in position will decrease the stress upon the spine and help to alleviate pain.

If the female is the one with back pain, positioning on your hands and knees with rear entry from the male allows the female to extend or flex the spine gently by tilting the pelvis, hunching or slouching the back into the most comfortable position. You also have the hands and knees for support, decreasing the demand on the lower back and abdominal muscles for strength and support. A pillow or cushion under the abdomen or hips can also give added support. A variation is to bend forward over a table with the feet on the ground — again a cushion or pillow under the arms or chest can help achieve a comfortable height.

Both men and women can also try lumbar supports (small pillows under the lower back) while lying on the bed, or bending forward from the hip when on top. Both these positions will help relax the spine and alleviate back pain.

Being sufficiently aroused is important. Adding lubrication makes movement smoother and requires less effort, thereby reducing strain on the back and causing less internal muscle tension.

Benefits

The benefits of sex go beyond the obvious pleasure and closeness it brings to a relationship. Arousal and orgasm lead to a release of endorphins, the body's natural pain-killers, which will temporarily help your back. In addition, the relaxation following orgasm can help reduce muscle spasm and assist sleep. Sex is a great stress-reliever, and given the close connection between chronic back pain and stress, this can only be of benefit.

The importance of a good relationship should not be underestimated in the patient with low back pain. A caring partner can provide daily support, encouragement, and constancy when, at times, it may seem everything else is going badly. Using your time with low back pain to nurture and develop that relationship is perhaps one of the positive aspects of the condition. However, it requires communication and effort, constituents lacking in many partnerships. The sexual relationship is only one part of this. Breaking through barriers in communication in this area will only lead the way to further progress.

Weight Management for Back Care

There is sufficient evidence that being overweight increases the incidence of low back pain to recommend a weight management program as part of an overall plan to prevent low back pain recurrence. A weight loss and weight management program should be implemented as part of a comprehensive rehabilitation and conditioning program, not only to contribute to the alleviation of back pain but also to increase general well-being.

Ideal Weight

There is much discussion as to what constitutes ideal body weight and how to calculate it. Unfortunately, as we all have different body types and different lifestyles, there is not an easy answer to this problem. The best-known technique to calculate the 'ideal body weight' is called BMI or Body-Mass Index. However, a better measure is a calculation of Body-Fat Percentage

✔ BACK FACTS

Medical research studies have shown that weight is a risk factor for chronic or recurrent back pain, that being overweight influences the progression of back pain from acute to chronic stages, and that increased body mass index (BMI) contributes to musculoskeletal pain, including low back pain and reduced mobility regardless of age. The value of weight loss in the treatment of both acute and chronic back pain, degenerative disc disease, arthritis, and many other conditions has also been demonstrated.

Body-Mass Index

The BMI scale was designed for a person of average height and build between the ages of 20 and 65 years old, doing an average amount of activity. It was formulated to give people a general idea about how their weight and size puts them at a relative risk for certain weight-related diseases like diabetes and heart diseases.

This is a ratio of height versus weight. However, it does

not take into account factors such as muscle mass, bone density and structure, or tissue hydration. In addition, it is not applicable to infants, teens, those over 65, body-builders, pregnant or breast-feeding women, or endurance athletes.

Body-Mass Index Calculation

For the average woman, the 'ideal' BMI is above 19.1 and below 25.8. For the average man, above 20.7 and below 26.4.

To calculate your BMI, you take your weight in pounds and divide this by the square of your height in inches. (To change your measurements from pounds to kilograms, take the number of pounds and divide it by 2.2. To change your height from inches to meters, take the number in inches and multiply that by 0.0254). For instance if a man was 5'10" or 70" tall and weighed 165 pounds, the calculation would be as follows:

Imperial Measure

$165 \text{ lbs} / (77 \text{ inches})^2 = 23.9$

Metric Measure

$165/2.2 = 75$ kilograms

$5'10" = 70$ inches $= (70 \times 0.0254) = 1.77$ meters

$75 / (1.77)^2 = 23.9$

Thus for this individual the BMI would be 23.9

Body-Mass Index Chart

You can also calculate your Body-Mass Index (BMI) using this chart.

BMI	19	20	21	22	23	24	25	26	27	28	29	30	35	40
Height (in.)							Weight (lb.)							
58	91	96	100	105	110	115	119	124	129	134	138	143	167	191
59	94	99	104	109	114	119	124	128	133	138	143	148	173	198
60	97	102	107	112	118	123	128	133	138	143	148	153	179	204
61	100	106	111	116	122	127	132	137	143	148	153	158	185	211
62	104	109	115	120	126	131	136	142	147	153	158	164	191	218
63	107	113	118	124	130	135	141	146	152	158	163	169	197	225
64	110	116	122	128	134	140	145	151	157	163	169	174	204	232
65	114	120	126	132	138	144	150	156	162	168	174	180	210	240
66	118	124	130	136	142	148	155	161	167	173	179	186	216	247
67	121	127	134	140	146	153	159	166	172	178	185	191	223	255
68	125	131	138	144	151	158	164	171	177	184	190	197	230	262
69	128	135	142	149	155	162	169	176	182	189	196	203	236	270
70	132	139	146	153	160	167	174	181	188	195	202	207	243	278
71	136	143	150	157	165	172	179	186	193	200	208	215	250	286
72	140	147	154	162	169	177	184	191	199	206	213	221	258	294
73	144	151	159	166	174	182	189	197	204	212	219	227	265	302
74	148	155	163	171	179	186	194	202	210	218	225	233	272	311
75	152	160	168	176	184	192	200	208	216	224	232	240	279	319
76	156	164	172	180	189	197	205	213	221	230	238	246	287	328

The levels of acceptable body fat differ for men and women. For a female, the normal range is considered to be 15% to 22%, and for a male it is slightly lower at 15% to 18%. There are risks to being outside this range on either side. The risks associated with having too low a percentage of body fat are abnormal menstrual cycles, osteoporosis, skin problems, thyroid problems, and sleep disturbances. The risks associated with being above this range are obesity, diabetes, heart disease, high cholesterol, and back pain.

Body Fat Percentage

A more accurate, though more complicated, way of looking at your weight and health is to calculate body-fat percentage. This measures the amount of fat versus muscle in the body. There are several ways to identify the ideal body fat percentage. The most simple is a body fat percentage scale. This measures the amount of body mass resistance using electrical sensors. It will differentiate the amount of water in both muscle and fat and calculate the percentage fat from this. However, like most fat testing methods, there are inaccuracies. If you are dehydrated, then the incorrect amount of water in the tissues alters the results and makes one appear to have a higher body fat percentage. If a female is close to or on her menstrual period, then the amount of fluid held in the body differs, or if you have eaten a meal high in sodium the night before, the results are again inaccurate.

Other ways to test body fat are by using calipers in what is known as the pinch test. These methods actually pinch the skin either with the hand or a tool to see how large the size of the pinch is and measurements are calculated from there. With this method, however, it is difficult to distinguish between skin and fat, and once again results are not that reliable.

The most reliable way of measuring body fat is in a 'dunk-tank', also called hydrostatic testing under water. This measures the amount of water displaced in a tank when one is immersed in it. This type of testing is not affected by alterations in tissue hydration, bone density, or increased muscle mass as seen in bodybuilding.

Diet Advice

It is important to remember that people can be healthy and not remain in the typical 'ideal' ranges. This may be due to lifestyle difference like athletics or genetics or individual variability and more. It is more important to focus on your overall health, your blood levels, your energy levels, and your ability to perform all your daily functions free of pain. Your health is more about how you feel than a specific number. When looking at changing your diet or losing weight, do it for the right reasons. Eat for your health, not just for weight, eat for energy, not because you are bored, be realistic with your goals, and make changes that you will be able to stick to in order to create healthy lifestyle patterns.

Diet Trends

Many different 'diets' have been developed over time to try to slow down or stop our ever-growing weight problem. Diet trends come and go, but, despite varying degrees of initial success, the calorie-deprivation, low-fat, and high-carbohydrate programs have *not* been shown to be consistently effective over time. Even the latest high-protein diets have some serious shortcomings.

Low Calorie Diets

Calorie-reduced diets flaunt their rapid weight loss, in some cases up to 5 pounds each week. This type of weight loss, however, causes other problems, which make maintenance of the reduced weight very difficult. Excessively rapid weight loss stimulates production of an enzyme known as lipoprotein lipase, forcing our bodies to store even more fat. Ultimately, this slows down our metabolic rate and therefore slows down weight loss. These diets mimic starvation and force the body to hold onto whatever food it is given. As well, the food groups chosen in these diets are imbalanced and disproportionately high in carbohydrates.

Low Fat Diets

The popularity of "low-fat" diets waned with the realization that not only did they dramatically increase hunger, they also reduced HDL ('good cholesterol') levels quite dramatically. Certain studies show that these low fat diets may even *increase* the risk of heart disease by lowering HDL levels too far. Removing 'good' unsaturated fats from our diet is also dangerous for our health, for these fats are integral to the construction of cell membranes and the regulation of hormones, among other essential bodily functions.

High Carbohydrate Diets

A diet high in carbohydrates seemed to be a logical solution to our weight-loss problem. These ingested carbohydrates are low in fat, low in cholesterol, and therefore lower in calories. So it made sense to eat carbohydrates primarily, such as pasta, rice, or potatoes, a regime promoted by *Fit for Life* and the Canada Food Guide, for example. Unfortunately, once the carbohydrates are ingested, this picture almost reverses due to the different hormonal secretion that occurs in response to a high carbohydrate meal.

There is, in fact, an increase in fat production and storage as well as a rise in blood triglyceride and cholesterol levels. These plain and simple carbohydrates become havoc-reeking substrates that damage the body. Sadly, this diet was advocated before any sound clinical data was collected. On paper, these foods looked good, but in reality they have only increased our weight problem, accentuating the process of fat storage that we are now trying to reverse. A high carbohydrate diet has also increased our risk of diet-related diseases.

In a study of the French population, which has far less obesity and cardiovascular disease than the North America population, Dr Michel Montignac first postulated that carbohydrate, rather than fat, is the crucial component in weight gain. Montignac's suggestion that the secretion of insulin could be tightly controlled simply by consuming only those carbohydrates with a low glycemic (sugar) index inspired Dr Morrison Bethea, Head of Cardiac Surgery at Mercy-Baptist Hospital in New-Orleans, to conduct studies on the insulin-cholesterol connection. By following a diet consisting of low glycemic carbohydrates, total cholesterol levels were reduced by 20% to 30% in most individuals. Dr Jennifer Marks at the University of Miami performed another series of studies on insulin resistance. She recognized that insulin resistance was characterized by glucose intolerance, an increase in cholesterol and triglycerides, high blood pressure, and obesity.

High Protein Diets

With the realization that carbohydrates were 'bad' came a revolution in dietary philosophy and the emergence of protein-based programs. Several high protein diets have become popular, such as the 'Carbohydrate Addict's Diet' advocated by Rachael and Richard Heller, Dr Atkins' 'New Diet', and the 'Protein Power Plan' diet developed by Michael and Mary Eades. These programs are biochemically well-grounded. Their shared premise of reducing insulin secretion so that we do not store our food as fat is sound. Nevertheless, they lack many nutrients and are quite deficient in such valuable carbohydrates as fruits and vegetables. In addition they can promote 'ketosis', essentially the body's emergency response to lack of food. Its purpose is survival at the expense of health.

Ketosis Dangers

Ketosis results in symptoms such as nausea, dehydration, light-headedness, and bad breath. Toxic effects to the body include kidney damage. Ketosis may be fatal to diabetics and to the fetus in pregnancy. With respect to weight reduction, ketosis results in weight loss due to dehydration and loss of muscle tissue. Not only is this harmful to the body, but it can ultimately cause weight gain through the conversion of amino acids to fat. Studies have also shown that ketogenic diets alter fat cells to make them hungrier for fat storage.

Naturopathic Diet

In order to achieve healthy and permanent weight loss, it is important not simply to deprive ourselves of fat or calories. What we need is a relatively simple and convenient diet that enables immediate weight loss and long-term weight management without potential damage to our health.

Naturopathic Diet Principles

The 'naturopathic' diet we have developed in our medical practice achieves these goals by training our body to use food as fuel rather than storing it as fat, leading to permanent weight loss and increasing our energy level. This is achieved with simple changes rather than with rigid dietary restrictions, in two stages, the weight loss stage, which adopts many of the clinically proven elements of popular protein diets, and the weight maintenance stage, which restores a truly natural balance to the diet. It is not a 'high-protein' diet but rather a balanced protein program with restrictions on high glycemic carbohydrates.

The Hypoglycemia-Hyperglycemia Connection

The key factor in a clinically sound and effective weight loss program is the control of a substance called insulin. Insulin is a hormone secreted by the pancreas. Its chief role is to keep blood sugar within a certain range. If the blood sugars get too high, insulin is produced to bring them back down. It does this by promoting removal of sugar from the blood and its storage as glycogen or fat. The other main hormone involved in blood sugar control is glucagon. This hormone is responsible for increasing blood sugars when they get too low. Together, insulin and glucagon maintain optimum blood sugar levels and stores for various metabolic demands.

*Hypo*glycemia is a condition in which blood glucose levels are abnormally low. This often occurs in reaction to *hyper*glycemia or high sugar levels, which follow a high carbohydrate meal. After the ingestion of carbohydrates, the breakdown of food into sugar is quite rapid. This sugar is then delivered to the blood and glucose levels rise. The faster the breakdown of food into sugar, the faster the delivery of sugar and the higher the blood sugar levels rise.

Due to the fact that the simple building blocks of carbohydrates are sugars and the bonds between them are weak relative to that of protein, a large amount of glucose is formed and delivered quickly to the blood after a meal rich in carbohydrates. It is here that insulin is called upon to scoop up all this sugar and carry it out of the blood. Glycogen stores are full and it is therefore deposited as fat. A few hours later, most of this meal has been stored as fat and our blood sugar levels are now too low, causing hypoglycemia. Our body senses this and we feel very tired, dizzy, and possibly nauseated. Then our body begins to crave foods that will release sugar into the blood quickly, such as a sweet treat or a starch. It is a rare individual who craves a piece of chicken when they are hypoglycemic! Most of us indulge in carbohydrates, once again raising our blood-sugar levels and starting the whole process anew. If you find that by 10:00 a.m. or 3:00 p.m. you are tired and hungry, take a look at your diet. Your breakfast or lunch was probably high in carbohydrates, creating this problem.

Insulin Resistance

Most North Americans have grown up on a diet that is high in carbohydrates. Cereal or toast for breakfast, a sandwich for lunch, and pasta for dinner. Over the years our insulin-glucagon system has been over-worked to the point of insensitivity. Our hormone responses have become exaggerated in order to achieve the same effect. Approximately three out of four Americans have a slight to serious problem with their blood-sugar level control mechanisms. This is known as insulin resistance, where there is a decreased reaction to insulin output, thereby stimulating extra insulin release. This extra insulin in our blood (hyperinsulinemia) acts as a barrier to using the existing fat in our bodies by blocking access to it.

If we need glucose or energy and cannot access our fat, we must look to alternate sources. Muscle is where our body turns, and slowly we eat away at our lean body tissue mass. Inside the muscle are mitochondria, the fat burning units, which are subsequently lost, thereby decreasing our potential to lose weight. In addition, it is the muscles that are responsible for supporting and protecting our joints.

For these reasons, it becomes clear that through a high carbohydrate diet it is almost impossible to lose weight while remaining in this biochemically undesirable state. Rising blood sugar levels stimulate the release of insulin, which ultimately stores the food we eat as fat. This is the process that has contributed to our society's weight problem; this is the effect we must reverse through our diet.

Naturopathic Diet Principles

The 'naturopathic' diet is not a change in eating habits that we make temporarily until we lose weight and then return to the bad eating habits we had before. Any diet change that is not a lifestyle change only results in temporary weight loss. There is no need to restrict ourselves completely from all the foods we love, though. By making a few additions to our diet (instead of restrictions), we will be able to eat almost anything we wish after we have lost the weight. We can return to a large variety of different foods without any fear of regaining the weight.

If we had maintained a balanced diet from childhood, we would not be trapped in the current nutritional crisis. Our bodies would not have developed insulin resistance and its attendant problems. Our goal is to retrain our bodies to a biochemical state similar to that of childhood. Once this is achieved, we can again enjoy a variety of different foods without gaining weight. To sustain this renewed metabolism and not undo or reverse the changes, balanced meals are still recommended.

Stage One: Weight Loss

The naturopathic diet progresses in two main stages. The first stage is the weight loss stage, lasting about 8 weeks. The diet here is protein-balanced and slightly carbohydrate restricted, especially complex carbohydrates. The second stage is the maintenance stage. Part of the maintenance diet is the addition of protein at each meal, but here the dietary choices expand, allowing us freedom to enjoy many different types of food. Weight loss ends but no weight is gained. If we return to a diet of high carbohydrates and low protein, though, we will undo all the metabolic changes that were brought about by the naturopathic diet.

For the first 8 weeks of this diet, we need to eat 15 to 25 grams of protein per meal. This size is approximately equivalent to ¾ the size of a hand. We may exceed this amount slightly but not go under it. We require this much protein to instruct the body not to secrete insulin at a high rate.

Good Protein Sources

Common protein sources are listed here. There must be one protein source from the list below at every single meal. Although there are other foods that contain protein, such as lentils or yogurt, they are not high enough in protein to be considered a protein source. Legumes, such as lentils and chickpeas, must be considered a carbohydrate because they are approximately 70% carbohydrate and 30% protein, so try to limit their use. Drink as much water as possible because the protein forces your body to pass more urine.

Restricted Carbohydrates

High-sugar carbohydrates need to be cut, including all breads or bread type products, such as bagels and muffins, all pasta, rice, bananas, potatoes, squash, corn, popcorn, yogurt, alcohol, and candy. This includes bread made with a grain flour other than wheat or rye, such as spelt and kamut flour, though a soy flour called 'Dr Atkins Bake Mix' can be used as a substitute. This flour has no carbohydrate and is high in protein and makes very nice pancakes and muffins.

Common Protein Sources

- Fish
- Chicken/Turkey
- Red Meat
- Tofu (extra firm, low fat)
- Eggs (3 egg whites to 1 yolk)
- Protein Powders (use a whey protein powder, as it will also stimulate the immune system, with at least 15 grams of protein and only 3 or 4 grams of carbohydrate)
- Protein Bars (use bars that are high in protein but low in carbohydrates and fat; two-thirds of a bar is all that is needed for the protein portion of a meal and the rest may be snacked on later)
- Low-fat Cottage or Ricotta Cheese (approximately ½ cup)

Limited Foods

Fruits need to be limited to a maximum of two pieces of fruit a day. Fruit is high in sugar and will force the body to secrete higher levels of insulin as well. It is important to note that one juice is equal to one piece of fruit.

All dressings, mayonnaise, butter, nuts, and cheeses are allowed but try not to use more than needed; for example, one slice of cheese and five nuts every other day. Do not replace the carbohydrates with fat.

You may have unlimited vegetables and salad including carrots, beets, and peas, but those that are high in carbohydrate, such as potatoes and squash, remain restricted.

Naturopathic Diet Stage One Summary

This stage lasts about 8 weeks.
1. Protein per meal 15–25 grams.
2. Unlimited salads and most other vegetables.
3. Two pieces of fruit per day maximum, no bananas.
4. No grains, rice, pasta, or starches.
5. Very limited high carbohydrate, low protein foods such as chickpeas and lentils.
6. Limited portions of dressings and condiments.
7. No alcohol.
8. Increased fluid levels by drinking more water.

Stage Two: Weight Maintenance

The maintenance stage of the naturopathic diet is a true lifestyle pattern that we can easily maintain for the rest of our life. Throughout this second stage, our energy levels will remain high, our weight stable. We can enjoy every food group and continue to protect ourselves against many food related diseases at the same time. These benefits will last forever as long as we balance our protein and newly introduced carbohydrates at each meal. The maintenance stage is thus not so much a stage as it is a permanent change.

Reintroduce Carbohydrates

During stage two we begin to reintroduce the some of the carbohydrates that were eliminated or markedly reduced in stage one. Now that our body has consolidated the protein/low glucose message, it is possible to add in carbohydrates at a higher concentration, along with the protein, without increasing insulin release. Blood sugar levels will not rise rapidly as they did before, the reason being that the protein we are combining with the carbohydrates will slow the delivery of the sugar into the blood. This in itself will reduce the amount of insulin released. In addition, the reversal of insulin resistance and hyperinsulinemia achieved by stage one will further reduce the insulin response. Overall, less insulin will be secreted than before we started the diet. This will inhibit weight gain. Slightly more insulin will be released during stage two than during stage one, and this will prevent further weight loss.

When we reintroduce the carbohydrates, we will stop losing weight. We will not regain the weight we have lost, but the stage one weight loss process will stop. We may never ingest carbohydrates at the rate we did before or we may wish to incorporate them at every meal. The choice is ours.

The order in which we reintroduce the carbohydrates is very important. We must slowly integrate them back into the diet in a particular pattern. The sequence of reintroduction is determined by the glycemic index and type of sugar found in each carbohydrate. Fructose, the sugar found in fruit, is the first to be introduced. Then glucose from whole grains and breads, followed by pasta and rice, then potatoes and squash, and finally candy and alcohol. Following this approach minimizes large jumps in blood sugar levels and allows for easy adaptation of the body to carbohydrates.

The amount of carbohydrate brought back into the diet is also very important. We should reintroduce a small amount of carbohydrate initially, approximately three parts protein to one part carbohydrate at each meal (for example, 21 grams protein with 7 grams carbohydrate). We should remain at this level of carbohydrate intake for four to five days. A typical meal would be half a slice of bread, a piece of chicken, and unlimited salad or vegetable.

Hyperinsulemia Signs

During this time period, we need to watch for signs of hyperinsulemia. Our body will become symptomatic when we ingest too many carbohydrates at once. We will feel tired shortly after the meal as our blood sugar levels drop too low. Several hours later or perhaps the next day we may feel bloated as our kidneys are not releasing enough salt. These signs will let us know that the ratio of carbohydrate to protein was too high and therefore insulin was secreted at a higher rate.

If none of these signs appear following the amount of reintroduced carbohydrate, then we can increase the amount consumed again. This time we might consider a ratio of 2:1 protein to carbohydrate. Again we need to watch for signs and symptoms of hyperinsulinemia. If they do not appear, we a can continue to increase slowly the amount and type of carbohydrate until we have reached a one to one ratio. Should the symptoms of hyperinsulinemia appear earlier, we have discovered our

Stage Two Carbohydrate Reintroduction Order

1. Fruits
2. Whole Grains, Breads, Cereals
3. Pasta
4. Rice
5. Potatoes and Squash
6. Candy and Alcoholic Beverages

limit of carbohydrate intake and must return to the proportion previously used where no symptoms occurred. While a final fixed ratio of protein to carbohydrate cannot be quoted because it differs from individual to individual, as a general rule, a ratio of one part protein to one part carbohydrate, excluding vegetables and salads, is a fairly good balance.

Naturopathic Diet Stage Two Summary

Once dietary balance is achieved, this stage becomes a constant weight management program.

1. Continue 15–25 grams of protein per meal.
2. Continue unlimited salad/vegetable.
3. Reintroduce carbohydrates:
   Type: Follow order in list above.
   Amount: Slowly introduce carbohydrates at a ratio of 3:1 protein to carbohydrate.
   Increase: Slowly increase this ratio to 1:1.
   Adjust: If symptoms of hyperinsulinemia return, reduce carbohydrate to the point where no symptoms occur.

Dietary Balance

This is our state of dietary balance — the ratio of protein to carbohydrate that we can ingest without changing our weight ever. At this balance between protein and carbohydrate, our blood sugar levels will remain steady and subsequently so will our insulin secretion and weight.

In order to maintain your ideal weight, it is important to ensure that the changes you make are permanent lifestyle changes. The addition of protein at each meal is a step that should never be forgotten. Vegetables, salads and fruits are always more nutritious carbohydrates than breads, pastas, and rice. This does not mean, however, that your life needs to be devoid of these other foods. Just remember, your health, your weight, and your back pain are all about maintenance and moderation.

Nutritional Supplements

There are several nutritional supplements that may be added to your dietary regime. These vitamins, minerals, and herbs cannot only help to maintain your weight loss but can improve the overall function of your body. They can aid in the repair of muscles and other tissues in the body, increase the enzyme reactions involved in anti-inflammatory and analgesic pathways, and help prevent further injury. If you are unsure about which supplements to take, or have other pre-existing medical conditions, ensure that you ask your health-care practitioner which supplements are right for you.

Natural Supplements for Back Care

Supplementation is the addition of vitamins, minerals, and herbs to the diet for preventive and therapeutic purposes. This philosophy of supplementation has gained greater acceptance over the past few years as we have become more aware of the deficiencies in our food.

Not only are our 'fast-food' food choices lacking in vitamins and minerals, even our supposedly fresh vegetables and fruit are nutrient depleted. Our farm soils are exhausted, no longer enriched with natural minerals. Supposedly fresh foods have usually spent many days in storage or transport before making it to our plates. Food storage and processing generally destroys over 50% of the vitamin/mineral content in that food, though variations exist between different nutrients within the food. Baking obliterates 100% of vitamin B1, for example, while processing damages 80% of vitamin B2. Given our over-processed, stale, nutrient-scarce diets, it is easy to see why nutrient supplementation has grown in popularity.

✔ BACK FACTS

Natural supplementation is just one weapon in a whole armory designed to help you beat your back pain, but it is also important to recognize that your back may need more aggressive treatment, such as pharmaceutical medicine, injection therapy, or surgery. Reference to our 'Red Flags' and guidelines will help you decide when to seek attention.

The use of natural supplementation in the treatment of low back pain is complex because the pain may arise from so many different conditions. Supplements applicable for arthritic back pain will be different from those for a lumbar strain, for example.

The following discussion will help as a guide, offering some of our recommendations for supplementation. Treatment, however, is individual, and if in doubt, you should consult your medical or naturopathic doctor.

Basic Terms

The term 'natural supplement' includes vitamins, minerals, enzymes and coenzymes, essential fatty acids, amino acids, and herbs.

Minerals

Minerals are essentially any inorganic substance found in the earth. Like vitamins, minerals must be taken in from an outside source and are necessary for proper bodily maintenance and growth. Minerals can be divided into two categories. 'Macrominerals' are those that the body needs in larger doses of milligrams or even grams. This includes such minerals as calcium, magnesium, phosphorus, and potassium. 'Trace' minerals are those that are required in much smaller amounts, in micrograms. This category includes iodine, selenium, and chromium, for example.

Vitamins

Vitamins are defined as any constituents in the diet other than protein, fat, carbohydrate, and inorganic salts that are necessary for normal growth and activity of the body. They must be obtained from external sources, and a deficiency may result in specific diseases, depending on the vitamin.

Enzymes and Coenzymes

Vitamins and minerals are essential components of enzymes and coenzymes. Enzymes are substances that stimulate different biochemical reactions in the body. Coenzymes aid the enzymes in this function. With proper nutritional supplementation, we can support certain enzymatic pathways to perform optimally, thereby speeding up certain reactions. If an enzyme is lacking a vitamin or mineral, it cannot function optimally and the process is slowed or halted. We must therefore ensure adequate nutrient supplementation to accentuate certain bodily functions.

Essential Fatty Acids

Most people try to stay away from fatty foods, and for the most part, this is a wise decision. However, there are some fats that are actually beneficial — indeed, essential to the body. Most people are approximately 70% to 80% deficient in essential fatty acids. The symptoms of a low dietary intake of essential fats are fatigue, dry skin and hair, constipation, depression, bloating, and arthritis.

Amino Acids

Amino acids are the component parts of protein molecules and are therefore needed for tissue repair, enzyme reactions, nerve and muscle function and recovery. Non-essential amino acids can be manufactured by the body, while essential ones need to be part of our diet.

Herbs

Herbal supplementation is the use of botanicals or natural plants as therapeutic agents. Over 70% of prescription drugs are based on plant formulas. It follows that by using the original plant we can achieve a similar result. Botanicals or herbs will often have the same physiologic effect as a drug. They will bind into the same receptors and produce similar outcome. The difference lies in strength. Generally, herbal medicine is much weaker, ranging from 1/100th to 1/1000th the strength of its pharmaceutical equivalent. Thus the natural medications require more time to have an effect. However, the benefit is that their side effects are generally minimal. Once again, by combining both forms of therapy, we can achieve a maximal effect with minimal side effects. This is done by decreasing the dose of pharmaceuticals and enhancing the therapeutic effect with natural supplementation.

Selecting and Combining Supplements

Taking every supplement indicated for a particular condition is never advisable. It is best just to choose a few different natural substances that work in different ways and to then take the most effective dose of each. Many people have the philosophy that more is better, and the greater the intake of supplements the greater the benefit. However, what usually happens is that people sacrifice a sufficient dose of one supplement in order to take several others. Then the dose of each supplement ingested becomes too small to have a proper therapeutic effect. It is also important to avoid the situation whereby the taking of multiple supplements becomes so cumbersome that doses are missed or forgotten. These are all reasons why it is better to choose only a few specific products.

BACK FACTS

Not all supplements will work equally well for everyone. We have found certain natural remedies to be more successful than others. However, if you do not achieve adequate relief, others can be tried from the following catalog of remedies. Just ensure you give them a chance to work, and do not change products too often. Natural supplementation for back pain usually takes 10 to 14 days before any significant effect is noted. It should not be compared to the rapid onset of action of an analgesic or NSAID, for example.

Supplement Quality

Few of the nutritional companies that offer products to consumers have the financial resources and infrastructure to guarantee absolute purity of raw material supply. It is not uncommon to find heavy metals, pesticide residue, and toxic micro-contaminates in products that consumers purchase. Our research has consistently led us to Jamieson Laboratories as one of only a few manufacturers in the world that integrates clinical protocols to guarantee the pharmaceutical purity of their raw material supply. Other suppliers felt to be reliable with respect to product quality include Sisu, Natura Pharm, Quest, Thorne, and Natural Factors. Many of these products are available at regular retail pharmacies, health food stores, and specialty natural supplement outlets. Remember, if the product you are looking for is not available, most pharmacies will special-order it for you.

Supplement Safety

It is important to discuss any new medication or supplement with your medical or naturopathic doctor, particularly if you are taking a number of different therapies. Supplements may be 'natural' but they can have side effects and interactions. Always let your treating doctors know every medication, natural or otherwise, you are taking. This is also vital before invasive tests or surgeries.

Minerals

Calcium

Calcium is the most abundant mineral in the body; in fact, it constitutes up to 2% of our entire body weight. The majority of calcium lies within the bones, but calcium is still essential for many reactions in the body that take place outside of the bone.

Calcium's best-known function is the role it plays in the prevention and treatment of osteoporosis, the thinning of the bones. Osteoporosis in the spine is common, causing fractures that can lead to life-long back pain. The main mineral lost from bone in osteoporosis is calcium, and without calcium, bone loses density and strength. Osteoporosis involves more than just a loss of calcium and affects many other joints. Since 15% to 20% of hip fractures result in fatal complications, the maintenance of bone density becomes very important.

Calcium Facts

In order to maintain strong and supportive muscles around the spine, sufficient calcium stores are required. Otherwise the structural framework of the back and spine weakens, leaving one more susceptible to harm and less likely to repair from injury.

Natural Supplements for Back Care

Type of Back Pain	Calcium Magnesium	Boron Manganese	Glucosamine, Chondroitin MSM, HA	Ginger	Capsicum	Curcumin
Sudden Onset						
Lumbar Strain						
Acute Phase 0–48 hours						
Pain worse with flexion	x			x	x	
Pain worse with extension	x			x	x	
Subacute Phase						
Pain worse with flexion	x		x	x	x	
Pain worse with extension	x		x	x	x	
Prevention	x		x			
Disc Herniation						
Acute Phase	x	x	x	x	x	
Subacute Phase	x	x	x	x	x	
Prevention	x	x	x			
Recurrent						
Acute episode						
Prevention	x	x	x			
Persistent						
Degenerative Disc Disease		x	x			x
Arthritis			x	x	x	x
Spinal Stenosis + Instability		x	x			

Calcium is also directly involved in muscle control and repair. Calcium works in tandem with magnesium to improve contractility and therefore muscle strength. It is necessary for proper nerve conduction to the muscle and the firing of the muscle fibers themselves. Without calcium, muscles may begin to fire or contract on their own. Alternatively, without sufficient calcium, muscles may not contract at all.

Safety: Calcium is generally a very safe mineral. When taken in very high doses for a long period of time (2 to 3 grams), there is a risk of developing kidney stones and calcium deposits in the muscle or soft tissues. As the parathyroid controls the movement and use of calcium in the body, individuals with a parathyroid disorder should consult their healthcare practitioner before supplementing with calcium. The absorption of calcium is decreased by caffeine, soda pop or other carbonated drinks, stress, high levels of protein and sugar, and increased exercise.

Back Care Use
- Involved in the control of muscle contraction and reduction of muscle spasm.
- Involved in muscle function, repair, and growth.
- Helps control proper muscle tone.
- Prevention and treatment of osteoporosis.

Dose
1000–1500 mg per day

This chart provides a convenient guide to the natural supplements most effective for treating specific back conditions. After reading further, you may find this chart convenient for planning a natural supplement program, ideally in consultation with your medical or naturopathic doctor.

Willow	Bromelain	Vitamin A, C, E & Selenium	Vitamin B Group	Essential Fatty Acids	California Poppy	Lavender, Hops, Valerian	Arnica
X					X	X	X
X					X	X	X
						X	X
						X	X
X	X	X			X	X	X
	X	X	X	X		X	X
		X		X			
					X	X	X
	X	X	X	X	X	X	
	X		X	X		X	
			X	X	X	X	

Common signs of magnesium deficiency are extreme fatigue, muscle cramping, mental confusion, irritability, and weakness.

Back Care Use

• Co-factor in many enzyme reactions in the body.

• Helps control muscle contraction in both skeletal muscle and smooth muscle like the heart.

• Involved in the production of energy or ATP in the body.

• Useful in chronic pain.

Dose

Supplementation of magnesium is often based on weight. On average, a safe and effective dose of magnesium is 5–10 mg of magnesium per kilogram (2.2 pounds) of body weight. In a very active individual, exercising regularly and utilizing magnesium stores for muscle contraction and repair, a higher dose (10 mg per kg of body weight) is recommended.

It is recommended that a combined magnesium-calcium supplement be used as the two minerals complement each other with regards to function. For calcium, the recommended dose is 1000–1500 mg per day.

Magnesium

Magnesium is the second most abundant mineral in the body. Approximately 60% of it resides in the bone, 26% in the muscle, and the remaining is distributed in the soft tissues and fluids of the body.

Low levels of magnesium in the body are associated with several diseases, including muscle cramping, high blood pressure, heart disease, kidney stones, and fatigue.

Magnesium functions in over 300 different enzyme reactions in the body. These reactions are involved in the production of energy, muscle contraction, regulation of electrolytes, and many more.

Magnesium is partly responsible for any reaction in the body requiring energy. Magnesium is used to produce ATP, the body's stored energy source. ATP is required to fuel or energize almost every reaction in the body, from muscle contraction to hormone production. Without sufficient magnesium, the use of ATP decreases greatly. A lowered ATP production can be seen in such symptoms such as chronic muscle spasticity to increased headaches, fatigue, and stress.

Anyone who has chronic back pain knows how tiring it can be. A deficiency in magnesium not only accentuates this through decreased ATP required to make the enzymes and hormones to heal the muscles and joints involved, but also to keep the overall energy level of the individual high. A low level of energy can result from chronic pain, adding to symptoms of depression. Supplementation of magnesium can help to avoid this side effect.

Magnesium is also used to help control muscle contraction. It works in conjunction with calcium to reduce spasticity and promote repair. While calcium is used to influence muscle contraction, magnesium is used in its release. Thus, if one is low in calcium, there is a tendency towards contraction rather than relaxation within the muscle. This occurs within any muscle, whether it is the shoulders and neck,or in the erector spinae muscles that run along the spine, creating further pain and inflammation.

Magnesium plays a large role in cardiac control and regulation. It is often referred to as nature's calcium channel blocker because of its ability to decrease vascular resistance, effectively opening up blood vessels and lowering blood pressure. Those with chronic back pain are often unable to exercise as they should, and this may increase their risk of heart disease. In addition, the heart itself is a muscle. Much like the skeletal muscles spoken of above, a deficiency in magnesium can lead to increased spasm and stress on the heart and ultimately cardiac damage. This includes hypertension, coronary artery spasm, abnormal heart rhythm, and sudden cardiac death. A low magnesium : calcium ratio increases vessel constriction and promotes formation of blood clots.

In athletes, magnesium supplementation reduces exercise-induced stress hormone release, indicating a protective and stress-modifying role for this mineral in acute stress.

Safety: Due to the powerful effects that magnesium can have on the heart and blood vessels, anyone considering magnesium supplementation should check with a healthcare practitioner for the correct dose. This becomes even more important if individuals are on calcium channel blockers or other cardiac medications. Outside of these restrictions, magnesium is considered very safe and well tolerated by most.

Boron

Boron is a trace mineral that has recently received a great deal of attention with respect to bone and joint maintenance. Boron is essential to the structure of plants, but it was not shown to be crucial to humans until the early 1940s. We now know that boron is essential in the metabolism of both calcium and magnesium in the body, minerals which greatly contribute to bone health.

Boron can be found in almost all fruits and vegetables. This mineral is taken up from the soil into the plant. The boron content in the plant is dependant upon the boron concentration in the soil, and in general our soil contains sufficient levels to ensure acceptable levels in produce. It has been shown that the average American ingests 1.7 to 7 mg of boron per day.

Boron does appear to have an analgesic effect in the relief or reduction of pain in arthritis, but further studies should be performed to determine its exact mechanism.

In one study of 20 patients with different types of arthritis, the patients taking boron reported a decrease in pain and took less acetaminophen over the course of the 8-week program. Another study looked at the effects of boron on pain in osteoarthritis. Patients received 6 mg of boron a day: 71% reported a reduction in pain as compared to only 10% for the control group receiving the placebo.

Side Effects: Nausea and vomiting have been seen at doses higher than 500 mg per day. Boron has also been associated with increased estrogen levels. It is also possible that it may increase testosterone, but this is still under scrutiny. Once again, the mechanism by which boron may increase these hormones is not completely understood. If you are in a high-risk category for any hormonally related cancer, it is best not to use boron in supplement form.

Boron Facts

A diet rich in fruits and vegetables should be enough to ensure adequate boron levels in the body.

Back Care Use
• Essential in the metabolism and use of both calcium and magnesium.

• Has analgesic, pain killing properties.

Dose
3–9 mg per day in general is good safe dose.

Back Care Use

• Involved in enzyme reactions that control the production of energy or ATP.

• Increases the production of free radical scavengers (SOD) to help reduce oxidative inflammatory damage.

Dose

For sprains, strains or other collagenous inflammatory conditions, it is important to start with a higher dose to help reduce the inflammation and break the inflammatory cycle. For 10 to 14 days, 50–150 mg a day with or without food can be taken. Following this, reduce the dose to 20 mg to prevent toxicity build up.

Manganese

For a long time, manganese was not considered an essential nutrient. This changed in the early 1930s when pregnant women deficient in manganese showed poor fetal growth and impaired repair of their own tissues. The symptoms of low manganese include impaired growth and repair, skeletal abnormalities, and weight gain. Offspring born to mothers who consumed diets low in manganese while pregnant displayed several different movement disorders upon birth, such as ataxia (lack of balance and coordination).

Manganese functions in various enzyme reactions, particularly those involved in energy metabolism and anti-oxidative reactions. By improving these reactions, more energy is available for repair, and the damage done to degenerate tissues by free radicals is reduced.

Manganese is used frequently for sprains, strains, and other inflammatory problems because of its ability to reduce the oxidative reaction in these tissues by increasing the production and activity of superoxide dismutase, one of the body's main free radical scavengers. It is often administered via injections in Europe to control pain and inflammation associated with various arthritides and joint inflammatory conditions.

Safety: The only known toxicity of manganese is a result of increased environmental exposure during mining, or in severely polluted areas. The result is a syndrome named "manganese madness" that is characterized by hallucinations, violent outbursts, and increased irritability. This has not been reported with dietary manganese or supplements containing manganese.

Supplements

Glucosamine Sulfate (GS)

Glucosamine sulfate is one of the primary building materials of cartilage and a vital component of the synovial fluid that lubricates a joint. Glucosamine sulfate is naturally produced by the body, but may also be taken in supplement form with a maximal absorption reaching approximately 90%. It has been used since the 1800s when it was isolated from chitin, a component in the exoskeleton of crustaceans, insects, and spiders.

Structurally, glucosamine is a molecule composed of glucose and an amine. The body uses this compound to make hyaluronic acid (HA) and proteoglycan (protein-glucose) substances known as glycosaminoglycans or GAGs. HA forms an essential part of the back disc nucleus pulposus as well as the matrix 'glue' that binds articular joint cartilage together, attracting water and giving it structural properties to withstand the forces of joint impact and motion. It is also a critical component of the lubricating joint fluid within the facets.

HA winds like a snake between the collagen fibers that give the cartilage its strength. Other molecules called proteoglycans branch off from the side to increase its volume and ability to hold water. Chondroitin sulphate is an important component of these branches. HA and the proteoglycans not only hold water, they attract the minerals, vitamins, and other nutrients that maintain the integrity of cartilage.

Glucosamine sulfate reduces pain and inflammation of the cartilage in the facet joints of the spine. Proteoglycans are also vital constituent of the intervertebral discs, specifically the nucleus pulposus, their size and quality decreasing as we age. This degeneration has a number of deleterious effects on the biomechanical properties of the disc leading to pain-producing problems discussed in previous chapters.

As we age, we lose the ability to synthesize sufficient levels of HA, and the HA that is manufactured is smaller in size and subsequently less structurally effective. This results in a loss of strength, resilience, flexibility, and shock absorption. Glucosamine has been shown to slow this disease process down. For this reason, it is known as a chondroprotective agent.

Further, the tendons and ligaments that support each vetebral joint consist of cartilage or collagen. When these become inflamed or weakened following a sprain or strain, supplementation with glucosamine sulfate is extremely beneficial.

A review of 16 randomized, controlled clinical trials from the literature found evidence to support the effectiveness and safety of glucosamine sulfate in all 16. In 13 trials where glucosamine was compared to a placebo, it was more effective in 12. In 2 trials, it was more effective than an NSAID (anti-inflammatory medicine), and in 2 was equally effective.

Safety: There has been no toxicity level of glucosamine sulfate reported to date. It is a very safe supplement with minimal side effects. The only reported side effects have been slight gastric irritation and diarrhea. These can usually be avoided by taking the glucosamine sulfate with a small amount of food. As glucosamine sulfate is derived from shellfish, anyone with an allergy to this should avoid this product.

Glucosamine Sulphate Facts

Glucosamine sulfate is the most widely researched natural therapeutic supplement used in the treatment of osteoarthritis and inflammatory pain.

Back Care Use

• Used to decrease inflammation, slow degeneration, and repair damaged tendons and ligaments, ultimately offering relief of pain while healing injury.

• One of the main ingredients that goes in to the synthesis of hyaluronic acid, a major building block of cartilage.

Dose

1500 mg per day, in 3 doses of 500 mg. Larger doses may be taken at once, but the risk of adverse side effects increases as the dose increases. To help prevent any adverse side effects, the glucosamine sulfate may be taken with food. However, when any substance is taken with a meal, the absorption decreases slightly. Pain relief usually begins anywhere from 2–4 weeks and reaches its maximal effect around 8–10 weeks.

However, there are many glucosamine sulfate supplements that are no longer derived from shellfish.

It has been suggested that glucosamine sulfate may induce insulin resistance and promote the development of diabetes and obesity when used long term. This theory was based on studies in which intravenous glucosamine was given to rats. The effect does not appear to apply to humans taking oral supplementation. Two long-term studies in humans using oral glucosamine have demonstrated blood sugar levels to remain normal or slightly lower than those of control subjects taking a placebo.

Chondroitin Sulfate

Chondroitin sulfate is another component of the intevetebral disc having a higher concentration in the nucleus pulposus than anywhere else in the body. It is a vital part of the matrix 'glue' that maintains the integrity of joint cartilage. Chondroitin sulfate is a glycosaminoglycan (GAG), composed of two different molecules. The first component is a substance called galactosamine, which is chemically similar to glucosamine sulfate, yet structurally differently. The second component is glucaronic acid.

In Europe, chondroitin sulfate is used as an injection directly into the joint. This procedure has been successful in the reduction of inflammation and pain. In North America, however, there are no such preparations available, so oral supplementation is used.

Unlike glucosamine sulfate, where the absorption is excellent, ranging from 90% to 95%, the absorption of chondroitin sulfate is limited, between 8% and 13%. Chondroitin sulfate molecules are simply too large to pass through the normal gastro-intestinal wall. The size of chondroitin sulfate can be up to 300 times that of glucosamine sulfate. If by chance a smaller molecule of chondroitin sulfate did pass through, it would still be too large to be delivered to the chondrocytes (cartilage cells).

Chondroitin sulfate appears to have the ability to reduce pain and inflammation in joints, as well as provide chondroprotective action. Chondroitin sulfate has been shown not only to stimulate cartilage repair mechanisms by offering partial building materials to the cartilage, but also to inhibit the enzymes that break down the cartilage.

Like glucosamine sulfate, the majority of the studies demonstrating the relief and repair of degenerative cartilage pain are on arthritic joints. However, as chondroitin sulfate plays such an important structural role in the disc, in addition to facet joint surfaces, it may be useful in low back pain, particularly degenerative types.

Chondroitin Sulphate Facts

Clinical studies demonstrate clinical benefit, with reduction of symptoms, following administration of oral chondroitin sulfate.

Back Care Use

- Inhibits the enzymes that break down cartilage in arthritis.
- Helps prevent further deterioration of cartilage.
- Offers structural building material with which to synthesize more cartilage.

Dose

400–500 mg, 2–3 times per day.

In a major double-blind, placebo-controlled study, 85 patients with osteoarthritis in the knee consumed 400 mg of chondroitin sulfate twice a day, or a placebo. Pain on motion was the main symptom that was examined, but the physician's overall impression was also considered. A more objective symptom was calculated, too — the time required for each patient to walk 22 yards was reported. After only one month of treatment, there was a 23% reduction in pain reported by those patients taking the chondroitin sulfate as compared to only a 12% reduction in the placebo patients. At the end of the 6 months, 43% of the chondroitin sulfate patients reported significant improvement in pain, and only 3% of the placebo patients declared a similar reduction. Similarly, a small change was noted in the speed of walking between the two groups, whereby the patients taking chondroitin sulfate walked slightly faster and with more ease. The physicians overall impression was that chondroitin sulfate did appear to have a beneficial affect on osteoarthritic joints.

There has also been radiological evidence for the benefits of chondroitin sulfate. Other studies have shown an increase in hyaluronic acid following oral administration of chondroitin sulfate. A double-blind, placebo-controlled study reported in the *Journal of the American Medical Association* showed that patients taking supplementation of glucosamine and chondroitin sulfate had more beneficial effects for up to 3 years without any adverse side effects than glucosamine alone.

Safety: No adverse reactions have been reported with chondroitin sulfate. As with any supplement, food, or medication, the possibility of allergic reactions exists. If this occurs, stop taking it immediately and consult a physician. If any gastric irritation occurs, try taking smaller doses more frequently and with food.

Methylsulfonylmethane (MSM)

Methylsulfonylmethane (or MSM, as it is more commonly called) is a naturally-occurring sulfur-containing compound used in the treatment of inflammation and degradation of cartilage. MSM contains approximately 34% elemental sulfur. MSM is a derivative of DMSO (dimethyl sulfoxide), which is converted to MSM when it enters the body. Only 15% of DMSO is converted into MSM, the active molecule. MSM is found in many foods, such as fruit, alfalfa, corn, tomatoes, tea, and coffee. Interestingly, the richest source of MSM is in mother's milk. MSM is quite volatile and therefore its therapeutic effect is lost when food is cooked, processed, or stored.

MSM Facts

Our MSM intake is generally low because we eat insufficient whole, unprocessed foods where the MSM has not been broken down, making it particularly important to supplement with MSM, especially with back and muscle pain.

Back Care Use

- Increases the production of SAM-e and NAC, which help to increase cartilage water content and increase shock absorption.

- Increases the production of glutathione, a major free radical scavenger, thereby decreasing harmful oxidative inflammatory damage.

- Provides sulfur as a building material for cartilage.

Dose

750–1500 mg per day.

Sulfur is needed to form connective tissue in the body and is essential for glycosaminoglycan (GAG) synthesis. It can be used to increase the production of s-adenosylmethione (SAM-e), glutathione, and N-acetyl cysteine. All of these substances individually influence the joint and cartilage structure and function. GAGs are an integral part of articular cartilage structure. Sam-e and N-acetyl cysteine, as seen later on in this section, contribute to the integrity of the cartilage matrix, attracting water and maintaining its shock-absorbing properties. Glutathione is one of the body's main free-radical scavengers, which decrease oxidation and inflammation. The role of oxygen free-radicals in the progression of disc degeneration and arthritis is expanding. Glutathione acts to 'mop-up' these damaging molecules. Sulfur plays a crucial role in the maintenance of cartilage, and its concentration is decreased by about one-third in diseased or damaged tissue.

Clinical studies thus far involving MSM are limited. One small investigation involved 16 patients with degenerative arthritis. Ten of these patients took 2,250 mg of MSM per day and the remaining 6 had a placebo pill. Eight of the 10 patients taking the MSM reported a significant relief in 6 weeks with no adverse side effects.

Side Effects: The only side effect reported with MSM is a garlic odor on the breath.

Hyaluronic Acid (HA)

HA forms an essential part of the matrix 'glue' that binds articular joint cartilage together, attracting water and giving it structural properties to withstand the forces of joint impact and motion. It is also a critical component of the lubricating synovial joint fluid. HA winds like a snake between the collagen fibers that give the cartilage its strength. In cartilaginous inflammatory conditions, HA is found with decreased concentration and the molecules are smaller in size. Injectable HA has been used for some time in both animals and humans and appears to have a beneficial effect in mild to moderate arthritis. Currently, most hyaluronic acid is administered through injection into the joint. It is theorized that an oral hyaluronic acid supplement may also stimulate cartilage to increase its synthesis of this essential molecule.

Side Effects: To date there is no know side effects with oral supplementation of hyaluronic acid.

Herbs

Ginger

There are several different species of ginger, the best known and most thoroughly studied being *Zingiber officinale.* Another well-documented species is *Alpinia galanga,* also known as greater galanga, the Siamese ginger plant. Both plants belong to the Zingiberacea family, which is comprised of well over 1300 different species. The rhizome (the underground stem, or root, as we call it) is the medicinal part of ginger.

Pharmacologically, ginger root contains several hundred active ingredients, but the most important constituent is a group of substances known as the 4-hydroxy-3-methoxyphenyl (HMP) compounds. This group includes the active ingredients gingerol and shogaol, both of which are types of oleoresins.

Ginger has many well-documented therapeutic uses, including anti-inflammatory and cholesterol-lowering properties. Several studies show that ginger is able to inhibit platelet aggregation by altering prostaglandin and thrombaxane synthesis.

Ginger operates in two different ways. First, when a tissue is injured, a group of immune modulators called cytokines are formed by the white blood cells. These cytokines, in particular interleukin-1 (IL-1) and tumor necrosis factor-alpha, give rise to the inflammation and pain. IL-1 and tumor necrosis factor (TNF) can damage the articular cartilage of a joint and inhibit the function of cartilage cells. In addition, tumor necrosis factor and interleukin-1 stimulate production of enzymes that destroy or degrade the articular cartilage. Ginger helps to combat this process is by preventing the white blood cells from liberating the cytokines at high rates. If there is less cytokine production, there will be less cartilage destruction, inflammation, and pain.

Ginger has another mode of anti-inflammatory activity. The balance of prostaglandins and leukotrienes in the body plays a very important role in the control of inflammation. There are various prostaglandins and leukotrienes that inhibit inflammation, while others promote it. Under normal circumstances, the body is able to monitor this balance and keep them in check. However, in inflammatory diseases or conditions, this balance is disturbed, resulting in an increase in the inflammatory prostaglandins, ultimately leading to the increased pain and swelling in the facet joints of the spine as well as the rest of the body. There are two major enzymes that control the production of inflammatory prostaglandins and leukotrienes:

Ginger Facts

For thousands of years, the ginger root has been used in Traditional Chinese Medicine to help decrease pain and inflammation. In recent years, research has demonstrated that the traditional use of ginger as a medication is both scientifically grounded and highly effective.

Back Care Use

- Decreases inflammation by controlling immune modulators such as TNF and ILs that cause inflammation.
- Reduces inflammatory prostaglandin synthesis.
- Reduction in pain comparable to pharmaceutical COX-2 drugs.

Caution

Ginger may interfere with other medicines related to blood clotting. As with any medication, natural or otherwise, let your doctor know you are taking this supplement, and check before starting it if you are on any blood-thinning treatment.

Dose

0.25–1.0 mg, three times per day.

cyclo-oxygenase 2 (COX-2) and 5-lipoxygenase. Ginger has an inhibitory effect on these enzymes, thereby decreasing the production of inflammatory prostaglandins and leukotrienes and subsequently their inflammatory effect on the body.

This is the same mechanism whereby the newest anti-inflammatories work. However, ginger does not appear to cause the frequent gastric irritation that the pharmaceutical anti-inflammatories do.

Clinical studies have demonstrated the effectiveness of ginger in the treatment of pain and inflammation. One randomized, double-blind study of 261 patients showed significant improvement in knee pain for those taking ginger extract as compared to individuals taking a placebo. A cross-over study (in which patients are tested with the ginger and the placebo) by the same group confirmed these results.

Side Effects: Occasional gastric irritation or dyspepsia has been reported in patients taking unencapsulated preparations.

Devil's Claw

Devil's claw (*Harpagophytum procumbens*) is a woody-barked plant indigenous to South Africa. The root has long been used for digestive and rheumatological conditions. Its analgesic and anti-inflammatory properties are often compared to those of phenylbutazone. Devil's claw contains a number of active ingredients, such as iridod glycosides, phenolic acids, and flavinoids. The primary active ingredients, however, are the iridod glycosides, specifically harpagide, harpagoside, and procumbide.

Despite the popularity of this herb and clinical trials depicting its benefits, there still is no known mechanism of action. Many have suggested that it possesses the ability to alter prostaglandin synthesis, specifically that of eicosanoids. Clinical evidence demonstrates that devil's claw may offer individuals a safe and effective form of treatment for back pain. Several studies have shown its effectiveness in controlling pain in the lower back. At the end of one study, over 50% of patients reported benefit with reduced pain, decreased consumption of other pain or inflammatory medication, and increased range of motion. In addition, very few side effects were seen.

Another study involved 43 arthritic patients, each consuming 500 mg of devil's claw three times a day. After only 8 days, symptoms had improved. Patients reported an overall 89% reduction in pain, an 84% improvement in range of motion, and an 86% reduction in time needed for stiffness resolution. Other double-blind, placebo-controlled studies have shown that patients taking devil's claw displayed a

Devil's Claw Facts

In the United Kingdom, 30,000 people were reported to be using devil's claw for arthritic symptoms as long ago as 1976. Today in Europe, the European Scientific Commission of Phytotherapy has declared that this herb might be useful in the treatment of arthritis and tendonitis.

Back Care Use

• Analgesic, pain killing action.

• Anti-inflammatory action.

Dose

500–1000 mg, 3 times per day.

statistically significant reduction in pain as compared to placebo patients.

Side Effects: Despite the fact that devil's claw has been compared to NSAIDs, it does not appear to have the same gastric effects that other NSAIDs do. Occasional loss of appetite and headache have been reported.

Capsicum

Capsicum is one of the most widely used spices in the world, with over 50 different species grown. We commonly see it in red, yellow, and orange peppers as well as paprika, cayenne, and chili peppers. Capsicum gives a 'hot' sensation to food when used as a spice. As an herbal remedy, capsicum has been used in Mexico and Peru since around 7000 BC to increase circulation and aid digestion, but is now used primarily for its analgesic and anti-inflammatory properties.

The active ingredients in capsicum are the capsaicinoids, primarily capsaicin, which has a direct effect on inflammation and pain in the body. It also mediates an inflammatory response by causing blood vessel dilation and the release of histamine from mast cells.

At first, capsicum actually increases the release of substance-P. This can be seen in the burning sensation that is experienced after eating a hot pepper. However, with continued supplementation with capsaicin, substance-P production greatly decreases, reducing the overall pain/inflammation response. It was originally thought that capsaicin only affected those fibers that conduct the pain message from the skin to the central nervous system, but it is now thought that it has a wider effect on all sensory nerves and plays a central role in the spinal cord where substance-P acts as a neurotransmitter for pain stimuli.

Most forms of capsicum are administered through a cream and applied topically over the affected painful area. The skin is supplied with many small nerve branches that then lead back to the main 'trunks' of the nerve. When capsaicin is applied to a nerve branch, substance P is depleted simultaneously in all connecting branches and thus has its effect on the joint.

Several studies have been conducted on the efficacy of capsaicin, primarily in a topical cream form. One such study examined 154 patients with back pain of a non-specific origin for at least 3 months. In this double-blind randomized study, the study group applied a capsicum pain plaster daily, while the control group applied only a regular emollient cream. After only 3 weeks, there was a minimum of 38.5% reduction in back pain from the study group, compared to

Shown to act through a specific receptor on pain fibers (the VR1 receptor), capsicum decreases the production and action of substance-P, a chemical released from nerve fibers in response to pain.

Back Care Use
• Analgesic control by decreasing substance P (substance Pain).
• Anti-inflammatory effects by decreasing histamine.

Caution
Do not use on damaged, inflamed or broken skin.

Dose
Creams generally range from 0.025% up to 0.075% of capsaicin. Due to skin sensitivity with these types of cream, it is wise to start with a lower concentration cream and slowly build up as needed. Remember, after the initial applications, the increase of substance-P will then reverse and that warm-to-burning sensation that may be experienced on the skin will deplete until it is no longer felt.

only 28% in the placebo group. In addition, only the study group showed a significant improvement in mobility and functional status.

Another study was conducted on 70 patients with osteoarthritis: 35 of these patients were instructed to apply 0.025% capsaicin cream a day, while the other 35 patients applied a placebo cream. After 2 weeks, 80% of subjects reported average pain reduction of 33%, significantly higher than the placebo group. In another study, topical capsaicin and glyceryl trinitrate were combined and compared to a placebo in a double-blind, randomized study. Pain scores and analgesic use were both significantly reduced in the treated group.

Side Effects: The main side effect experienced with capsaicin is a redness, irritation, and initial burning of the skin. This generally only lasts for a few minutes after application, and will subside with each following application until it is no longer experienced.

Curcumin

Curcuma longa, otherwise known as turmeric, is a perennial herb that belongs to the ginger family and naturally grows in Southern Asia and throughout the Caribbean. The useful parts of the plant are the rhizomes, or roots, from which volatile oils are extracted. This herb has culinary use as a flavoring agent, especially in curry dishes, but also medicinal use for the treatment of inflammation and pain as well as an aid in the digestive process.

Several different mechanisms have been shown whereby curcumin decreases inflammation in the body. The best documented is through the reduction of prostaglandin and leukotriene synthesis, achieved through the inhibition of, or interference with, the enzymes that control the production of these inflammatory mediators (the 5-lipoxygenases).

Curcumin also acts in a variety of other ways. It has been hypothesized that curcumin inhibits the breakdown and metabolism of cortisone by the liver. This would increase the amount of circulating cortisone in the body and prolong its effect. Curcumin also appears less active in experimental animals without adrenal glands, indicating that the herb may also work by stimulating the release of adrenal corticosteroids. Further studies support a role for curcumin in the sensitization or priming of cortisone receptors. Cortisone is a powerful anti-inflammatory agent, and it might therefore be expected that these actions would increase its activity to reduce inflammation in arthritis.

Another mode of action that curcumin has been shown to possess is the inhibition of tumor necrosis factor (TNF) and interleukin-1 (IL-1). As seen in the section on ginger, tumor necrosis factor not only damages and breaks down the cartilage in the joints, but also increases the production of interleukin-1. Interleukin-1 increases the production and action of the enzymes that degrade cartilage. By decreasing the production of both of these cytokines, inflammation, pain, and joint damage will be reduced.

One study comparing the effects of curcumin to that of phenylbutazone (an NSAID) showed that patients improved equally, independent of which therapeutic supplement they were given. Arthritic patients in this study were given either 400 mg of curcumin three times per day or 300 mg of phenylbutazone per day. Symptoms such as joint swelling, stiffness in the morning, and walking speed were monitored. Patients in both groups displayed equal relief and improvements in symptoms.

Side Effects: Curcumin does not appear to have any adverse side effects. However, it may cause slight gastrointestinal upset with prolonged use. As turmeric has been shown to increase production and flow of bile, those with common bile duct blockage or gallstones should avoid this herb.

Willow

There are several species of willow, all of which belong to the family Salicaeae. The most common members of this family are crack willow or *S. fragilis*, black willow or *S. nigra*, white willow or *S. alba*, and purple osier willow or *S. purpurea*. Crack willow and purple osier willow contain up to 10% and 8% active ingredient, respectively, whereas the white willow contains slightly less than 1%. Despite the fact that the crack willow and the purple osier willow contain the highest concentration of active ingredient, the white and black willows are most commonly used in North America.

The bark of the willow is the part of the plant that is used medicinally. The bark of young branches is particularly rich in medicinal substances, particularly a glycoside known as salicin. However, salicin's anti-inflammatory effect is quite weak, requiring metabolism in the gastro-intestinal tract liver to reach its final form, salicylic acid (ASA or aspirin). This conversion takes time, so willow has a slower onset of action than salicylic acid itself, but the therapeutic effect of salicin appears to last longer than salicylic acid.

Willow Facts

Willow or salix has one of the longest histories of use in medicine, primarily for fever, gout, and inflammation. It has provided the foundation for many of the anti-inflammatory drugs used today.

Back Care Use

• Anti-inflammatory action similar to ASA.

• Reduces fever and muscle pain.

Dose

20–40 mg of salicin, 3 times per day; or 1–2 ml of liquid extract, 3 times per day. This is equivalent to approximately 7–10 grams of dried herb, 3 times per day.

To speed up the onset of action of salicin and to increase its potency, a German chemist in 1835 created acetyl salicylic acid, aspirin, now one of the most regularly used anti-inflammatory, analgesic, and antipyretic (fever-reducing) medicines.

Side Effects: Despite the great success of salicylic acid (Aspirin), it does have adverse side effects. Salicylic acid is very irritating to the lining of the stomach, where it can induce pain, nausea, and ulceration. In addition, salicylic acid decreases the blood's clotting ability by reducing platelet aggregation.

Salicin, however, does not appear to irritate the stomach. Very few people experience digestive upset or nausea with the use of willow alone. Salicin does have a mild effect on platelet aggregation, so its use should be discussed with your doctor. Due to the mild inhibition of platelet aggregation, willow is not recommended in any one with a bleeding disorder, young children, pregnant women, or those with serious kidney diseases. In addition, willow can interact with other drugs, so it should be avoided in those people taking anti-coagulants, methotrexate, phenytoin, probenecid, spironolactone, and valproate.

Bromelain

Bromelain contains enzymes naturally found in pineapple that have proteolytic properties, meaning that they help breakdown proteins into smaller units known as peptides. Other such enzymes include pepsin, trypsin, rennin, and chymotrypsin. Several beneficial results have been achieved by using these proteolytic enzymes as anti-inflammatories in diseases such as laryngitis, bronchitis, and pneumonia, as well as in sports injuries. Today, they are used extensively in the treatment of inflammatory joint disease such as arthritis.

There are several ideas postulated as to the anti-inflammatory mechanism behind bromelain. The most popular postulates that it is mediated through the breakdown of fibrin. During inflammation, fibrin encourages the formation of matrix that walls or blocks off the inflamed area. This then leads to a build up of blood and edema around that area as it cannot be adequately drained. Bromelain promotes the degradation of fibrin, thereby allowing proper blood flow into the area and subsequent removal of inflammatory by-products that further injure the inflamed area.

It has also been shown that bromelain may block the production of the substances that are produced during an inflammatory reaction. These substances are known as

Bromelain Facts

Bromelain is a non-toxic substance that can be used in doses up to 1500 mg a day without fear of adverse effects.

Back Care Use

• Decreases inflammation by inhibiting the formation of fibrin.

• Decreases inflammation by decreasing the production of kinin which increases swelling.

Dose

150–300 mg per day.

kinins. By decreasing kinin production, there will be less swelling and inflammation and therefore less pain within the joint.

Studies have been performed to compare the use of oral enzymes in arthritis with that of traditional anti-inflammatories. One such randomized, single-blind study evaluated 50 patients with osteoarthritis in the knee over a 7-week period. Patients received either 2–3 enzyme tablets three times a day or 50 mg of the NSAID, diclofenac sodium. At the end of the study, a reduction in pain, joint tenderness, and joint swelling was seen in both groups. However, the reduction in pain was greater in those taking the enzymes ($p<0.05$). A slight improvement in range of motion was also observed in the group taking enzyme therapy.

Side Effects: In some individuals, loose stools and mild blood thinning can occur. For this reason, those people already on blood thinners should not take high doses of bromelain.

California Poppy

California poppy (*Eschscholtzia californica*) has traditionally been used as a mild sedative and hypnotic for anxiety, stress, and other psychological disorders. Clinical studies reveal statistically significant anxiolytic actions in mice when placed under stressful laboratory tests. The amount of anxiety reduction was dose dependant and no toxicity level was observed.

This poppy has proven to be one of the most effective natural spasmotics known in botanical medicine. Local Indians have been using this for colic and other cramping and spastic conditions for decades. It is now regularly used for the control of muscle cramping, spasms, and inflammation in all areas of the body. It is of particular use in reducing the pain and inflammation in joints and skeletal muscle, such as back pain, muscle strains and tears. The California Poppy can also be mixed with sedating herbs such as valerian or chamomile to help induce a better sleep.

Safety: The safety of the poppy is extremely high. Unlike the Opium poppy, the California poppy is non-addictive, and can therefore be used for prolonged periods of time. Despite no evidence to the contrary, it is best not to use during pregnancy.

California Poppy Facts

California poppy has several other beneficial effects that are medically significant. The flower has powerful anodyne, analgesic, or pain reducing effects on both skeletal and smooth muscles.

Back Care Use
- Natural anti-spasmotic for muscles.
- Encourages production of relaxing hormones that decrease pain and inflammation.
- Powerful anodyne (pain killer) for both skeletal and smooth muscle.

Dose
1000–1500 mg raw herb or 50–150 mg extract.

Vitamins

Vitamin E

Vitamin E Facts

Vitamin E It is an essential vitamin for fat metabolism and may help with recovery from nerve inflammation such as occurs in sciatica.

Back Care Use

- Helps prevent further degradation of cartilage and promotes repair of cartilage.
- Stimulates the growth of chondrocytes (cartilage cells).

Dose

400 IU per day. It can safely be increased to 800 IU per day (the usual dose for hot flashes). However, as an anti-oxidant, 400 IU is sufficient, particularly if it is combined with vitamin C because they have a synergistic effect.

Vitamin E is a fat-soluble vitamin, whose main function is that of an anti-oxidant. Vitamin E is a constituent of every cell membrane, where it helps to stabilize the structure of the cell and protect it from free radicals. Vitamin E has a variety of other functions, including enhancement of the immune system. Of importance to arthritis is the role it plays in cartilage as it appears to inhibit the breakdown of cartilage and stimulate the growth and production of new cartilage cells (chondrocytes).

Vitamin E is available in different forms, either natural or synthetic. The natural forms are d-alpha-tocopherols and the synthetic versions are the dl-alpha-tocopherols. It has been shown through several studies that the natural version has a greater absorption and biologic activity than the synthetic version.

Side Effects: Because vitamin E is fat soluble, it can build up in the tissues if the dose is too high. This generally does not occur unless individuals are chronically taking more than 1600 IU per day. Vitamin E also has blood-thinning properties. It should not be combined with any other anti-coagulants, such as warfarin (coumadin), heparin, aspirin, or vitamin K. In addition, this vitamin should be stopped 10 to 14 days prior to any surgery. As with all medicines, let your doctor know if you are taking it.

Vitamin C

Vitamin C Facts

Vitamin C does appear to have a potential role in the treatment of back pain and arthritis, primarily in helping to build and repair collagen.

Back Care Use

- Decreases free radical oxidative inflammation and pain.
- Increases collagen repair by stimulating the production of structural proteoglycans.

Vitamin C or ascorbic acid is a water-soluble vitamin. Vitamin C was first isolated in the late 1920s for the treatment of scurvy. New roles for this important vitamin continue to be found. Vitamin C is an important free-radical scavenger in the body. Free radicals are known to mediate some of the damage and inflammation in arthritis. Blood levels of vitamin C are reduced below normal in patients with rheumatoid arthritis and levels within joint fluid are even lower.

Vitamin C increases the binding together of amino acids to help support the structure of the collagen, an important structural component of cartilage. These amino acids are proline and hydroxyproline. Vitamin C has also been shown to increase the production of proteoglycans, also structurally important molecules in cartilage. Several studies have been performed supporting this. One such study evaluated guinea pigs with osteoarthritis. Cartilage erosion was decreased when the pigs were given high doses of vitamin C.

Side Effects: When vitamin C is taken in too high of a dose, loose stools or diarrhea results. Otherwise, there are no adverse reactions with vitamin C.

Vitamin B Complex

The B vitamin complex is a group of structurally similar but not identical compounds. B vitamins are used in many different areas of the body, including nerves, muscles, liver, skin, and brain. They are involved in many co-enzyme reactions (helping an enzyme reaction take place) and thus are crucial to the function of the body. There are several different B vitamins, and although they are often supplemented together and do have similar actions, some of the B vitamins have unique properties. For this reason, we have broken down each B vitamin separately.

Studies out of Japan show that B vitamins supplementation enhanced not only overall nerve health, but also helped repair existing nerve damage and increased the efficacy of nerve signaling throughout the body. In addition, German scientists found that B vitamins were very beneficial in the relief of nerve pain. This effect can be seen as early as 8 weeks following supplementation. Their role in treating chronic pain includes improved energy, reduction of stress, and resistance to depression.

Vitamin B-1 (Thiamin)

Vitamin B-1 or thiamin is a water-soluble vitamin. It is a constituent of an enzyme called thiamin pyrophosphate and is required for oxidative decarboxylation of alpha-keto acids. This aids the body by releasing energy from the carbohydrates more quickly. Thus fewer carbohydrates are needed and consumed and a stable blood sugar level is maintained more easily. What this actually means is that vitamin B-1 helps to breakdown carbohydrates creating energy. It also has a specific role aiding nerve cell function. Thiamin is crucial in helping transmit a particular nerve impulse along a nerve fiber and in repairing nerves. Vitamin B-1 is also important for brain function and memory. B-1 helps to increase the production of neurotransmitters or brain chemical messengers. It has been shown to mimic the important neurotransmitter acetylcholine, thereby increasing the overall function of the brain.

Safety: No toxicity levels have been seen with B1. Magnesium increases the efficacy of B1 by helping to convert thiamin into its more active form. Alcohol, diuretics, and dilantin have been shown to decrease the effect of thiamin on the body.

Vitamin B Complex Facts

The B-group of vitamins provides a number of vital functions in the body with direct impact on the spine, its nerves, and brain function. It is recommended particularly in sciatica and stenosis where nerve injury or inflammation occurs.

Vitamin B-1 Facts

Back Care Use
• Increases nerve impulses along the nerve fibers to help maximize nervous transmission.

• Helps to repair damaged nerve fibers.

Dose
50–100 mg per day.

Vitamin B-2 Facts

Back Care Use

- Helps with the growth and repair of the myelin sheath (insulating coating around the nerve).
- Decreases inflammation by increasing the production of the free radical scavenger glutathione.

Dose

50–100 mg per day.

Vitamin B-3 Facts

Back Care Use

- Helps to regulate the entire nervous system aiding in nerve repair, transmission, and growth.
- Helps to increase the formation of ATP energy from food, supplying more fuel to the body for repair.

Dose

30–80 mg per day.

Vitamin B-2 (Riboflavin)

Vitamin B-2, also known as riboflavin, is also a water-soluble vitamin. Riboflavin is the vitamin that is responsible for the florescent yellow color of your urine upon ingestion of a B complex vitamin or a multivitamin with B vitamins included. Riboflavin is necessary for the growth and repair of the insulating coat around a nerve known as the myelin sheath. Without B-2, this myelin sheath is more prone to injury and inflammation and recovery from insult is impaired.

In addition, B-2 is also required for the production of energy and the burning of fat as it helps to increase mitochondrial output. Mitochondria are the components in muscle that are responsible for breaking down fat and generating both heat and energy, so this vitamin is important in weight regulation. Mitochondrial output also appears to affect migraine development. Clinical studies show significant benefit to migraine sufferers through B-2 supplementation.

Apart from these metabolic benefits, vitamin B-2 is also involved in recycling glutathione, the main free radical scavenger in the body. Free radicals mediate the cell damage caused by ingested and environmental toxins. Glutathione and other molecules mop up these free radicals and protect us from damaging pollutants. Low levels of riboflavin have been associated with certain cancers, especially esophageal cancer.

Safety: No toxicity has been seen with B-2. No interactions have been seen with riboflavin and other vitamins or minerals or pharmaceutical drugs.

Vitamin B-3 (Naicin)

Vitamin B-3 or niacin is used in the maintenance of blood sugar levels, in detoxification, and in the production of energy. It functions as part of two enzymes, NAD (nicotinamide adenine di-nucleotide) and NADP (nicotinaminde adenine di-nucleotide phosphate). These enzymes are part of the glycogen cycle, in which glucose and fatty acids are oxidized into energy. Thus B-3 or niacin is used in the production of energy from our food. As we have seen previously, unstable glucose levels and energy production can alter both the function and health of the nerves.

B-3 has also been shown to help regulate the general enzymatic control of the nervous system, thereby aiding in transmission of particular messages, and in repair of damaged nervous tissue.

Niacin has been used to help lower LDL, the bad cholesterol and other lipoproteins in the blood. Its effects are also quite long lasting, and studies show that niacin actually can provide better overall results as compared to meds such as lovastatin.

Safety: Liver toxicity may be a side effect of too much B-3, but this has been seen only in doses ranging from 2–6 grams per day. The most common side effect is skin flushing or heat rash and nausea. In order to decrease this side effect, a time-released B-vitamin complex is now available. Another version of niacin exists, known as niacinamide, which is a non-flushing version of niacin with no effects on the liver when used in appropriate doses.

Vitamin B-6 (Pyridoxine)

Vitamin B-6 or pyridoxine, like the other B vitamins, is a water-soluble vitamin. This vitamin has been studied extensively and is now considered one of the most important vitamins available. It is utilized in many different bodily processes, including the production of hemoglobin, cellular turnover, and all new protein manufacture. For this reason, B-6 is very important in pregnancy, nervous system function, immune regulation, and skin and mucous membrane turnover. B-6 also been shown to help in the control of diabetes and plays an integral role in the function of the immune system. A deficiency in B-6 results in decreased production of antibodies and immune cells such as lymphocytes.

Vitamin B-6 also greatly helps with stress, anxiety, and depression, which can greatly aggravate any type of back pain. Vitamin B-6 helps to regulate nerve conduction and combats depression, as it is necessary for the production of serotonin, our body's 'happy' hormone. For this reason, vitamin B-6 is known as the anti-stress vitamin or anti-depression vitamin, used extensively in both depression and pre-menstrual syndrome.

B-6 goes into the production of serotonin and GABA, the neurotransmitters involved in preventing depression and stress and promoting relaxation. In addition to the effects directly on the stress receptors, B-6 helps relieve anxiety and depression, particularly in women with high estrogen or on the birth control pill. Estrogen depletes vitamin B-6 in the body. Women who take the birth control pill or hormone replacement therapy have increased circulating levels of estrogen and therefore lower levels of B-6. Studies carried out over a 15-year period across several different countries reveal that increased estrogen leads to increased excretion of B-6 and subsequent depression, decreased libido, decreased glucose tolerance, and anxiety. Administration of only 40 mg per day of vitamin B-6 restores the biochemical values back to normal and relieves the associated psychological symptoms.

Vitamin B-6 Facts

Back Care Use
- Helps to decrease glycosylation of proteins that causes nerve damage.
- Decreases stress and stress related pain by increasing the production of serotonin and GABA.

Dose
50–100 mg per day.

Safety: Vitamin B-6 has been shown to express signs of toxicity when taken in large quantities and over long periods of time. Ironically, toxic symptoms include nerve damage and loss of muscle coordination. This is seen at levels higher than 2 g per day.

Vitamin B-12 (Cyanocobalamin)

Vitamin B-12, also known as cyanocobalamin, functions primarily as a coenzyme. Vital for production of new DNA, it is essential for the growth of all new cells but particularly those involved with the blood, immune, and nervous systems. B-12 is therefore is an integral part of any therapeutic program involving these areas. B-12 is also important for lowering homocysteine levels in the blood. Homocysteine is an independent risk factor in heart disease, and when elevated, greatly increases the risk of stroke.

Deficiency of B-12 can lead to anaemia (*Pernicious anaemia*) and is associated with gastric upset and peripheral nerve dysfunction. Spinal cord involvement results in impaired sensation and movement disorder. B-12 is essential for brain function, acting as a methyl donor to many compounds in the body and is thus involved in neurotransmitter production. This is one of the methods of nerve damage repair, making B-12 essential to health and function of the entire nervous system.

Safety: No toxicity levels have been seen with B-12. B-12 is intimately linked to folic acid such that a deficiency in one will lead to a deficiency in the other. Treatment is usually combined.

Vitamin B-12 Facts

Back Care Use

• Essential for the production of all DNA and cellular growth and repair.

• Donates methyl groups used as a substrate for nerve repair.

Dose

50–100 mcg per day.

Essential Fatty Acids

There are several different types of fatty acid. All fats, whether they are good or bad fats, have a similar basic structure; that is, a molecule of glycerol and three fatty acids. Fatty acids come in a variety of different shapes and sizes, and they perform a multitude of different functions in the body. For instance, fats surround each cell in the body and act as a barrier, protecting the cell from metabolic toxins and allowing hormones and enzymes to bind to it. Fats are also an energy source for the body.

Types of EFAs

The fats that are actually good for us are known as essential fatty acids (EFAs). There are four main types of essential fatty acids: omega-3, omega-6, omega-7, and omega-9. These are unsaturated fats, meaning they have one or more double bonds connecting their chemical structure. It is this double bond property that allows them to interact with other substances in the body.

Omega-3 Essential Fatty Acids

Omega-3 fats are broken down into three different groups. The first are alpha-linoleic acids, found in flax seeds, hemp seeds, canola, soy, walnuts, and dark green leaves. The second group are stearidonic acids, found in blackcurrants. The final group, eicosapentaenoic acids, are found in cold-water fish like salmon, mackerel, sardines, and trout.

Omega-6 Essential Fatty Acids

Omega 6 fats are also broken down into three different groups. The first group is the linoleic acids or LAs, found in safflower, sunflower, hemp, soybean, pumpkin, and sesame. The second group, gamma-linolenic acids or GLAs, are found in borage oils, evening primrose oil, and blackcurrant seed oil. The final group of omega-6 fatty acids are the arachidonic acids found in meats and other animal products.

Omega-7/9 Essential Fatty Acids

Omega-9 fats are also called oleic acids and are widely abundant in olives, almonds, avocados, peanuts, cashews, and macadamia oils. Omega-7 is found in coconut and palm oils. These fatty acids do not play a crucial role in the treatment of inflammation, back pain, and arthritis.

Effects of EFAs

The relative ratio of EFAs fats in the body is crucial in determining which prostaglandins will be produced. Prostaglandins are hormone-like substances that are important in the regulation of many bodily functions, such as blood pressure, pain, inflammation, swelling, allergic reactions, blood clotting, and more. Inflammation is mediated by such chemicals as prostaglandins and leukotrienes. The body also produces 'good' prostaglandins that moderate inflammation and have other important protective functions.

The role of essential fatty acids in the treatment of back pain is to limit the availability of arachidonic acid, the base molecule from which prostaglandins are manufactured. They seem to promote the preferential manufacture of 'good' prostaglandins. While some fats, like those found in animal products, promote the synthesis of inflammatory ('bad') prostaglandins, the omega-3 and 6 fatty acids lead to the production of the more beneficial molecules.

The main goal of essential fatty acid supplementation is to decrease the production of arachidonic acid and increase the production of eicosapentaenoic (EPA) and dihomo-gamma-linoleic acids (DHGLA). These latter two are the final products

Essential Fatty Acids Facts

Essential fatty acids are also of vital importance in the maintenance and integrity of the myelin sheath that covers most nerves. They are therefore recommended in back pain associated with nerve irritation or damage such as sciatica or spinal stenosis.

Back Care Use

• Decrease nerve pain and inflammation by repairing the myelin sheath.

• Decrease inflammation by regulating the production of prostaglandins.

Dose

The dose of essential fatty acids that is of most benefit is approximately 4–5 g per day with food. The ratio in general should be around a 4:1 omega-6 to omega-3 fatty acids.

of omega-3 fatty acids and omega-6 fatty acids, respectively. Several studies have been performed using essential fat supplementation and measuring the relative levels of EPA and DHGLA. For example, when a diet rich in omega-6 fatty acids was followed (1.5 tablespoons/day of flax oil), the levels of EPA rose significantly in the participating individuals.

Omega-3 to Omega-6 Ratio

The important issue then becomes achieving the correct balance of different fats in the body in order to decrease inflammation. The most favorable ratio of omega-6 to omega-3 essential fatty acids is approximately 4:1. However, it is important to note that most dressings and oils in the grocery store contain omega-6 oils. Thus, many people are already consuming it in high quantities. In fact, many people are consuming a ratio of 15:1 of omega-6 to omega-3 fatty acids. The most viable solution is to increase the omega-3 fatty acids. This is easily achieved by consuming more flax seed oil, which has a relative ratio of 1:3 of omega-6 to omega-3 fatty acids.

In order to determine which fatty acid supplementation is best for you, it is important to consider all the different fats already in your diet. If you generally follow a very low fat diet, then you should consider a mixed essential fatty acid supplement that contains both omega 6 and 3, with a slightly higher concentration of omega-3 to counteract the hidden omega-6 fatty acids that will undoubtedly exist in your diet.

There is some clinical evidence for the efficacy of essential fatty acids in the reduction of inflammation associated with arthritis.

Safety: Essential fatty acids are very safe. There is no real toxicity level associated with essential fats. However, they can cause some gastro-intestinal changes, such as belching, after consumption and loose stools when the dose is too high. If you already have loose stools, it is advisable to drop the dose in half.

Many essential fats come from cold water fish so it important to ensure that you are not allergic to these sources. Fish oil supplementation can have an effect on blood clotting. In high dose, it can slightly thin the blood and should therefore be used with caution if you are taking blood-thinning medication, such as warfarin, heparin, or high dose aspirin. If you are predisposed to easy bleeding and are on high doses of other vitamins that can contribute to thinning of the blood like vitamin E and C, then you should consult a healthcare practitioner to determine the correct dose for you before starting essential fatty acid supplementation. You should stop taking EFAs a few weeks before any surgical procedure.

Additional Supplements for Stress, Anxiety, and Depression

Stress and anxiety can contribute to back pain, and back pain can be accompanied by depression.

The following supplements have been found useful in managing stress, anxiety, and depression disorders. However, self-medication is not recommended with some of these due to the difficulty in making an accurate diagnosis and the numerous interactions these products have with other medication. Discussion should be carried out with your physician or naturopath as to whether these supplements are appropriate for you.

Lavender

Lavender or *Lavendula angustifolia* — which literally means to cleanse, from the Latin root *lavare*, meaning to wash or clean — has been used extensively for its aromatic fragrance in soaps, shampoos, and sachets for scenting clothing drawers. Traditionally, lavender was used medicinally for its impressive healing qualities that stems from the natural antibiotic and antiseptic (cleaning) qualities of this herb. Lavender is also one of the most versatile herbs used in an essential oil form extracted from the flowering tips of the evergreen shrub. Essential oil of lavender can be a powerful tool against stress, anxiety, and depression.

Although there is little scientific data to support the benefits of lavender, there is a great deal of subjective evidence. One study examined 17 patients with cancer, all of whom were in hospice. These patients were treated with the essential oil of lavender infused in a humidifier on 3 different days prior to treatments. They were assessed from levels of pain, anxiety, depression, and sense of well-being, as well as physical changes such as blood pressure and pulse. The results demonstrated a positive, although small, change in blood pressure and pulse, but a large change in anxiety, depression, well being, and pain as compared to the days where only water was administered in the humidifier.

Similar studies reveal alterations in brain wave activity following the use of lavender oil extracts. One study examined the EEG activity, alertness, and mood of 40 healthy adults. The participants were given mathematical equations to perform before and after a 3-minute treatment with lavender. As a control, one group received a 3-minute placebo treatment. The group receiving lavender displayed increased beta wave activity on the EEG. This indicates increased sedation and relaxation. This was confirmed by their verbal

Lavender Facts

Lavender has been shown to improve and promote sleep, decrease the activity of the nervous system, reduce anxiety and depression, and improve moods.

Back Care Use

• Decreases stress and stress-related pain by regulating the activity of the nervous system, in particular, depression and anxiety.

• Can help promote a better sleep to allow the body more time for optimal repair and recovery.

Dose

Lavender is most often used topically in an essential oil. It is best to use 1 to 4 drops of oil in a tablespoon of oil, then massage into the skin. When used as an inhalant, 2 to 4 drops may be added to 3 cups of boiling water and infused in a vaporizer. As a tincture (liquid oral form), 20 to 40 drops up to 3 times a day in warm water may be sipped upon.

reports of feeling less depressed, more relaxed, and generally better over all. In addition, their math scores were better when treated with lavender as they were more relaxed. Not only did they complete the mathematical equations faster, but they were also more accurate with their computations.

Side Effects: Although side effects are rarely seen with lavender oil, some people may experience a topical allergic reaction on the skin to the oil. This usually only occurs if the dose is too strong or the oil is applied directly to the skin without blending it with a neutral massage oil. In very rare cases, nausea, headaches, and chills have been reported. It is not clear whether lavender is safe during breastfeeding or pregnancy, so it should be avoided during these times, for fear of uterine stimulation. Due to the fact that lavender can affect the central nervous system, those people taking medications that also affect the same area, such as diazepam and lorazepam, should consult a healthcare practitioner before extensive use with lavender oil.

Trypsic Hydrolysate Milk Peptide

There has always been a strong bond between a mother and her infant, but is that bond more than just genetics? When infants are stressed, they often look around the room for their mother or cry out until she arrives. Is this just her face? Research would say differently. When children suckle on the breast, they are quickly relieved of agitation.

Milk contains a high concentration of peptides or chains of amino acids that children and adults break down differently. An infant's enzyme system is very immature and has only a trace amount of pepsin, the enzyme that breaks down many of these peptides. As they do not break them down, they are left with larger peptide chains. There is one particular sequence of amino acids that is 10 units or amino acids long found in milk, the trypsic hydrolysate decapeptide, which has been shown to possess strong anxiolytic properties. This peptide in adults can be broken down more readily with naturally higher levels of pepsin. If you increase the concentration of this peptide in adults, they too will benefit once again from the stress reducing or calming effects of milk they once enjoyed as a child.

Like many anti-anxiety drugs, trypsic hydrolysate decapeptide specifically binds into the GABA receptor. The GABA receptors are responsible for negative feedback or inhibition in the nervous system. This is the opposite to cortisol or the catecholamines that stimulate the HPA axis or act with positive feedback. GABA will inhibit the stimulation of the HPA axis, thereby decreasing the stress response and increasing relaxation and calmness. However, the pharmaceutical drugs used to produce this effect are usually accompanied with sedation.

It has been speculated that the binding into the GABA receptor is not complete. It does not fill the entire receptor at all sites. The sites that are not filled are the sedation sites. This is why, unlike a benzodiazepine such as diazepam where sedation is a large factor, there are no such symptoms with the protein peptide.

Side Effects: To date there are no side effects known with these protein decapepetides.

5-HTP

5-HTP or 5-hydroxytryptophan is one of the most important neurotransmitters in the brain. Normally, 5-HTP is synthesized from tryptophan, an amino acid or breakdown product of protein, with the help of vitamin B-3. A further step under the influence of vitamin B-6 then completes the conversion to 5-HTP. However, tryptophan is readily broken down by the liver or used as a protein building block for hormones, muscles, and other tissues in the body. Only what is left over is then converted into 5-HTP. If an individual is deficient in protein or tryptophan, there is a subsequent deficit in 5-HTP, and depression and anxiety can easily ensue.

5-HTP can be taken orally and therefore by-pass the conversion steps and ensure a better effect. 5-HTP easily passes through the blood-brain barrier, a filter-like wall at the base of the brain that acts as a protector barrier. It will only allow certain substances through, while others are 'turned away'. This again ensures a better response as this 5-HTP neurotransmitter is utilized in the brain. Tryptophan does not pass the blood-brain barrier, so using this as a 5-HTP precursor is not efficacious.

Over the past two decades, scientists have displayed that serotonin is a day neurotransmitter responsible for mood (anxiety and depression), impulse control, pain control, and obsessive behaviors. Serotonin is also the precursor to the production of our sleeping hormone, melatonin, by the pineal gland. Human clinical studies have revealed that not only does a decrease in serotonin induce a poor sleep but that sleep patterns are greatly improved following supplementation with 5-HTP. The rate of improvement is far superior to that of tryptophan for the reasons mentioned above.

5-HTP helps to induce relaxation through the increased production of dopamine and the suppression of noradrenaline activity. Because 5-HTP is very useful in promoting proper sleep and relaxation and decreasing the stress reaction

5-HTP Facts

A close relative of serotonin, our happy hormone, 5-HTP aids in well being, relaxation, and stress relief.

Back Care Use

• Increases the production of serotonin, which decreases pain and promotes happiness and a sense of well-being.

• Suppresses the production of noradrenaline and increases the production of melatonin to promote a better sleep and therefore recovery from injury.

Dose

50–100 mg, 2 times per day (for general relief of anxiety).

through noradrenaline suppression, it is has been said that it may be more useful in the treatment of insomnia and anxiety rather than true depression. However, as increased stress hormones decrease serotonin and therefore increase depression, 5-HTP offers relief from both anxiety and depression at once. Several other studies reveal similar conclusions with the supplementation of 5-HTP and the reduction of anxiety.

Side Effects: Despite the fact that 5-HTP already exists in the body naturally, occasional upset stomach or increased abnormal euphoria can be seen at high doses (200 mg twice a day). It should be noted though that 5-HTP can interfere with MAO inhibitors, tricyclic anti-depressants and SSRIs such as Prozac, Paxil, and Zoloft. 5-HTP supplementation should be avoided when on these medications.

St John's Wort

St John's Wort has several different properties, but the two main actions it possesses are as an anti-depressant and as an anti-viral. There are two main active ingredients responsible for these effects: hypericin and isohypericin. St John's Wort has a clear pharmacological effect on a number of neurotransmitters in the brain. It prevents re-uptake of serotonin, GABA (gamma-aminobutyric acid), dopamine, and noradrenaline, potentiating the effects of these chemical messengers. It has been proved effective in the treatment of mild depressive states in a number of clinical studies, is well tolerated, and has few side effects. There are, however, significant interactions with a number of pharmaceutical drugs and anaesthetics.

Clinical studies reveal that St John's Wort is useful in the treatment of mild to moderate depression and anxiety. This is achieved without the common side effects experienced with many psychotropic drugs. It is important to note, however, that St John's Wort has only been studied on mild and moderate anxiety and depression and not severe or suicidal depression.

Side Effects: Although there are very few incidences of reported side effects with St John's wort, a few symptoms have been seen after prolonged use at high doses (over 6 months with 500–600 mg, 4 times a day), including photosensitivity, constipation, dry mouth, and gastric irritation. St John's wort should not be used in conjunction with other pharmaceutical drugs as it may alter their action or efficacy, including the MAOIs, SSRIs, dibenzazepine derivatives (like amitriptyline), the sympathomimetics (like amphetamines and ephedrine), and foods high in tyramine.

St John's Wort Facts

St John's Wort (*Hypericum perforatum*) is used extensively for its effects on mood and emotion.

Back Care Use

- Prevents the uptake of serotonin, promoting decreased pain and anxiety and an increased sense of well-being.

- Regulates the uptake of GABA, allowing for a more sedative and restful sleep.

Dose

250–400 mg, 3 times per day, when the extract is standardized to 0.3% hypericin. It is best to take St John's wort on an empty stomach as food will decrease the rate and amount of active ingredient delivered to the body.

Hops

Hops (*Humulus lupulus*) has been an essential part of the brewing industry for decades, making it by far the most commonly used herb ever! Much of the sedating and relaxing effect of beer is due to hops.

Hops contains a resinous component called 2-methyl-3buten-2-ol, which possesses sedating and hypnotic actions. It has been shown to induce a deeper, more consistent sleep by increasing the slow wave activity of the brain seen in 'deep' stage 4 sleep.

Safety: Hops is a fairly allergenic herb and has resulted in acute respiratory distress and skin rashes in those sensitive to it. It should not be given to people with depression due to its hypnotic effects. Hops has also been shown to have a slight estrogenic effect and therefore can disrupt menstrual cycles. It should not be used in pregnant women or those with estrogen sensitive cancers.

Valerian

Valerian (*Valerian officinalis)* has been traditionally used as a sedative, an anti-convulsant, and a muscle relaxant. Research has shown its effect to be mediated in part by interaction with the GABA and serotonin neurotransmitter pathways in the brain. Valerian also appears to inhibit the breakdown of GABA, increasing availability of this relaxing chemical. It may react with the GABA-A receptor, the site of action of benzodiazepines such as diazepam (Valium).

There is good clinical evidence to support use of valerian as a hypnotic-sedative, improving relaxation and sleep without the 'hangover' and lasting drowsiness of pharmaceutical medicines. There is also some research to support its role as an anxiolytic or 'stress-reliever'.

Safety: Valerian is contraindicated in children under 3 years of age, and should not be used in pregnant women. Valerian should not be used in combination with other pharmaceuticals effecting GABA such as the benzodiazepine family, or other central nervous system depressants. Always advise your doctor, surgeon, or anesthetist if you are taking this supplement.

Hops Facts

Back Care Use
• Increases a deeper sleep with greater body repair by altering the nervous system and allowing the body to remain in stage 4 or "deep" sleep longer.

Dose
250–500 mg, before bed.

Valerian Facts

Back Care Use
• Anti-convulsant and anti-spasmodic effect to ease muscle pain and spasm.

• Increases the production of serotonin and GABA to promote better relaxation and sleep and therefore help with recovery from injury.

Dose
500–800 mg, before bed.

Medications for Back Care

When a muscle or tissue is inflamed, the immune system has a difficult time clearing away the inflammatory by-products and bringing in new healthy nutrients to repair the area. Pharmaceutical medications can help quickly alleviate this and get you back on the road to recovery with less discomfort and damage.

This does not mean that one has to use only pharmaceuticals on their own. In fact, your body will often reach optimal repair more quickly by using pharmaceutical drugs and natural supplements. The natural supplements can offer more long-term, slower anti-inflammatory and wound healing properties, while the quick and strong acting pharmaceuticals can offer acute relief to an area and provide more pathways for the natural supplements to get into the injured area and take effect. Natural supplements can allow you to stop medication sooner or reduce the dose.

✔ BACK FACTS

Quite often when one is in acute pain, the pain becomes so debilitating that it can actually create further problems. For example, trying to remain active during the acute stages of low back pain has been to shown to be extremely beneficial in promoting recovery, immobility due to pain being detrimental. In such cases, stronger medication is useful. It can be used to help break that pain/inflammation cycle and offer a faster route to relief and recovery.

Painkillers (Analgesics)

Painkillers are the first line in the medicinal treatment of low back pain, although in the presence of one of the more systemic inflammatory arthritis diseases, such as rheumatoid arthritis or gout, other medications will be necessary. For the basic symptoms of back pain, a simple analgesic, such as ASA (acetylsalicylic acid, aspirin), Tylenol, or Acetaminophen, is extremely useful. However, Acetaminophen and ASA should be used only intermittently for pain. ASA has more anti-inflammatory action but is less well tolerated, particularly in older individuals. Neither drug should be used excessively on a long-term basis. Pain requiring such prolonged use likely needs an alternative medication and further investigation.

ASA

Because of its more significant anti-inflammatory activity, ASA is likely more effective at reducing swelling and inflammation than Acetaminophen but has similar pain killing properties. Gastric side effects are more frequent, including indigestion, gastritis, ulcers, and bleeding. ASA also reduces the ability of the blood to form clots, increasing risk of bleeding. ASA should not be used in the presence of active stomach ulceration, and its use should be reconsidered with a prior history of this condition, especially if associated with bleeding. ASA treatment should be stopped 10 days prior to any surgery due to its effect on blood clotting, and not be used in individuals with a history of clotting problems.

Acetaminophen

Acetaminophen has painkilling activity equal to ASA but does not have such anti-inflammatory activity. It is not associated with bleeding from the stomach and does not interfere with blood clotting, two of the possible side effects of ASA. Excessive use of Acetaminophen, however, can have significant effects, with possible damage to the liver, and can interfere with blood-thinning medicines.

Non-Steroidal Anti-Inflammatory Medications (NSAIDs)

Non-steroidal anti-inflammatory medications are a group of drugs that include ASA and have a specific affect at controlling inflammation. By blocking an enzyme involved in the production of inflammatory chemicals (prostaglandins), NSAIDs, like ASA, can have a dramatic effect on reducing and controlling inflammation. These beneficial effects are not without a risk to other areas of the body, however. The most significant of these is the possibility of causing ulceration and bleeding in the stomach.

Recently a new type of NSAID has been developed, the so-called COX-2 NSAIDs, and include Rofecoxib and Celecoxib. The enzymes responsible for the production of chemicals mediating inflammation (prostaglandins, leukotrienes, etc) are the cyclo-oxygenase or COX enzymes. There are two types. The COX-2 enzyme is particularly involved in arthritis and inflammation, and has been shown to greatly increase its activity during acute episodes. The COX-1 enzyme, which is constantly present at certain levels in all tissues, appears to produce similar chemicals that are of value to the body and protect it particularly in areas such as the stomach. The older anti-inflammatories did not distinguish between these two enzymes, and as a result, side effects were more frequent. The

NSAIDs have proven benefit in the management of low back pain, but with regards to efficacy, no one anti-inflammatory has proven to be superior to another or indeed to ASA. However, there does seem to be a tremendous variability in tolerance to these medications and in how well they work for different individuals.

Back Care Contraindications

• Not be used in patients with active ulceration or bleeding (a history of this condition in the past is a relative contraindication to their use).

• Risk increases with age over 60 and smoking.

• Older NSAIDs also affect blood clotting and should not be used with a history of bleeding disorder or at the same time as use of anti-coagulants.

• Stop use 10 days prior to surgery.

• Avoid use in patients with kidney disease or heart failure.

COX-2 NSAIDs have less stomach irritation and do not interfere with blood clotting.

Doctors will usually prescribe an NSAID they have administered before with success for patients in your situation. The prescribed medication should be tried for about 2 weeks. If at that stage it is not working or there are intolerable side effects, then it can be changed. Factors such as cost, pill size, frequency of medication, effectiveness, and side effects are all factors in choosing the right NSAID.

Side Effects: All NSAIDs are associated with rare side effects, such as skin rash, liver and kidney problems, asthma, dizziness, and headaches. The main side effect is indigestion or stomach ulceration and bleeding. About 1% (or one in one hundred) of patients who take anti-inflammatories for one year will develop an ulcer, and about half of those will get bleeding problems. Unfortunately, not all ulcers cause symptoms of heartburn or indigestion, and the first sign of trouble may be bleeding, causing black tar bowel movements, low blood count, dizziness, and fainting.

It is possible to prescribe a stomach protective agent as an additional medication. Some NSAID preparations actually include this. Problems, however, can still occur. The highest risk comes from continued use of anti-inflammatories. This may well be minimized by intermittent use. Even chronic low back pain is usually periodic nature. NSAIDs can be used quite effectively during these 'acute' periods and then stopped once the discomfort settles down.

Rofecoxib and Celecoxib do have their own set of side effects. Celebrex cannot be taken if you have an allergy to sulpha. They affect the kidney and can cause fluid retention in susceptible individuals, which may cause an increase in blood pressure. There has been recent concern as to whether COX 2 medications increase the risk of heart attacks. Although the risk is slight, it appears primarily due to the fact that the COX-2 NSAIDs, unlike ASA and COX-1, do not have a blood thinning effect on the clotting cells or platelets. While this is beneficial in reducing bleeding episodes and making reversal easier for surgical procedures, it likely removes the protective effect on the heart. It has been suggested, therefore, that in susceptible individuals aspirin treatment in low dose be continued along with the COX-2 NSAIDs.

Stronger Analgesics (Narcotics)

There are numerous and conflicting opinions about the use of narcotic-based analgesics for the management of low back pain. These medications include prescriptions containing codeine (Tylenol #3, for example), percocet, morphine (MS Contin, for example), and Fentanyl (transdermal Duramorph). No one opioid analgesic has proven to be of superior benefit to the others, and their use is generally dictated by physician comfort and patient tolerance.

Tolerance to narcotics, the need for progressively stronger doses, is not supported by clinical studies of groups as widespread as low back pain and cancer. Generally, the need for higher doses indicates progression of the disease and a physiologic increase in 'pain'.

Side Effects: Most patients taking narcotic analgesics will experience side effects to a certain degree. Most bothersome can be somnolence and altered mental capacity making complex tasks, including driving or operating machinery, unadvisable. Interestingly, chronic pain can inflict similar dysfunction and use of appropriate narcotic analgesics in these individuals may actually *improve* mentation. Nausea is common as is constipation and further medication may be required to relieve these. Some natural alternative remedies are listed below. Reduced libido may be a problem but is also affected by chronic pain and depression.

The main concern surrounding the use of narcotic analgesics is the risk of dependence, the physiologic state whereby stopping the medication leads to 'withdrawal' and addiction, a psychological condition in which compulsive use of the drug leads to ill health and social malfunction. While there is little evidence that using opioid analgesics for pain leads to addiction (except in those with a pre-existing addictive condition), dependence can be a problem.

Narcotic Analgesic Facts

The use of narcotics in acute or recurrent, non-specific low back pain is not generally supported. A number of studies have found no benefit of these medications over a combination of simple analgesics and anti-inflammatories in these individuals. Their role in chronic pain, however, is important, with studies showing pain relief in over 75%, with similar numbers reporting improved function, including return to work.

Back Care Use

• Use only to treat specific, pathology-related pain.

• Use for pain consistent with clinical findings.

• Use only when aggressive rehabilitation and simple analgesia has failed.

• Do not use with history of psychological illness or addiction.

• Use medication only as directed.

• Make regular follow-up visits to prescribing physician.

• Use only one prescribing physician.

• Do not renew prescription by telephone.

Complementary Natural Medicines for Reducing Side Effects from Analgesics

Several natural remedies can be used in conjunction with analgesics for gastritis, constipation, and nausea side effects. For back pain due to degeneration or arthritis, use of a natural arthritis supplement may allow you to reduce the frequency or dose of NSAID and thus the potential side effects.

Slippery Elm, Marshmallow and Cabbage

These are all demulcent, emollient herbs that help to soothe irritated and inflamed mucous membranes such as the stomach and bowel. They are useful in reducing the gastric side effects of regular anti-inflammatory medications.
Dose: 350–500 mg of each can be used 3 times per day without food.

Zinc

This mineral is used to help stimulate cellular turnover and wound healing, and to reduce irritation from NSAIDs.
Dose: 25 mg per day with or without food.

Acidophillus

Acidophillus (*Lactobacillus acidophilus*) is the 'good' bacteria that normally inhabits the bowel and helps to maintain the normal bacterial floral balance, prevents yeast and fungal infections, and helps to regulate bowel movements.
Dose: 1–3 capsules per day with 1 billion bacteria per cap on an empty stomach.

Essential Fatty Acids (Omega-3, -6, -9)

These EFAs are natural anti-inflammatories and natural stool softeners. They help to regulate bowel movements, softening the stool, allowing for easier more fluid evacuation without straining.
Dose: 3–6 grams of fatty acids with food.

Cascara Sagrada

Cascara Sagrada or *Rhamnus pushiana* is the most gentle natural laxative available. Unlike other natural or pharmaceutical laxatives, this herb is non-addicting and helps to increase bowel movements without spaciticity, cramping, or urgency. Some people may be more sensitive than others and therefore require a smaller dose. If irritation occurs, discontinue its use.
Dose: 200–400 mg before bed.

Senna

Senna is a stronger and more addictive laxative that works by slightly irritating the surface of the bowel, causing increased contractions of the muscles of the bowel. With long-term use, the bowel may become tolerant to this herb, so do not use for more than 10 to 12 days in a row.
Dose: 300 mg before bed.

Aloe Vera Gel

Aloe vera gel is a natural laxative and wound healer. Aloe, when taken internally, gently increases bowel stimulation and contraction, while soothing the lining of the mucous membrane itself. When taken in high doses, it can have a purgative (vomiting) effect.

Ginger

Ginger or *Zingiber officinalis* is a natural gastric anti-spasmodic. It helps to relieve nausea and upset stomach. It works locally, rather that through the central nervous system like many of the pharmaceutical anti-nausea formulations. It can be taken in tea form or in capsule.

Dose: In tea, infuse fresh ginger (1 tsp) in hot water and drink as needed; in capsule form, 200–400 mg as needed.

Peppermint

Peppermint or *Mentha piperita* is a natural anti-spasmodic, anti-emetic, and anti-septic herb. It helps to decrease spasm and nausea without stimulation and irritation, while offering natural anti-microbial support. It may be taken in tea of capsule form.

Dose: In tea form, use peppermint infused tea bags as needed; in capsule form, use 150 mg in an enteri- coated capsule as needed.

Acupuncture

Acupuncture is very useful for nausea and constipation. There are specific points around the wrist to help relieve nausea of any nature, and specific points around the umbilicus and lower legs to help stimulate bowel contraction and bowel movements. For acupuncture treatment for the relief of side effects, it is necessary to consult a practitioner of acupuncture.

Muscle Relaxants

Despite their name, there is little evidence that 'muscle relaxants' actually act by specifically reducing muscle activity or contraction. Based on the notion that pain is secondary to 'muscle spasm', they are often prescribed in the acute phase of non-specific low back pain. Their mechanism of action is unknown and they have significant side effects, including drowsiness and dizziness. Although shown to be more effective than placebo, there is no evidence they are any more effective than analgesics or NSAIDs. Nor do they appear to provide additional benefit to these medications. A short trial of muscle relaxant may be considered if standard analgesic and NSAID combinations have been unsuccessful in relieving pain.

Muscle Relaxant Facts

Muscle relaxants should not generally be used for first-line management of low back pain, except where an individual reports previous significant value. Use in chronic low back pain is unjustified due to the mental side effects.

Anti-Depressant Medication

Tricyclic anti-depressants (TCAs), such as nortriptyline (Pamelor) and amitriptyline (Elavil), have substantial efficacy against pain, predominantly through their ability to block re-uptake of the neurotransmitter norepinephrine at nerve

Anti-depressant medications have an important role in the treatment of chronic low back pain, especially for treatment of pain itself, particularly nerve pain, and also aid management of sleep disturbance and clinical depression associated with chronic pain.

endings. In addition, they are valuable for the treatment of depression and sleep disorder, although not as good as some of the other anti-depressants in this regard. Significant side effects, including sedation, fainting, and dry mouth, often limit their use.

Selective serotonin reuptake inhibitors (SSRIs), such as fluoxitine (Prozac), sertraline (Zoloft), and paroxitine (Paxil), act centrally to reduce re-uptake of serotonin, the neurotransmitter primarily responsible for mood. Though not as effective at pain control as the TCAs, they are highly effective at treating depression. Their effects on sleep vary and therefore the choice of specific drug should be correlated to the patient's symptoms. Side effects are less prevalent than with TCAs but may include sedation and insomnia.

Natural Supplements for Liver Support and Minor Allergic Reaction

The liver is the major site of drug breakdown in the body. High doses of pharmaceutical medications can put a strain on its function, leading to headaches, nausea, poor skin, and altered sleep.

Milk Thistle
A liver protective and liver detoxification herb, milk thistle helps to soothe, protect and clean out the liver.
Dose: 500 mg, 2 times a day on an empty stomach.

Lemon Balm
This herb directly stimulates the detoxification processes in the liver.
Dose: 1 tsp per day in warm water, preferably first thing in the morning.

Globe Artichoke
This herb helps to break down uric acid crystals and helps both the gall bladder and liver clean and re-cycle metabolic bi-products.
Dose: 250 mg, 3 times per day on an empty stomach.

Quercitin
Known allergy to any drug is a contraindication to its use. A severe reaction requires emergency treatment. Lesser degrees of allergic reaction such as mild itchiness or skin rash can be minimized by use of Quercitin, a bioflavinoid that acts as a natural anti-histamine by binding to the cell that produces histamine (mast cell), decreasing its production and release of histamine. It takes 2 to 3 weeks to be effective.
Dose: 600 mg, 2 to 3 times per day on an empty stomach.

Florazone Cream
This natural homeopathic cream is useful for the treatment of minor skin rashes and itchiness.
Dose: Rub gently into affected skin, 3 to 4 times per day.

Medicinal Treatment of Inflammatory Arthritis

Medicinal management of rheumatoid arthritis remains the mainstay of treatment for this form of the disease. It becomes increasingly important as the severity of the disease progresses, not only to control the pain and swelling around joints, but to reduce the involvement of other areas such as the eyes, lung, and heart.

Initial treatment may involve the analgesics and NSAIDs. However, the more acute and severe the presentation of the arthritis, and the more extensive the involvement of other tissues and organs, the more likely it is that other drugs may be incorporated. Full discussion of this subject is outside the scope of this book but further information can be found in one of our other books, *Healing Arthritis: Complementary Naturopathic, Orthopedic, and Drug Treatments*.

Rheumatoid and Inflammatory Arthritis Treatments

- Simple Analgesics

- NSAIDs

- DMARDs (disease modifying anti-rheumatic drugs)
  These include oral steroids, anti-malarials, sulfasalazine, gold compounds, penicillamine, methotrexate, and azathioprine. These powerful drugs reduce disease activity, although their mechanism of action is often unclear. They have significant side effects and numerous drug interactions.

- Biologic Response Modifying Drugs
  These include Tumour Necrosis Factor Antibody (Infliximab – Remicade), Etanercept (Enbrel), Leflunomide (Arava), and Anakinra (Kineret). These new drugs are still largely experimental but have shown tremendous promise in the control of inflammatory conditions such as rheumatoid arthritis. They require injection and have significant side effects.

- Antibiotic Therapy
  While no specific transmissible infectious organisms have been identified as a pathogenic cause of rheumatoid arthritis, treatment of the disease with antibiotics such as minocycline and rifamycin has shown limited success.

Injection Therapy

Injection therapy in low back pain attempts to bridge the somewhat lengthy gap between non-surgical management, such as physical therapy, and surgical intervention. Not surprisingly, many patients who find their back pain has not resolved with time and an appropriate rehabilitation program are keen to explore the potential of this non-operative option.

 BACK FACTS

Injection therapies can play a vital role in the diagnostic workup of low back pain. The therapeutic extrapolation of these techniques has offered a valuable treatment alternative. In the absence of contraindications to an injection procedure such as reduced blood clotting, infection, or allergy, certain individuals may be considered suitable for one of the three principal treatments: epidural steroid injection; facet joint steroid injection; or facet joint nerve ablation.

Epidural Steroid Injection Facts

The aim of the epidural steroid injection is to reduce local inflammation and swelling, thereby removing the nerve sensitization and reducing pain. Epidural steroid injection should be considered an integral part of low back pain management, particularly that associated with disc herniation.

Epidural Steroid Injections

Pressure on a nerve root does not automatically cause pain — try pressing on your own ulnar nerve as it runs behind the bony prominence on the inside of your elbow. Disc herniations are seen on MRI in perfectly normal, pain-free individuals despite impingement on the spinal nerve roots. Symptoms of sciatica subside in most individuals over 2 to 4 weeks, despite the fact that the disc herniation remains the same size. Furthermore, sciatic nerve pain can persist in the absence of clear nerve compression or after surgical decompression.

There must be other factors at play in the development of a painful nerve root. The unifying factor is nerve sensitization, the process by which a normal nerve becomes hyper-sensitive and more likely to cause pain when compressed. One of the most important sensitizing mechanisms is that of local inflammation. Chemicals released locally as a result of this cascade of activity result in changes within the nerve, allowing it to be stimulated more easily and produce a painful sensation rather than regular feeling. Additional factors include the pressure associated with disc herniation and inflammatory fluid which compromise the blood supply to the nerve and have a direct chemical effect of the disc material itself.

The technique of epidural steroid injection was developed in the 1950s and '60s and is now carried out under X-ray guidance by an experienced practitioner using contrast dye to ensure accurate needle placement and avoid injection into a blood vessel. The injection, usually of local anesthetic and steroid, is placed around the exiting nerve root and its covering layers in an attempt to reduce local inflammation. In effect, it aims to speed up or enhance the natural healing process, which would normally follow a similar, though slower, path.

Most patients obtain benefit from one injection but the technique should not be considered a 'failure' until three have been tried.

Effectiveness

Despite the lack of conclusive evidence of their effectiveness, their use is endorsed by the North American Spine Society. A number of the better studies show a significant benefit of epidural steroid injections over placebo (simple salt water injection). Some studies have shown a response rate of 90% with results lasting over 3 years in almost 80% of subjects. In another study, epidural steroid injections followed by physiotherapy resulted in over 50% pain-relief in 75% of patients at 18 months.

Epidural steroid injections have been shown to reduce the likelihood of progression to surgery. In one study, 86% of patients who had injections after 4 months of radicular pain were improved without operative intervention at one year. In another study, 70% of the epidural steroid injection group elected not to have surgery as opposed to 30% in the placebo group.

In common with other injection therapies, epidural steroid injections allow sufficient temporary improvement in pain to allow increased function and participation in a therapy program, as other studies have shown. Future studies may further clarify the indications to include back-dominant pain related to other neurogenic pain pathways.

Despite these finding, a review of completed trials in *Pain Digest* in 1999 found an equal number of studies for and against epidural steroid injection as an effective treatment. The value of the procedure remains controversial.

Safety: Many people have a fear or distrust of cortisone or steroid injections. While there are some cautions, the medication generally acts simply as a local anti-inflammatory agent.

Indications

- Patients who may be suitable for a trial of lumbar epidural steroid injections have predominantly leg pain, typically radicular, associated with signs of nerve root irritability on clinical testing.

- Although back pain may be present, the pain is leg-dominant, typically in the sciatic distribution down into the calf or foot.

- The patient will have failed an initial course of therapy or remain unable to participate because of pain.

- The presence of nerve dysfunction such as numbness or even weakness is not considered a contra-indication as long as there is no evidence of cauda equina syndrome.

- Positive EMG (electromyography) tests or selective nerve root blocks along with correlating disc herniation on CAT scan or MRI are found to improve outcome.

Contraindications
• Reduced blood clotting ability due to disease or medication.
• Presence of infection either at the proposed injection site or systemically.
• Allergy to local anesthetic or steroid.

It is similar to the anti-inflammatory pills you take every day but it is actually getting directly to where it is most needed. The bad effects on the body associated with taking steroids by mouth do not occur with these injections, and unless repeated frequently at the same site, there is no good evidence that they cause local damage.

Side effects of cortisone injection are infrequent, generally mild and temporary. Complications of the injection itself are uncommon, with more serious risks being extremely rare in the hands of an experienced injectionist using X-ray and contrast guidance. Factors found to reduce the benefit of epidural steroid injection include protracted symptoms, back-dominant pain, and smoking.

Cortisone Steroid Injection

Effect on Inflammation
• Inhibits enzymes that manufacture prostaglandins (inflammatory chemicals).
• Impairs function of inflammatory cells (neutrophils, eosinophils and monocytes).
• Reduces production of inflammatory cytokines by T-cells.

Side Effects (temporary, rarely longer than 5 days)
• Facial Flushing
• Difficulty Sleeping
• Agitation or Anxiety
• Mild Fever
• Temporary Increase in Blood Sugar (diabetics)

Risks
• Up to 5% risk:
  • Headache
  • Temporary numbness or weakness in the legs
  • Injection into a blood vessel
• Rare complications:
  • Spinal blood clot
  • Infection
  • Nerve root injury
  • Persistent scarring/irritation of nerve root

Facet Joint Injections

The lumbar facet joints (also called the zygoapophyseal joints) are the paired joints at the back of each vertebra. These synovial joints, like the knee or the hip, are supplied by branches of the dorsal sensory nerve, the main trunk through which peripheral sensation reaches the spinal cord. Each facet is supplied by two nerves, one from its own level and one from the level above. The capsule of the joint is densely supplied with sensory endings, responding to pressure and stretch. It also contains specific pain fibers.

Mechanical stimulation by chronic or acute strain of the joint capsule can give rise to painful sensation, particularly in the presence of sensitization by local factors such as inflammation or by central mechanisms described earlier. The presence of nerve endings within the synovial tissue lining the facet joint provide an additional source of painful stimuli.

Facet joint damage or inflammation resulting in chronic pain with peripheral and central sensitization sets up a cycle of pain that is hard to break. The reflex protective muscle spasm associated with pain increases forces across the facet joints, further contributing to damage and discomfort. Prolonged spasm leading to damage and inflammation within the muscle will cause further sensitization, as well as inducing pain sensation from the muscle itself. It is reasonable to conclude that effective pain relief by intra-articular facet injection may help break this cycle.

The use of injected steroid to reduce inflammation within the facet joint employs similar reasoning to injection therapy for other joints such as the hip or knee. Just as systemic anti-inflammatory medication, such as aspirin and non-steroidal anti-inflammatories (NSAIDs), reduce pain and swelling, intra-articular (into the joint) injection of cortisone acts locally at the specific joint into which it is placed. While the predominant site of action is on the inflamed lining of the joint (the synovium), the small size of the facet joints and the dense innervation of the capsule may provide a secondary site of pain relieving activity.

Effectiveness

Facet joint injections may be considered in back-dominant pain, worse with extension of the spine and without leg radiation or other features to suggest disc herniation or nerve compression. The technique should be particularly helpful in inflammatory arthritis where the disease process is active within the facet joints. However, evidence for this is lacking and most studies indicate the most beneficial outcomes in recent onset pain. The use of properly performed diagnostic facet block tests and correlation with SPECT bone scans are shown to improve the reliability and effectiveness of facet blocks.

If following the injection pain relief lasts for a few weeks, a repeat injection may be carried out. A third injection can be performed if longer relief occurs, but this is generally considered to be the maximum. Partial success or recurrent pain warrants discussion about medial nerve blocks.

The reported results of lumbar facet joint injection with steroid are variable and the procedure remains controversial. Pain relief in some studies occurs in as few as 20% of individuals, while others report values nearer 60%. A controlled study in patients with chronic low back pain reported in the *New England Journal of Medicine* in 1991 found no value for the procedure, although their inclusion criterion was only one positive facet block. Clearly, for this technique to be of use, patient selection has to be highly specific.

Medial Branch Neurotomy

Medial branch neurotomy aims to provide long-term pain relief by disrupting the nerves that carry pain sensation from the facet joints. In the lumbar spine, these nerves are small branches from the large dorsal sensory nerve trunk entering the spinal cord. There are generally two of these 'medial branch' nerves for each facet joint.

The technique of medial branch neurotomy involves placement of a needle under X-ray guidance adjacent to the nerve, followed by ablation of the nerve using heat, cold, or chemical techniques. Use of cold (cryotherapy) or chemical (phenol) has largely been abandoned in favor of 'radiofrequency neurotomy', which uses a high-frequency alternating current to create local heating.

Effectiveness
Results of radiofrequency neurotomy, as with facet injections, are improved the more selective the criteria for patient inclusion and the more specific the spinal level treated. A recent study in the journal *Spine* found 60% pain relief at one year in subjects selected according to back pain and diagnostic block criteria. This study also evaluated the effectiveness of the treatment in ablating the medial nerves, showing the importance of accurate technique. This procedure appears to offer lasting, though not permanent relief, and may be most valuable in allowing sufficient pain reduction for the patient to attend an zygoapophyseal joint pain active therapy program.

Radiofrequency Neurotomy Facts

Indications
- Similar to those for facet joint cortisone injection, specifically back-dominant, extension type pain.
- Facet joint diagnostic blocks providing over 80% pain relief appear to predict patients likely to benefit most from the neurotomy procedure.

Botulinum Toxin (Botox) Injections

Botulinum toxin is a product of the bacterium *Clostridium botulinum*, which is now commercially manufactured under trade names such as 'Botox'. While commonly recognized as a panacea for aging skin, its applications within medicine are becoming increasingly widespread. Its ability to prevent muscle contraction has resulted in successful use for spasticity secondary to nervous disorders, facial twitches, and torticollis (neck muscle spasm). More recently, these injections have been utilized for the treatment of myofascial pain, fibromyalgia, headaches, and chronic low back pain.

The rationale for the use of botulinum toxin in low back pain involves its ability to reduce tone or tension in chronically painful muscles. This allows improved motion and activity of non-involved muscles. However, the benefit of botulinum toxin may not just be through the relief of muscle spasm. First, it is likely that by diminishing spasm, sensory nerves supplying the muscle will convey fewer pain messages, reducing the overall central sensitization that accompanies low back pain. Second, botulinum toxin appears to reduce activity in the lumbar sympathetic nerves responsible for the deep-seated 'visceral' component of lumbar pain. Third, the toxin seems to be able to mitigate part of the inflammatory response, reducing the concentration of pain-transmitting chemicals such as substance-P.

Botulinum Toxin Facts

The use of botulinum toxin in chronic low back pain remains largely experimental, but appears to offer tremendous potential as another weapon in the armory to attack this ubiquitous and refractory condition.

Effectiveness

Studies assessing the benefit of botulinum toxin in chronic low back pain are limited at present. The most reliable research, a randomized, placebo-controlled study in 2001 found significant improvement in pain and function in the botulinum group at 3 and 8 weeks with no side effects. Other studies have shown improvements in pain, mobility, and function lasting up to 12 weeks.

Sacroiliac Joint Injections

The sacroiliac (SI) joints are at the back of the pelvis. They are large synovial type joints between the lateral mass of the sacral vertebrae and the posterior part of the pelvic bone, the ilium. Stabilized by thick, strong ligaments, movement is very limited in keeping with the tremendous forces they endure suspending the spine and torso on the pelvis and legs. The incidence of SI joint pain in the chronic low back population is reported to be as high as 30%, but identification of this patient subgroup has remained elusive.

Effectiveness

Injection of local anesthetic and steroid into the SI joint has been used as a treatment for low back pain. Access is difficult and requires careful X-ray guidance. However, SI joint injection has not been demonstrated to have any significant benefit in the management of low back pain, except in cases of sacroiliac inflammation in inflammatory disease such as ankylosing spondylitis. As with other injection techniques, the problem may be more in the identification of appropriate patients than in the technique itself.

Chemonucleolysis (Chymopapain Injection) for Disc Herniation

Chemonucleolysis is a technique, more popular in Europe than in North America, in which an enzyme (chymopapain, derived from the papaya plant) is introduced into the intervertebral disc via a needle and X-ray guidance, in order to dissolve the nucleus pulposus. It is considered a less-invasive alternative to surgical discectomy.

The intervertebral disc consists of a tough outer shell or annulus fibrosus and a soft inner core called the nucleus pulposus. A weak spot in the outer shell can allow the nucleus to protrude or become herniated, allowing pressure and irritation on adjacent nerve roots. This typically results in leg pain or sciatica, possibly associated with numbness of weakness. The concept of chemonucleolysis is that the injected enzyme 'melts' the nucleus, reducing the herniation and thus the nerve pressure.

Effectiveness

Use of chemonucleolysis as a treatment for the herniated disc declined rapidly after a report was published on its complications in 1993. However, refinements in technique and more specific guidelines as to patient suitability have provided the basis for increased acceptance in recent years, supported by large clinical studies. Patients who seem to do the best with chemonucleolysis are generally younger with short duration, leg-dominant pain and well-localized correlating disc pathology on imaging (MRI or CT scan). Immediately following the injection many patients get some relief from their pain, although the majority do not see full benefit for about 6 weeks. Reported results in appropriately selected individuals are comparable to surgery with 75–80% pain relief lasting long term 5 to 20 years. Complication rates are reported as 5 to 10 times less than surgical discectomy.

A review summary from the *Mount Sinai Journal of Medicine* in 2000 reports that "chemonucleolysis using chymopapain is the least invasive technique used to treat a herniated lumbar pulposus. After 37 years of clinical experience, multiple clinical trials, a national multicenter, double-blind study mandated by the Food and Drug Administration, and heated controversy in the scientific community, the injection of chymopapain to treat herniated discs has (in appropriately selected patients) proven as successful as laminectomy, with fewer complications and the advantage of considerable cost savings."

Safety: There are some specific contraindications to chemonucleolysis using chymopapain, in particular an allergy to papaya present in 0.3% of the population, which should be tested for before the procedure.

Chemonucleolysis

Indications
- Leg-dominant sciatic-type pain.
- Increased pain on straight leg raise test.
- Patient 18 to 50 years of age.
- Short duration of symptoms.
- Well localized disc herniation on imaging studies.
- Imaging studies correlate with symptoms.
- Soft, protruding disc.
- No calcifications.
- Other conservative treatments have failed.
- Patient wishes to avoid surgery.

Contraindications (using chymopapain)
- Allergy to papaya.
- Pregnancy.
- Cauda equina syndrome or progressive nerve deficit.
- Sequestered (completely detached) disc fragment.
- Spinal tumor.
- Spinal instability.
- Spinal stenosis.
- Neurologic disease (e.g., Multiple sclerosis).
- Multiple failed back surgeries.

Intradiscal Electrothermal Coagulation (IDET™)

Intradiscal electrothermal coagulation (*IDET™*) is a relatively new technique that has developed out of research evaluating the effects of thermal energy on tissue collagen. A fine heating probe is introduced into the disc under X-ray guidance to deliver thermal energy at temperatures around 60° to 70° Celsius to the nucleus and annular wall.

The principle of intradiscal electrothermal coagulation is the cauterization of nerve fibers supplying the annulus, thought to be responsible for much of the pain associated with disc degeneration. In addition, small blood vessels that have grown into the disc as part of the degradative process are coagulated. The thermal energy shrinks the collagen protein, thereby improving the strength and biomechanical properties of the disc.

The procedure is performed as an out-patient procedure, with return to office work in about 2 weeks. Heavier jobs may require more intensive post-procedure rehabilitation and a few months off work. This technique spares the disc rather than sacrificing it as with fusion, an important factor when looking at long-term impact on other areas of the spine.

The complication rate for intradiscal electrothermal coagulation is reported to be low, although research is currently limited. The only clear contraindication is obesity, which increases side effects and reduces success rate.

Effectiveness

Early results are encouraging with up to 80% of patients reporting good relief of pain even at 2 years. However, it has been pointed out that all new technology produces initial high success and the true test of this technique will come with the results of controlled, randomized studies. There are no long-term follow up studies to indicate whether this procedure has lasting benefit or induces biomechanical failure. Needless to say, intradiscal electrothermal coagulation is not a panacea for all back pain. Its indications are quite restrictive and will likely become even narrower as research accumulates. However, it provides another exciting prospect for the treatment of disc-related low back pain in the future.

Intradiscal Electrothermal Coagulation Facts

Intradiscal electrothermal coagulation provides a minimally invasive option in patients with internal disc derangement. The only other option in these individuals, if they fail conservative management, is fusion, so disc coagulation is certainly worth investigating.

Spinal Surgery

Michael H. G. Ford, MD, FRCSC

Dr Michael Ford is an orthopedic spine surgeon at Sunnybrook and Women's College Health Sciences Center. He was trained at the University of Toronto. He has a special interest in adult degenerative and deformity problems of the cervical, thoracic, and lumbar spine.

There are many myths surrounding spinal surgery. Some people believe that it should be avoided at all costs. Some think that it is a treatment of 'last resort'. Some people firmly believe that there is large possibility that you can end up paralyzed and in a wheel chair after spinal surgery. That being said, it should also be recognized that spine surgery has specific indications and significant limitations. There are many wonderful things that we can do and many more that we cannot. It is the ability to recognize the difference that sets our limitations and allows us to establish the role of surgery in the management of low back pain.

BACK FACTS

Surgery is not a last resort. Indications are very specific and it must be recognized that there are limitations. Individuals with very specific, surgically-reversible lesions can truly benefit from an invasive procedure with reduction of symptoms and a markedly improved quality of life. Surgical procedures should be undertaken with a solid understanding of the risks versus the benefits and equal expectations of outcome for both patient and surgeon. While many spine problems can be prevented or treated successfully with conservative measures, some individuals, despite best efforts, continue to have pain and disability. For this group, surgery may provide an answer.

Back Surgery Basics

General Indications for Back Surgery

All surgeries are either 'absolutely' indicated or 'relatively' indicated. If an individual has an absolute indication for surgery, this means that failure to have surgery can result in loss of life or limb or a very important bodily function. This is the only situation when a surgeon will say that the patient absolutely needs to have the surgery. The surgeon will recommend surgery and explain the potential consequences if the operation is not performed. However, this scenario is actually quite rare in spinal surgery. The vast majority of cases where spinal surgery is absolutely indicated are emergent in nature and decisions need to be made very quickly. An example is if someone has a massive disc herniation compressing the nerves that supply bowel and bladder function (cauda equina

Surgical Procedures

- **Decompress:** removes pressure from nerves and spinal cord
- **Stabilize:** restores spinal stability
- **Straighten:** corrects deformity
- **Strengthen:** restores the strength of vertebral bone
- **Replace:** disc replacement still considered experimental

Elective Back Surgery Facts

Indications

- Non-operative treatments have failed.

- There is a surgically amenable problem.

- The problem is responsible for the patient's symptoms.

- There is a high probability that the surgery will be successful.

- The benefits of the surgery outweigh the risks.

- The patient is willing to cooperate with post-operative care.

- The patient is fully informed of the above.

- The surgeon and the patient have the same expectations.

syndrome). In this case, a decompression procedure is absolutely indicated. Most reasonable individuals faced with this situation readily accept this as their only answer.

The surgery is explained to the patient along with the potential benefits versus the potential risks. Patients then make an informed decision as to whether or not they wish to proceed. The surgeon may provide recommendations or advice and may even answer the age-old question, "What would you do?" The final decision, however, rests with the patient.

Most elective surgeries, those that are booked on a scheduled basis, are being carried out for relative indications for those individuals experiencing problems secondary to degenerative change or disc herniation. Depending on the symptoms and presentation, varying periods of conservative treatment will have been tried before considering surgery. Those individuals who, despite having undergone comprehensive rehabilitation, experience persistent symptoms that are not tolerable are candidates for elective surgery.

Surgery is indicated in those individuals who have a well-defined, surgically reversible lesion, which, after careful evaluation, is felt to be responsible for their symptoms. A patient may have a huge disc herniation at the L4-5 level on the right side on MRI, but if the symptoms indicate a lesion on the left at L5-S1, surgery may not be the answer. Surgery should be contemplated only if it has a high likelihood of success. Most would agree that 50–50 is not a good basis for operative intervention, but the ideal ratio is dependant on the symptoms and the patient. In addition, the benefits of the surgery with respect to relief of symptoms and improvement in function should far exceed the risks. Risk of loss of life or important bodily function should be extremely small.

Many patients with low back pain seem anxious to have surgery, believing it is the Holy Grail of therapy, a panacea for all ills of the spine. This type of expectation needs to be identified and corrected before embarking on any operative procedure. It is vitally important for the patient to know why the surgery is being performed, what it hopes to achieve, and what it will not rectify. If it aims to eliminate leg pain and numbness but is likely to leave some back pain, the patient who expects a completely pain-free existence after the procedure is going to be sorely disappointed.

Finally, the surgeon needs to be sure that the patient understands all these aspects of surgical care and is willing to cooperate with whatever post-operative regimen is recommended to ensure an ideal outcome.

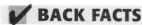 **BACK FACTS**

The vast majority of spinal conditions that come to surgery do not potentially threaten life or bodily function. Most spinal surgeries are relatively indicated, that is, their goal is to improve quality of life.

Basic Procedures

There are basically five things that can be done in spinal surgery:

Decompression

Pressure on nerves or the spinal cord produces symptoms including back pain, leg pain, numbness, and weakness. Pressure can arise secondary to pathology such as herniated disc material, bone spurs from arthritis, bone fragments from fractures, and invasive tumors. Surgical decompression aims to remove the structures causing compression, allowing the nerves to recover.

Stabilization

The spine can be stabilized. Fractures, a tumor, or severe degenerative changes may have compromised components of the spine that normally ensure stability. Regaining stability is typically carried out with the use of bone graft and instrumentation such as screws and rods in a procedure called a 'fusion'.

Straightening

Spinal deformity can be corrected. Deformity can result from abnormal growth, such as childhood scoliosis, or adult problems, including degeneration, fracture, infection, and tumor. This procedure involves straightening the spine and fusing it, again with the use of bone graft and metal hardware. Such surgeries may be extensive, requiring release of soft tissues that are preventing the correction of the deformity and removal of part of a vertebra.

Strengthening

Surgery can strengthen the bone by injecting bone cement. This is known as a vertebroplasty, used following collapse of a bony vertebra from osteoporosis or tumor.

Replacement

Disc replacement surgery shows great potential for back surgery but for now is still considered experimental.

Candidates for Back Surgery

There are some things that cannot be fixed with spinal surgery. An individual who has back pain resulting from degenerative changes at multiple levels is someone for whom we currently do not have a surgical answer. The elderly osteoporotic woman with multiple compression fractures and severe deformity secondary to old untreated scoliosis is also not someone we can help with an operation. In these individuals, successful outcome cannot be predicted and the risks far exceed the potential benefits.

Similarly, someone who has a surgically treatable problem, but has a serious medical condition, such as unstable heart disease or poor lung function, is also considered a poor candidate for surgery, because, once again, the risks far exceed the benefits. The individual who has had multiple surgeries but continues to experience severe ongoing back or leg pain with an MRI that demonstrates just a small amount of post-operative scarring is not someone who can be helped with additional surgery either.

Surgery can be of benefit, however, to reasonably healthy individuals who have distinct symptoms or patterns of pain secondary to readily identifiable pathology on X-ray, CT, or MRI that correlate well with their clinical presentation. Many people who have disc herniations on CT or MRI have no symptoms. By the same token, many people who have back pain have relatively normal imaging studies. The individual who has severe leg pain extending down to the foot, with accompanying numbness, and who demonstrates a well-defined focal disc herniation compressing a nerve root on the appropriate side is someone who has a surgically reversible lesion.

Disc Herniation

A disc herniation in an individual complaining of leg dominant pain is a surgically reversible lesion. A fragment of disc tissue, which looks and feels like crab meat, can be readily removed from the spinal canal and pressure taken off the nerve, resulting in dramatic relief of leg pain.

Spinal Stenosis

Older individuals who have severe leg pain when they walk most often have nerve compression secondary to spinal stenosis, again a surgically treatable lesion. Removal of bone spurs and disc material with decompression of the nerve roots results in reliable relief of lower extremity pain in well over 80% of individuals. Both of these procedures are relatively small, with a very low complication rate. Therefore, the essential criteria of benefit far greater than risk is readily met.

Disc Herniation Facts

Studies show that 95% of individuals who undergo surgery for disc herniation experience relief of most of their severe symptoms.

Degenerative Spondylolisthesis

Low back pain and leg pain made worse by walking secondary to what is known as a degenerative spondylolisthesis is also amenable to surgical intervention. This condition is most common in the older female. Wear and tear changes in the disc and the small joints allow the L4 vertebrae to slide forward on the L5 vertebrae, resulting in narrowing in the canal. Decompression and fusion is indicated. In the correctly selected patient, the benefits exceed the risks.

Surgical Techniques

Each of the various surgeries that are currently employed for the management of those individuals with surgically reversible lesions is presented here. For each surgery, indications, risks, benefits, and a typical post-operative course are discussed.

Discectomy

The indications for a discectomy are very specific. The majority of disc herniations resolve with the passage of time and conservative care. The NP material in the herniation dries out and shrinks in volume, some of it being absorbed by the body's immune system scavenger cells. However, approximately 25% of individuals with a disc herniation do not recover within a reasonable period of time. Those who get better on their own typically do so within 6 to 12 weeks. For those who still have severe disabling leg symptoms beyond that period of time, surgery is relatively indicated. Following discussion of the risks versus the benefits, most people opt for surgery. Studies have in fact demonstrated that in long-term follow-up at 1 to 4 years, those who opted for surgery did better with regards to pain and function than those who did not.

Procedures

There are different ways to achieve this. It can be done with a very large incision and removal of a significant portion of bone forming the posterior arch of the vertebrae. This older technique was successful most of the time but resulted in protracted rehabilitation. Newer techniques typically utilize a much smaller incision with reduced recovery time. Interestingly, despite this obvious advantage, the overall success rate has not improved with these newer methods. The currently accepted standard technique is the micro-discectomy, with or without use of the operating microscope.

Discectomy does not mean removal of the complete intervertebral disc. Rather, it refers to the removal of the portion of the central part of the disc or nucleus pulposus (NP) that has been extruded into the canal so as to compress a nerve root. With this procedure, the reliability of producing a positive outcome is quite high.

Indications

Within first 6 weeks:

• Disc herniation with cauda equina syndrome.

• Disc herniation with progressive nerve deficit.

After 6 weeks:

• Leg pain with/without numbness.

• Herniated disc on MRI/CT that correlates with clinical findings.

• Severe leg pain unresponsive to conservative treatment.

• Little or no back pain.

Percutaneous and endoscopic techniques with or without laser are being used extensively throughout the world with very little evidence that they are superior to the micro-discectomy. While most disc herniations can be treated by these so-called 'band-aid' procedures, large masses of extruded disc are not amenable to removal using these techniques. It should also be recognized that many of these procedures have not generated the success rates of the micro-discectomy, which is now the 'gold standard'. The drive to continue to use these 'band aid' techniques is primarily patient and market driven rather than scientifically proven. Private clinics, especially in the United States, offer these procedures for anywhere between $20,000 and $50,000. This kind of monetary reward, however, can result in the expansion of indications, resulting in the procedure being offered to individuals who are not candidates for any form of decompressive procedure. I have seen many people with back dominant pain, secondary to multi-level degenerative changes, making a pilgrimage to these clinics, returning with nothing more than a thinner wallet and, in some cases, an increase in their back pain.

A micro-discectomy is typically carried out through a 2.5 centimeter incision. The muscles are gently stripped off of the spine on the same side as the disc herniation. A small window is made in the ligamentum flavum, the yellow-tinged tissue between adjacent bony laminae. Little or no bone is resected. The nerve root that is being compressed by the disc is gently lifted off of the protrusion. A disc herniation looks somewhat like a giant pimple coming off the back of the disc. This pimple is burst and the crab-meat like NP material is removed. In cases where the herniated NP has separated and become sequestered, a more extensive exposure may be required to locate it.

Results

Removing the herniated disc takes pressure off the nerve and relieves the typical leg-dominant pain. Studies have shown that 95% of individuals report that the surgery is beneficial and has improved the quality of their life. Rarely does any operation make someone completely pain free forever. Approximately 15% of individuals report intermittent episodes of low back pain, although these are rarely severe enough to affect day-to-day function and most patients find they can cope with them.

This is not a complication of the surgery, but rather a manifestation of the disease process that caused the disc herniation in the first place. Ongoing degenerative changes in the disc or other discs may be the source of intermittent low back pain. Some individuals may be left with residual areas of numbness that again do not interfere with function.

Many discectomies can be carried out on an out-patient basis. Those who do not leave hospital the same day are typically discharged the following day. The surgery does not weaken the spine in any way, and patients are encouraged to assume all activities as quickly as possible. There is no need to impose any restriction to any activity. I recently had two patients who resumed competitive mountain biking and volleyball, one week after surgery!

Reports evaluating the outcome of surgical discectomy report success rates from 75% to 98% with respect to long-term pain relief and normal function. Interestingly, these figures are much lower in legal cases and workers' compensation injuries, with only 26% to 43% returning to work post-surgery. This demonstrates the impact of psychological and social issues on this condition. Overall recurrence rates following disc surgery are in the region of 5% to 8%.

Risks

With respect to the risks, any time an incision is made in the skin there is always a risk of infection. Bacteria from the air, even in an operating room, can enter the wound. A wound can also become seeded by bacteria from the patient's own blood stream. The infection rate for this procedure, however, is very low, rated at less than 0.5%. Most of the time it presents as a superficial wound infection that recovers quickly with oral antibiotics. Notably, 1/500 to 1/1000 cases develop a disc space infection or discitis. This is best managed with further surgery to clean out the infection along with intravenous antibiotics. Again in most cases, a positive outcome ensues without any serious long-term sequelae.

During spinal surgery there is always a risk of injury to the nerve root. If this were to happen, then one may be left with a focal area of numbness and weakness in a specific muscle group. Despite 'folklore' to the contrary, this does not result in paralysis and a life spent permanently in a wheel-chair. The risk of a serious nerve root injury occurring is less than 1/1000.

Recurrent disc herniation can occur. At the time of the surgery we do not attempt to remove the entire nucleus or center of the disc. We only remove the material that is herniated or detached. However, as time passes, further disc degeneration can result in the expulsion of more of the nucleus. In most cases this settles with conservative care, but if not, it is again amenable to surgical intervention. The success rate of surgery for recurrent disc herniation is equally high.

Micro-Discectomy

Positive Predictors for Success Following Surgery
- No work-related injury.
- No or minimal back pain.
- Pain extending to the foot.
- Leg pain with SLR (straight leg raise).
- No back pain with SLR.
- Size of disc herniation.
- Good social/family support.

Spinal Stenosis Surgery

The two procedures carried out for spinal stenosis are 'decompression', the removal of any bone, disc or ligament compressing nervous structures, and 'decompression with fusion', in which vertebrae are fused together (joined with bone) in addition to the decompression. The decision as to which operation to perform is based on an evaluation of the 'stability' of the segment of spine being operated upon.

In the absence of instability, such as spondylolisthesis, there appears to be no benefit to performing a fusion. Studies comparing decompression/fusion surgery with decompression alone in patients *without* instability show that outcomes were identical, with 80% getting good results regardless of whether or not fusion had been performed.

Decompression

This surgical procedure involves the removal of bone, disc material, or ligament that may be compressing nervous structures. Pre-operative CT or MRI will demonstrate those areas of significant narrowing. Surgery addresses the areas that are clinically relevant; there needs to be a good match between the imaging studies and the patient's clinical presentation. Original surgical technique involved removal of a large amount of bone, including the spinous processes as well as the laminae. We now know that this may in fact be too extensive and may result in instability and chronic low back pain. Recent studies have demonstrated that more conservative bone removal still results in excellent outcome without the potential problems of more expansive resection. The average length of stay in hospital is also lower with this type of procedure.

Procedure

Typically a mid-line posterior incision is made measuring 3 to 10 centimeters in length, depending on the number of vertebral levels involved. In most cases, the muscle is stripped from just one side of the spine and small port-holes are made in the bone, removing only those elements that are compressing the nerves. This reduces the amount of post-operative pain, improves recovery time, and minimizes blood loss.

Results

Overall, decompression for degenerative spinal stenosis results in over 80% of individuals reporting significant post-operative reduction in walking-related leg pain. Again, one must have reasonable expectations. Walking tolerance may not be completely unlimited and other medical conditions may play a part in this. Most report, however, that their quality of life has been significantly improved. A degree of ongoing low back pain may persist, especially if this was a major feature pre-operatively. Generally, however, it is tolerable compared to the lower extremity symptoms experienced pre-operatively.

The post-operative course is typically one of early mobilization and most leave hospital within 1 to 3 days. Again, there are usually no medical restrictions to activity, and patients are strongly encouraged to regain normal physical strength and flexibility through an active program of exercise post-operatively.

Risks

With respect to surgical risk, there is always a risk of infection rated at 0.5% superficially and 1/500 for a deep wound. There is always a risk of injury to the nerve, but this risk is low. Some individuals do not experience any neural recovery despite an adequate decompression and these individuals may continue to have lower extremity symptoms. Although spinal stenosis does not typically paralyze an individual or put them in a wheel chair, the more profound the weakness and sensory loss in the extremities, the more difficult it is for full recovery to occur.

Decompression with Fusion

In the event that there is spinal instability associated with the stenosis, either a degenerative spondylolisthesis or a symptomatic isthmic slip in a younger individual, decompression is combined with fusion.

Degenerative spondylolisthesis most often results in the forward slip of L4 on L5. This results in narrowing of the canal and can produce a secondary spinal stenosis. These individuals typically experience both back and lower extremity pain when they walk or stand for prolonged periods of time. For many individuals, the symptoms are at a nuisance level, and obviously there is no indication for any aggressive intervention. For some, however, it can severely affect quality of life. For the patient, this is technically a more physically demanding surgical procedure than micro-discectomy or simple decompression for stenosis. Therefore, it is indicated only in those individuals who are medically healthy and expected to go through the procedure without any medical complications. Chronological age is not necessarily a limiting factor but one's 'physiological' age is. The obese smoker with severe coronary artery disease would not be a good candidate for this procedure, regardless of age.

Fusion Facts

Fusion or arthrodesis means joining two mobile spinal segments together so they no longer move. This is achieved by using bone graft to create a bony bridge between the vertebrae. Metal hardware may be used to fix the vertebra until the bone has knitted together.

Procedure

The operation involves a mid-line incision, typically with stripping of the muscles on both sides of the spine. The spinous processes and laminae are removed. Most often screws are placed into L4 and L5 and linked together by rods. This prevents any further slipping of L4 and L5 after removal of the bone compressing the nerves. Bone graft is then packed on either side of the spine. This can be obtained from the pelvis or it can be the local bone that is removed as part of the decompression and ground into small particles. Small titanium cages can be placed into the disc space packed with bone graft to further increase the likelihood of achieving fusion. This is known as a posterior lumbar inter-body fusion. Surgery typically takes 2 to 3 hours. The patient is in hospital anywhere from 3 to 5 days, and again early post-operative mobilization is encouraged. Aggressive physical activity is refrained from for approximately 3 to 6 months until the surgeon is happy that bony union has occurred.

Results

Studies show that 80% to 85% of individuals are pleased with the relief of symptoms. Invariably, there are residual symptoms, but at a level that most can cope with compared to their pre-operative symptomatology.

Risks

The risks of the surgery again include infection rated at 0.5% superficially and 1/500 chance of developing a deep wound infection. Nerve injuries are relatively rare, rated at much less than 1%. Depending on the techniques used, the chances of the bone graft not healing is anywhere from zero to 10%. Using metal instrumentation increases the likelihood of healing while smoking reduces it considerably. This latter factor is so important your surgeon may refuse to perform the procedure unless you quit. If the bone graft does not heal, the screws will eventually loosen and break, or if inter-body cages are used they too may also loosen or migrate. However, these cases are unusual, and the vast majority go on to fuse uneventfully.

Decompression with fusion is a much bigger procedure than decompression alone, and as there is a significant component of post-operative pain, recovery can be more protracted. Certainly for the first 6 weeks, most patients are somewhat grumpy, although they may notice an early improvement in their leg symptoms. Usually by the 3-month mark, patients are a little bit happier that they have had the procedure done, but it can really take a full year before they ultimately plateau with respect to their recovery. In the interim, however, they are active, mobile, and independent in self-care.

At the 3-month mark, if all is well radiologically, and evidence of bony union is occurring, then a more aggressive exercise program is usually instituted. The patient at this point will be stiff and weak, and the exercise program is aimed at reversing that. Many are able resume all the activities that they were able to participate in pre-operatively. The surgery does not in any way weaken the spine; in fact, the area that is fused with instrumentation can be compared to re-inforced concrete. I always tell patients that if they were to be hit by a bus, in all likelihood they would fracture the areas above and below the fusion. This, of course, is only to reassure them that although they have had surgery, they are not fragile!

Spondylolytic Spondylolisthesis Surgery

The younger adult with symptoms related to vertebral instability most often has a condition known as a spondylolytic spondylolisthesis. This most commonly occurs at the bottom of the spine, with L5 slipping forward on the sacrum (S1), as opposed to L4 on L5 in the degenerative type. This is usually due to a developmental condition that we know is genetic.

Many people inherit a genetic weakness in the back portion of the L5 vertebrae. Typically, around the age of 5 or 6 years old, this area of the vertebrae can break much like a fatigue fracture that occurs when one continually bends an area of a coat hanger. Most children do not experience any symptoms. During their growth spurt, because this fracture has not healed, the front of this vertebrae can separate from the back and slip forward on the sacrum below. Again, many children do not experience any symptoms, but as they grow older this may accelerate degenerative changes at that level, producing pain in adulthood. That pain may be initiated by a minor event or may come on spontaneously.

Some children have quite severe forward slippage of L5 and S1 and they are typically symptomatic at a younger age. Again, surgery may be indicated in those individuals, especially if it is apparent that they may be predisposed to further slip, although it should be borne in mind that most children have reached maximal slip at the time of clinical presentation.

Procedure

The surgery for this condition is quite similar to the surgery described for degenerative spondylolisthesis. A mid-line incision is made with muscle stripping on both sides, typically with the insertion of screws into L5 and the sacrum, which

Spondylolytic Spondylolisthesis Surgery Facts

In many cases of spondylolytic spondylolisthesis, the pain can be controlled with an aggressive exercise program and by maintaining a high level of physical fitness. For those individuals who, despite this, have on-going symptoms that are disabling, then they may again opt for elective surgical stabilization with an understanding of the risks versus the benefits.

Indications
• Low back pain associated with spondylolisthesis not relieved by non-surgical treatment.

• Spondylolisthesis associated with nerve compression.

are then joined by rods. Again, bone graft is placed on either side of the spine, and intra-body cages may or may not be used. Bone graft may be obtained from the back of the pelvis or it may be local bone that has been removed.

Results

Studies show that 80–90% of patients report relief of the pre-operative symptoms, including severe low back pain and, in most cases, referred pain to the lower extremity on prolonged walking or standing. The post-operative protocol is similar to that described for degenerative spondylolisthesis. This group, however, tends to be younger individuals and may rebound faster. Again, once recovery is complete, resumption of normal activity is strongly encouraged with no need for imposed restrictions.

Spinal Fusion for Degenerative Disc Disease (DDD)

Second only to the controversy surrounding the diagnosis of degenerative disc disease (DDD) as a cause of low back pain is that concerning surgery for this condition. Of the 10% of patients with acute back pain who develop chronicity, about 40% are found to have DDD as evidenced by examination, MRI, and discography. Of these about 30% do not respond to conservative measures. That leaves about 1 in 100 individuals in this age group who develop acute back pain as eventually being a candidate for surgical fusion. With a population of 15 million adults in the age bracket 20–50 in Canada, for example, and an incidence of acute back pain of 50%, that makes about 90,000 patients per year eligible for surgical consideration! This figure is both impractical and improbable. A marked reduction in this number results from both patients unwilling to consider surgery and patients not suitable for any number of reasons.

Indications for surgery include chronic, disabling back pain unresponsive to an adequate trial of conservative treatment. There should be no evidence of disc herniation, and positive degenerative MRI findings should correlate with discographic symptoms and the overall clinical picture. In addition, there should be no underlying significant psychological factors because these should definitely be addressed prior to any surgical intervention. Of course, these indications are only guidelines, and each case should be taken on its individual merits.

Procedure

The most common procedure for fusion in DDD is postero-lateral decortication (removal of hard surface bone to expose soft inner spongy bone) and bone grafting with or without metal instrumentation. This is similar to the technique described above for 'decompression with fusion', although in this case the decompression is not generally required. Newer techniques approach the fusion from the front of the spine via the abdomen and may use open surgical exposure or laparoscopy (small incisions with fiber-optic visualization). These so-called 'anterior interbody fusions' often employ metallic hardware or 'cages' filled with bone graft to achieve fusion.

Results

Although the techniques to achieve fusion have improved and have become extremely reliable, we have not been able to demonstrate a reliable reduction in low back pain with this procedure. A study in 2000 found no clear scientific evidence to support decompression or fusion for treatment of DDD. Individual studies, however, have found it to benefit a high proportion (nearly 90%) of carefully selected patients; it is likely that this selection process is the key. For example, fusion is a very useful option for individuals with isolated, severe degenerative changes at L5/S1 and with the remainder of the spine looking quite healthy.

Although between 55% and 90% of individuals report initial relief of symptoms, recent literature indicates that this number may deteriorate over the course of a few years. Some may go on to develop degenerative changes at adjacent levels. Whether or not this is secondary to the fusion itself, or merely a manifestation of the natural history of the disease process, is unknown. The relevance of this finding is also controversial. One paper compared patients who had spinal fusion for DDD to those who had other, non-fusion surgery. They found that 20 years later, although disc degeneration above and below the level of the fusion was twice as common in the fusion group on X-rays, there was no difference in clinical outcome.

Nevertheless, there is a role for spinal fusion in DDD. Research over the next few years should more clearly define its role and the specific group of patients it is likely to benefit.

Artificial Disc Replacement

Although spinal fusion remains the most popular and accepted surgery for degenerative disc disease (DDD), it is not ideal. It alters motion, biomechanics, and stress across the remaining spine and may induce degeneration at other levels. Fusion at other joints, such as the hip and the knee, was originally popular but has now been almost abandoned due to the success of joint replacement arthroplasty. It is hoped that this may also be the future for disc degeneration.

Artificial disc replacement is an exciting field but is still very much at the experimental level. Despite a long list of implant prototypes, few have made it as far as animal studies and even fewer to human implantation. Ongoing clinical studies in Europe, South America, the Middle East, and North America are evaluating a number of these techniques and products.

Procedure

There are basically two distinct types of artificial disc: the 'true' disc replacement and the 'nuclear' replacement. Surgery for the true disc replacement involves complete removal of the disc via an approach through the abdominal cavity. The replacement is designed with two metal discs and an intervening plastic component, much like that seen in artificial hip or knee replacements. The nuclear replacement involves removal only of the central part of the disc, typically via a small posterior approach, and the implantation of a hydro-gel, which absorbs local water and swells, thereby partially rebuilding a degenerative disc, improving its overall load bearing capabilities.

Results

Preliminary results from Europe suggest a 70–80% success rate for both procedures, but unfortunately many complications have been described. The most significant complication is migration of the implant out of its position in the spine. The technique is currently applicable only to individuals with single level disease, not for the person with wear and tear changes at multiple levels or with previous back surgery. Artificial disc replacement is currently only available in a few select centers and then only as part of a clinical trial. A very extensive informed consent must be understood and agreed to by the patient before undertaking in any surgery.

With further study and improvements in both implants and technique, this procedure may very well be available for widespread clinical use one day. However, as with any back surgery, the indications will be limited and patients will have to be carefully selected to ensure good results. While a useful tool in the surgical armamentarium, no one expects this to be the 'cure' for back pain. Its use will be in the individual with focal, single-level disease. This comprises only a minority of individuals with spinal problems.

Vertebroplasty

In the early 1980s, a French surgeon described the injection of bone cement into the vertebrae of a woman with an osteoporotic compression fracture who had abnormally persistent pain. This resulted in the marked relief of her symptoms and the technique of vertebroplasty was born. This technique has gained popularity in North America as a means of treating the increasing number of compression fractures in an aging population. There are an estimated 700,000 per year in the United States, 85% of which are related to osteoporosis. One third give rise to chronic pain.

While many osteoporotic compression fractures improve over the course of 6 to 12 weeks, they may take as long as a year to recover fully. Some individuals may experience ongoing, disabling pain, and there is some evidence that in certain cases this is due to inadequate healing or progressive deformity. The functional impairment this condition imposes upon already-frail individuals results in significant morbidity.

For those with an isolated, one-level fracture or even fractures limited to less than three levels, vertebroplasty may be

Vertebroplasty Facts

The results of vertebroplasty are encouraging with rapid pain relief (within 24 hours) in 90% of patients and significant improvements in function and mobility.

a treatment option. Although attempts have been made to perform this procedure at more than three levels, they have not proved effective. Similarly, results in patients with compression fracture due to tumor have only met with limited pain relief.

Procedure

The vertebroplasty procedure is carried out under local anesthesia by an interventional radiologist. Under X-ray or CT guidance, a hollow metal tube is inserted from the back, through the pedicle of the vertebrae and into the vertebral body. Bone cement (PMMA or polymethyl methacrylate), the same material used to fix hip and knee replacements, is then injected under pressure. This helps make the vertebra stronger and stiffer, resulting in pain relief in most individuals.

Results

Vertebroplasty provides an excellent option for elderly patients and may substantially reduce hospitalization and disability for this growing orthopedic problem.

Risks

There are a number of potential risks associated with this procedure. There is a risk of cement extrusion into the spinal canal causing significant nerve compression. Management of this complication may involve a surgical procedure to remove the cement. The cement gets very hot as it hardens, which may cause thermal injury. Cement particles can get into the bloodstream through vessels in the spine and cause problems in the lungs. Overall the complication rate is approximately 6%.

Kyphoplasty

Kyphoplasty is another technique developed over the past few years to treat osteoporotic compression fractures. While vertebroplasty is able to restore strength to the fractured vertebra, it does not correct deformity caused by the bony collapse. In addition, vertebroplasty requires the cement to be injected at high pressure, which increases the risk of extravasation (leakage into areas it is not wanted). In one recent paper, although serious consequences were extremely rare, leaks occurred in 30–80% of all procedures.

Procedure

Kyphoplasty involves insertion of an inflatable balloon into the vertebral body using a similar X-ray guided technique to that of vertebroplasty. The balloon can be inflated, thus restoring vertebral height and correcting deformity. Once this is achieved, cement can be injected at low pressure.

Results

Early results of this relatively new technique are promising with pain relief equal to or better than vertebroplasty and significant reversal of deformity as long as the procedure is performed within three months of the fracture occurring. While kyphoplasty appears to offer advantages over vertebroplasty, to date there have been no randomized clinical trials comparing the two techniques.

External Fixation for Low Back Pain

An external fixator is a rigid device used to link two bones or parts of a bone (in the case of fracture) together, thus preventing movement. The frame is attached to the bone via heavy pins that penetrate the skin, while the main device sits on the surface. These constructs are used quite extensively in fracture care, where it is impossible or inadvisable to use internal fixation devices such as plates and screws that normally lie under the skin. The external fixator holds the bone fragments until they are healed, at which point the entire frame and pin system is removed.

 BACK FACTS

The original concept of external fixation in low back pain was to immobilize two adjacent vertebrae reversibly in order to determine whether the particular disc or motion segment between them was causing pain. If it was, then more formal immobilization could be performed using a spinal fusion. Despite the attractiveness of this theory, external fixation has not proved practical and is no longer used.

Dr Charles Gregory is a psychiatrist and specialist in neurosurgery. He founded the Pacific Centre for Human Development as well as the Columbia Center for Integrated Health Services.

Chronic Pain Management

Charles Gregory, MB, ChB, FRCP(C)

During the past 40 years, more advances have been made in our understanding of the mechanics of nerve transmission of what are still called pain impulses than in the past two millennia, but the fundamental question has not been definitively answered, 'What is pain?' Nor have we found the final answer to preventing pain, though we have made great advances in managing its effects, notably in the management of back pain.

What Is Pain?

Since Rene Descartes in the 17th century — and for probably a long time before — the predominant belief about pain has been that physical events happening in the body from some tissue damage are somehow detected and this information is somehow transmitted to the brain. Concerning this detection and this transmission, the current opinion is split. One theory holds that events happen in the body that are detected by pain receptor nerve endings, which transmit the information to the brain via the spinal cord, which is registered by the cortex merely as mental representations of the pain stimulus in the periphery. In this definition of pain, a pain stimulus leads to pure sensation, which then leads to perception.

Traditional Pain Definition Limitations

The traditional definition of pain as a simple stimulus-sensation-perception process is limited, for several reasons:

Injury can occur without causing pain

This is seen most clearly in those who have a congenital inability to feel pain no matter how destructive the changes in the tissues. But it is also true that normal people can suffer injury without feeling pain, at least for some minutes or hours afterwards. A study in Montreal found that 37% of the people arriving at the emergency clinic of a large general hospital with a variety of injuries, including amputated fingers, minor lacerations, and fractured bones, reported that they did not feel any pain for varying lengths of time following the injury.

Back Pain Treatment Strategies

Pain can occur without injury
Again, this phenomenon is seen most clearly in congenital disorders, but also in those without physical pathology to support the complaints of pain.

Experienced pain may be totally disproportionate to the degree of injury to the tissues
There are such things as the 'exquisite' pain of gout or of passing a kidney stone. In the latter case, the ureter (tube from the kidney to the bladder) through which the stones pass is very poorly innervated, and it sends relatively few messages to the brain. Yet the pain is excruciating.

Phantom limb pain is real
There is a very puzzling phenomenon that often occurs after amputation of a limb — the feeling that the limb is still there, but without any sensory input from the limb itself. This is called 'phantom limb pain,' not ' phantom pain,' for it is the limb that is a phantom — the pain is all too real. This can happen very soon after an operation or injury but is often delayed. Frequently, quite severe pain can develop in the 'phantom limb'. This is somewhat more puzzling than the phantom sensation itself, for our classic interpretation of pain is tissue injury and clearly in this instance there is no tissue to act as a source of input.

There are great variations in the experience of pain from person to person and culture to culture
Stimuli that may produce excruciating pain for one person will be easily tolerated by another. Similarly there are wide differences between cultures in the way they cope with and express pain.

Pain perception changes with the meaning of the situation
As a result of observations during the Second World War, one doctor discovered that that "there is no simple direct relationship between the wound per se, and the pain experienced. The pain is very largely determined by other factors and, of great importance here, is the significance of the wound. In the wounded soldier the response to injury was relief, thankfulness at his escape alive from the battlefield, even euphoria. To the civilian, surgery was a depressing, calamitous event." Thus the civilian demanded five times the amount of narcotic medication and made many times more complaints about severe pain than did soldiers with comparable injuries.

Suggestion and placebos reduce pain
About 35% of patients in one study and even up to 50% in another reported marked relief after being given placebo (a substance which is biologically inert and exerts no direct effect on tissues). This is striking because morphine relieves severe pain in only 75% of individuals, even in very high doses. Another interesting fact is that placebos always demonstrate 50% of the effectiveness of the particular drug under study, even in double-blind experiments. The major factor operating here appears to be the expectation of the individual receiving the placebo, and again this exemplifies the fact that pain is not simply a sensation anchored in the body tissues.

Hypnosis reduces pain
These effects can be very dramatic, and even major surgery has been performed using only hypnosis as the anesthetic. The most celebrated example is that of Victor Rausch, a dentist from Waterloo, who had his gall bladder removed under self-hypnosis and immediately after the operation climbed down from the table and walked down the corridor with the surgeon and the observing, but inactive, anesthetist on either side. The whole performance was recorded on videotape and played over the TV networks.

Another theory is based on the definition of pain proposed by the International Association for the Study of Pain (IASP) as "an unpleasant sensory and emotional experience associated with actual or potential tissue damage or described in terms of such damage. Pain is always subjective ... This definition avoids tying pain to the stimulus." In this definition, the word 'pain' covers several dimensions — sensory, affective, and emotional. Pain is seen as something much more complex than stimulus and response.

The relationship between the stimulus, whether applied externally or whether due to tissue damage, and the experience of pain is highly complex. There are obviously many factors involved in the cause of pain not necessarily related to the presence of injury. There are equally as many factors involved in managing pain.

The word 'pain' is best used for any kind of noxious or harmful experience. This experience doesn't necessarily have to come from bodily injury. It can arise from any other set of events that evoke a similar experience, and one of the most frequent examples of this is the profound pain that a depressed

Characteristics of Acute Pain vs Chronic Pain

Physiological

Acute	Chronic
Primary	
Symptomatic evidence of dysfunction with or without evidence of tissue damage	Increasing dysfunction, pathological changes and complications
Tissues involved tend to remain localized	Tendency to involve ever wider areas
Duration limited with gradual return to normal	Duration uncertain and may be permanent
Secondary	
Generally reversible	Not usually reversible
General level of conditioning approximates to demands of daily life	Poor general condition consistent with minimum physical activity Obesity — rarely weight loss

Psychological

Acute	Chronic
Anxious	Anxious+++ Depressed
Oriented to the world	Oriented towards possible exacerbating events and possible sources of relief
Cognition and abstract reasoning unaffected	Often seriously impaired

person experiences. Individuals who have attempted suicide often express the pain they were suffering. But pain can happen to some after, say, a love affair gone wrong. Pain is a metaphor that we apply to experiences that have the quality that a physical injury would create but without the injury.

The traditional approach to understanding pain, which insists on finding the specific causes and applying specific remedies, is overly simplistic and often highly erroneous, especially when applied to chronic pain. One of the most pernicious consequences of the belief that pain is a sensation felt in the tissue where it happens is the 'logical' step to the proposition that there cannot be any pain without tissue damage. This view has led to chronic pain being dismissed as not being 'real' because the sensation or tissue damage cannot be detected or traced.

Acute vs Chronic Pain

Acute and chronic pain conditions are two entirely different phenomena. In themselves, both conditions are also complex.

Sociological

Acute	Chronic
Confined by nature of tissue damage	Less social contacts not related tissue damage
Eagerness for social contact after initial shock	Increasing withdrawal from all forms of social activity
Family relations may be impaired	Steady deterioration with increasing dependency and disability
Sexual activity limited only by nature of specific disability	Reduced and often absent

Treatment Response

Acute	Chronic
Medical and surgical methods usually very effective	Often ineffective or at best palliative
Side effects temporary	Can be detrimental

Vocational

Acute	Chronic
Dominated by immediate situation	Consider themselves unemployable

Spiritual

Acute	Chronic
Self-image intact	Despairing, helpless, defeated
World seen as actually or potentially pleasurable	World seen as a source of suffering

Acute Back Pain

Concerning acute back pain, Dr R.A. Deyo has commented in *Scientific American* that "the prospects for patients with acute back pain are quite good. The bad news is that recurrences are common. Fortunately, these recurrences tend to play out much as the original incidents did and most patients recover again quickly and spontaneously." Dr W.H. Kirkaldy-Willis likewise describes the on-again, off-again nature of acute back pain in his book *Managing Low Back Pain*, based on his personal as well as his clinical experience. "The writer has had three attacks of moderately severe low back pain over a period of 25 years," he notes. "On no occasion was he aware of more than minimal trauma. On two occasions he had been under tension and stress. This parallels the experience of may people with low back pain." These are two excellent accounts of recurrent acute pain. Often the onset of acute pain follows trauma, but case histories often show that patients who develop low back pain have often been under stress before experiencing pain and that the episode of trauma resulting in pain is minor. An interval of hours or days may intervene between the perceived episode of trauma and the onset of pain.

Many who have had one bout of acute back pain have occasional recurrences, often after considerable lapse of time, but what defines this as acute recurrent and not chronic is that after an acute episode is over, there is no 'hangover' of physical or emotional symptoms. Management of these acute episodes is successful in preventing the development of chronic pain.

But not all patients are so lucky, as Dr Simon Carette observes. "Acute back pain is usually self-limited and the majority of patients do not seek medical advice," he notes. "Of those who do, more than 90% improve and are back to work within two months. The 5% to 10% of patients who remain disabled after this time present a difficult challenge due to the influence of psychological and social factors on the continuation of pain. This small percentage are responsible for more than 75% of the total costs of low back pain to our society, estimated to be more than $50 billion in the U.S. in 1990." Thus, chronic pain syndrome is much more difficult to manage than recurring acute back pain.

Chronic Pain Syndrome

Chronic pain syndrome commonly starts off with an injury, the severity of which may vary enormously and may not have any direct relationship with the development of chronicity.

Typically, following an accident, an individual will be examined and investigated. A diagnosis will be made and conveyed to the patient, who not only is in severe pain but also in the throes of an acute traumatic reaction and intensely anxious over the uncertainty of the outcome, not only as it has a personal impact but also as it has an impact on the patient's family. This all adds to the intensity of the experience of pain.

Traditionally, various medications are prescribed, and the patient is either admitted to hospital or sent home with strict instructions, possibly to rest and to avoid movements that cause pain. However, the worst possible instruction is to avoid movement when it is precisely that immobility that puts the first foot on the slippery slope to chronicity.

The admonition not to move, added to all the other sources of anxiety, conspire to create an increase in tension. Shortening of the muscles develops, creating pressure on the blood supply, which along with the vasoconstriction produces 'trigger point zones'. These have the microscopic appearance of tissues subjected to experimental ischaemia — the deliberate starving of blood to muscular tissues. Many patients fail to believe that pressure could produce such pain, but they often reconsider when it is explained that the universal experience of muscle cramps (a 10 out of 10 pain on anyone's scale) is due to inadequate blood supply to muscle tissue.

Acute Stress Response

The acute stress response is the body's natural response to threatening internal or external change — the 'fight or flight' response. When the emergency is over, the body returns to its former state. Imagine you are at home watching television when suddenly there is a shout from the kitchen: "Fire." You jump up, dash into the kitchen, grab a fire extinguisher, and put out the flames arising from burning fat in the frying pan, after which you ensure that everyone is uninjured and the damage caused only slight. You settle down to relax again.

During such emergencies, the entire body is transformed so as to provide energy in the form of glucose and oxygen needed for the emergency. There is a fast shift in the distribution of the blood to carry energy to the lungs, muscles, and brain. The immune system is inhibited, the thought processes speed up, sensitivity to external events increases, and the experience of pain may be dulled. These are very dramatic changes. If they had to be sustained for a long period, sooner or later exhaustion would set in. Once the emergency is over, the whole system settles down and returns to a balanced state. There is no persistence of this 'fight or flight' overactivity.

This 'acute' stress response is perfectly normal. The ability to perform like this is a condition of survival any time an emergency arises.

Chronic Pain Syndrome Facts

The development of a chronic pain syndrome has an identifiable course into which one can slide with deceptive ease.

Stress Response

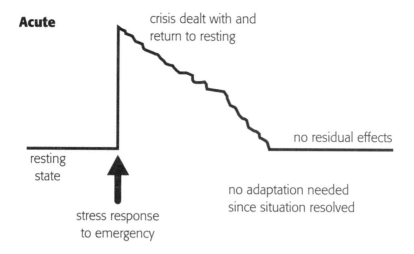

Acute

resting
state

stress response
to emergency

crisis dealt with and
return to resting

no residual effects

no adaptation needed
since situation resolved

Chronic

situation unresolved (e.g. job, relationship)
no full return to resting
accumulated stress
adaptation to breakdown

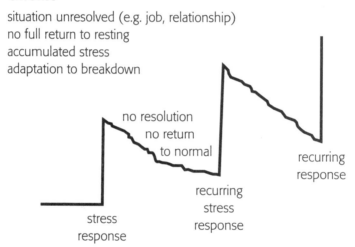

no resolution
no return
to normal

stress
response

recurring
stress
response

recurring
response

Exhaustion

85% of us die of chronic illness
15% from accidents homicides suicides

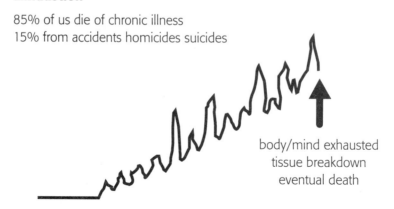

body/mind exhausted
tissue breakdown
eventual death

Chronic Stress Response

The 'chronic' stress response is a very different process altogether. Instead of returning to a balanced state after the emergency, the body remains in a state of stress. Much of our life is spent dealing with situations that do not resolve, cannot be controlled, and recur. Whether these involve balancing rigorous and unmanageable work and family schedules, wrestling with financial worries, or struggling with relationship problems, they all show little hope of rapid resolution. Instead of intermittent respite from this stress, your body simply keeps raising the level of ongoing tension. Your health begins to deteriorate — stomach troubles, migraine headaches, menstrual irregularities — everything seems to conspire to drive you into the ground. Anxiety and depression can follow.

This is more the rule than the exception. In industrial countries, 85% of us die of a chronic disease. We are all training very hard to acquire the illness that will kill us. This chronic stress response is a huge factor in the development of chronic pain.

Pain-Tension-Anxiety (PTA) Cycle

The result is the creation of a PTA (pain-tension-anxiety) cycle that defines chronic pain. Once the first increase in tension begins, every aspect of living becomes a potential source of yet another stress response. Possible loss of a job leads to economic anxiety and fear of what the future holds. Physically there is general deterioration, maybe weight gain or loss, insomnia, poor general conditioning. Profound changes in family relationships, withdrawal from external social contacts, onset and deepening of serious depression are almost inevitable. Contacts with agencies that are supposed to help with any of these developments seem to go sour and institutional red-tape and inertia simply intensify the frustration. Continued use of increasingly potent medication or even certain therapy modalities may result in dependency. Add to all this the fact that the pain does not seem to go away and indeed often gets worse. The individual is on a downward spiral of deterioration and desperation.

Until the 1960s, the outlook for anyone caught in this devastating process of chronic pain was grim. Despite the considerable advances that have been made in both understanding the nature of the chronic pain process, these have not yet become the accepted basis of clinical practice.

Pain-Tension-Anxiety (PTA) Cycle

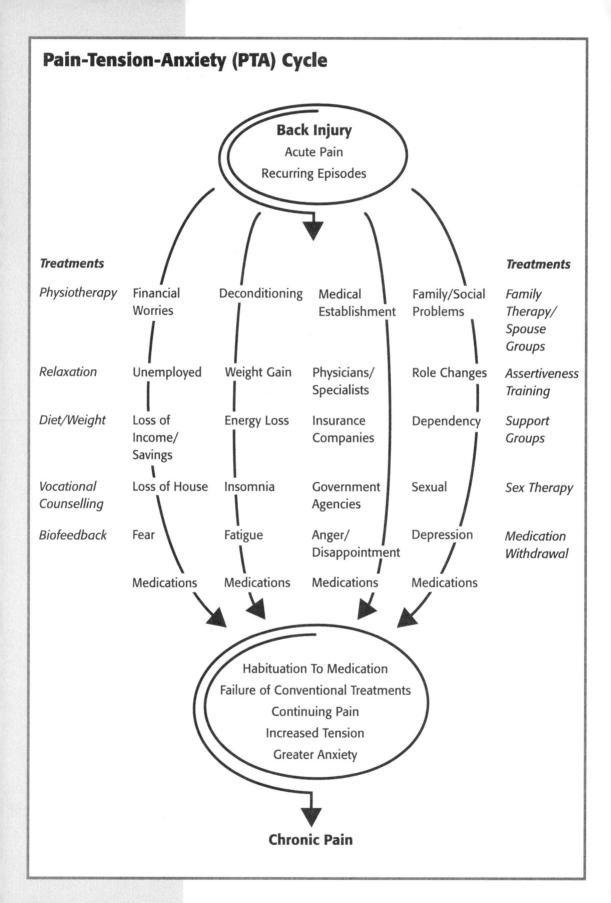

Back Injury
Acute Pain
Recurring Episodes

Treatments

Physiotherapy — Financial Worries — Deconditioning — Medical Establishment — Family/Social Problems — *Family Therapy/ Spouse Groups*

Relaxation — Unemployed — Weight Gain — Physicians/ Specialists — Role Changes — *Assertiveness Training*

Diet/Weight — Loss of Income/ Savings — Energy Loss — Insurance Companies — Dependency — *Support Groups*

Vocational Counselling — Loss of House — Insomnia — Government Agencies — Sexual — *Sex Therapy*

Biofeedback — Fear — Fatigue — Anger/ Disappointment — Depression — *Medication Withdrawal*

Medications — Medications — Medications — Medications

Habituation To Medication
Failure of Conventional Treatments
Continuing Pain
Increased Tension
Greater Anxiety

Chronic Pain

PTA Cycle Case History

This case exemplifies almost all of the aspects of the PTA cycle and the all-encompassing process chronic pain can become:

A 42-year-old married woman with one child had been injured in a car accident 9 years earlier. The injuries were to her lower spine, and although there were no actual fractures, she apparently had a prolapsed intervertebral disc. An operation was done which only made things worse — more pain, more limitation of movement, more medication — and eventually she wound up in a wheelchair. The painful physical experiences were accompanied by the reverberations of items on the PTA cycle, especially those of deterioration of family relationships.

This was a woman was highly competent, an excellent employee, highly regarded in the community, the dominant member of the family who ran it like a naval commander, with a profound belief in herself and her ability to deal with any kind of problem. Within two months of the accident she had begun the process of deterioration, which included an inability to return to work, a consequent lowering of the family's financial status, withdrawal from social and church activities, and dramatically changed family relationships. She had gone from being the rock on which her husband and 6-year-old daughter depended to being increasingly dependent on them.

The surgery, several months after the accident, merely accelerated the decline, until she had to use a wheel chair. This led to her husband building ramps and other devices to facilitate her ability to move around the house, which they called their 'paraplegic house'. Her daughter had to do all the housework and by the girl's 15th birthday, she had gone through 9 years of living with a seriously disabled mother and had missed much of what a young girl would normally have experienced. Father had eventually given up his job to become nurse to his wife with the previous dependency status being completely reversed.

Inevitably, her self-image was shattered, her confidence gone, and her fears of a future — it only looked like more of the same — or worse. By this time she was profoundly depressed.

Eventually, someone suggested she be referred to our clinic, and we decided to interview her despite the dismal history. I recall that while she was sitting in the wheel chair after we (the orthopedic surgeon, the physiotherapist, and I) had discussed her case, she looked at us in disbelief when we said, "We will accept you into the program on condition that you are able to get up out of the wheel chair and move on your feet — with assistance, of course."

She didn't believe this was possible. However, we were convinced that she could, and after some further discussion, she decided to give it a try. Six weeks later this woman was able to touch her toes with ease, to stand and walk with an erect back. She had blossomed like a tropical flower. So far so good.

She returned for several follow-up sessions over a period of 4 months and grew progressively confident and optimistic about her future. But then problems began to surface in the family during the weekly spouse groups we held with patients and their 'significant other'. Her husband had no job now and she didn't need or want any dependency on him. In fact, she wanted a return to her former status, and he simply couldn't handle this. He found it difficult to find a job, and without care-giving he no longer had purpose in life, so he became increasingly depressed. Her daughter, who was in many respects more mature than her years, felt that her relationship with her mother had now deteriorated as her mother took over all the responsibilities the daughter had performed for so long. So 6 months after mother's dramatic recovery, father was being treated for major depression and they all were attending the clinic for family therapy.

Multi-Disciplinary Treatment

The typical way of dealing with chronic pain is to visit a physician, who goes through the routine of history, examination, investigations, advice, prescriptions for medication, and sometimes referral to a 'back' specialist, a physiotherapist, a rheumatologist, or a back surgeon. But there is also a need to involve multi-disciplinary professionals trained in sociology, social work, psychology, and vocational rehabilitation in dealing with chronic pain. Unfortunately, there is little awareness of the possible therapeutic contribution these non-medical disciplines can make and the probability of referrals to them is low.

How does this work out in practice? The following answers are valid whether you are an individual attempting to manage your own chronic pain, are consistently involved with one of more varied professionals on an ongoing basis, or are part of a program at a multi-disciplinary pain center. This is not a static program that does not vary: it is a dynamic day-to-day schedule of activity in which any or all of the stressors (events that evoke a stress response) recur with varying frequency. At every juncture there are increasing levels of stress responses, which are steadily adding to the intensity of

Multi-Disciplinary Treatment Facts

Because the chronic pain process is so complex, involving every aspect of a person's life, a wide range of healthcare professionals may need to be consulted.

the bodily changes. This destructive process just doesn't stop unless there is an effective interruption, but with so many interacting factors, if intervention is confined only to one or two of these factors, then the chances of significant reversal are poor.

It is therefore important to identify all the contributing factors and to form a therapeutic plan that aims at each part of the downward spiral. This includes, most importantly, the spouse or partner, other members of the family, close friends, and possibly colleagues at work or employers.

Pain Clinics

By the time your back pain becomes chronic, you have often resigned yourself to the belief it will not go away. You may have exhausted many forms of treatment, and now you feel you are on your own. Your concern has changed from resolving the pain to learning how to manage it.

If you are to be successful in learning how to control your pain, it is important to start by understanding the dynamics of the process, preferably from a group of multi-disciplinary experts with experience in treating severe chronic back pain. For difficult or unremitting cases, a pain clinic should be considered. These clinics will offer the multi-disciplinary approach needed to resolve chronic pain.

Group Therapy

Groups are the most powerful therapeutic tool available, for much more can be achieved by the sharing of common problems, with the recognition that you are not alone and the realization that your problems are not as uniquely devastating as you had thought. Watching another person begin to change from a 'pain victim' back to normal, finding comfort from a fellow pain sufferer while going through a particularly bad patch yourself, learning how to communicate and cooperate in ways you have not done before — this is all part of the value of group therapy.

Physical Methods

Physiotherapy
Physiotherapy is typically carried out in groups, but with individual attention given to each participants. All of the usual physiotherapeutic techniques are used. Other physical therapies — dance and movement, for example — may be added.

Relaxation Training
Given the role that changes in muscle spasm play in causing chronic pain, this is an important preventive and therapeutic tool. The effects include an improved sense of well-being, combined with a sense of being able to exercise control over the body.

The common sense belief is that we have to try hard to relax: if you are not succeeding, it is because you're not trying hard enough. The situation is not so simple. While we do have a nervous mechanism that enables us to move voluntarily, we do not have such a mechanism to instruct ourselves to relax.

So how do muscles relax? It is a simple mechanism: we simply stop instructing our muscles to move. The normal 'default' condition is one of relaxation, so the muscles automatically relax themselves.

You can check this out by trying hard to relax — the harder you try, the tighter you become. The key to relaxation is to learn to let the muscles themselves do it.

✔ BACK FACTS

One of the most effective methods for learning how to relax is Jacobson's Progressive Relaxation training, which involves deliberately increasing the tension in the muscles, holding it for 10 seconds, and abruptly letting it go. This method is simple but effective, especially if — as happens frequently — people don't know experientially the difference between contraction and relaxation.

Hypnosis

Although hypnosis can be very useful in acute pain conditions, it does not work well in chronic states. Learning self-hypnosis is difficult while in pain, but is well worth trying.

Biofeedback

This is a method of learning a limited but useful degree of control over the autonomic nervous system using electronic devices. The most effective types are raising skin temperature and controlling muscle activity.

The rationale for gaining the ability to raise your skin temperature is that it can counteract an over-active sympathetic nervous system conducive to feeling tense and anxious. Use of temperature control was discovered accidentally during experiments when a patient announced that when warming her hands her migraine headache had vanished. It is still useful sometimes in this kind of headache but the results are not really predictable.

By observing changes on the dial of a machine that measures activity in a particular muscle it is possible to learn how to allow the muscle to achieve relaxation itself with little difficulty.

Psychological Methods

Group Psychotherapy

My remarks above about the efficacy of group work applies powerfully in psychotherapy. In fact, I much prefer working with groups than with single patients, although a combination is probably the best option. Better results can be obtained in much shorter times than individual therapy alone. The ideal group number is about 8, plus or minus one.

Spouse Groups

Spouse groups should be an indispensable part of any program, for it is by far the most effective way for 'significant others' to learn how their own behavior compares with that of other couples. It is far better than marriage counseling at improving interpersonal communication.

Behavior Modification

Most patients acquire habits that are counter-productive as part of a therapeutic program, such as avoiding movement when experiencing back pain. Patients may use their disability in order to get attention from others, and they may not be willing to stop this behavior when it is no longer appropriate. This behavior may persist even when treatment has become effective. By a system of rewards and punishments (nothing traumatic, such as withdrawal of attention by staff or family members), these behaviors can be changed.

Assertiveness Training

This is a tried and true method for learning how to assert oneself. There are many people who simply don't understand how vital this ability is in all aspects of life. In any situation in which there is a disagreement, it cannot be successfully resolved if an agreement is made that depends on one person not being willing to assert his or her own views. The agreement simply won't last. If one individual in a relationship persistently refrains from being assertive, there will be a succession of failed agreements, a sure way of breaking a relationship of any kind — interpersonal, familial, or business. The alternatives to assertion as the usual way of conducting your life are to be aggressive or to be passive — as habitual behavior, both attitudes create serious problems. This applies even more powerfully in the life of a sufferer from chronic pain.

Sex Therapy

Sexual activity and low back pain are not easy to reconcile. This is often a major factor in chronic pain and particularly so when the back is involved. It is sometimes essential for a sex therapist to be consulted and should be available in any effective pain center.

Vocational Counseling

Chronic back pain sufferers are often are unable to continue in their previous employment. It is a devastating experience to be faced with a completely unfamiliar way of earning a living. This often means accepting a lower salary, with little chance of promotion or advancement. Efficient and compassionate vocational counseling is essential for patients trying to put their life together. This should be done as soon as possible: hanging about in limbo is one of the worst scenarios that develops from a serious injury or chronic pain.

Self-Confidence

Self-confidence and personal awareness invariably suffer greatly after a while in the process of developing a chronic pain syndrome. The most effective aspect of a chronic pain management program is for all therapists to reinforce the positive features of a patient's personality and to encourage patients to express themselves as often as possible in their daily encounters with others.

Self-Help

Failing the availability of such treatment programs, usually found at a pain treatment center, you may need to find appropriate information by researching health books, medical journals, and relevant internet sites. Other important resources are the various groups that have emerged during the past 10 years or so that are aimed at some aspect of illness — diabetic, cardiac, arthritic, and low back pain conditions. They may supply sound information and advice to anyone who asks for it, free of charge. These self-help groups encourage more involvement with the outside world, which helps in recovery from chronic pain, for one of the most destructive consequences of chronic pain is depression in the form of withdrawal from social activities.

Self-Managing Chronic Pain

Restore physical function and return to as normal a life as possible

Generally the level of physical health has deteriorated drastically and every aspect needs to be dealt with, including exercise for strength, flexibility, and endurance, weight loss or gain, sufficient sleep, and ability to relax. An exercise schedule is aimed at graduated improvement in movement, recognizing that it will be necessary to push through pain. Pain is not going to harm you unless there is some structural reason, like a fracture, for avoiding it. This should be decided upon in conjunction with the your physician. Common sense should tell you when to stop and to avoid overdoing it.

Control use of medication

Your objective should be to stop using medication. However, this may not be possible, so it is best to work at reducing usage to reach the lowest amount needed. Most drugs are toxic. Side effects are the rule, not the exception. Ensure that you find the medication with the least injurious potential. It is always a balance between the drug and the side effects: do the beneficial effects exceed the harmful side effects? Couple this with personal idiosyncrasies and finding the right medication is an arduous pastime with possible serious outcomes if due precautions are not taken in assessing dosage.

An important consideration is the manner in which morphine type compounds are used. The conventional attitude of taking a dose when the pain worsens or the effects of the last dose have worn off is entirely the wrong way to manage chronic pain. It should be time-based, in the sense that a dose should be taken on a regular, scheduled basis. The object is to maintain a steady concentration in the blood stream. If taken only on an irregular, pain-level basis, the blood level falls too far and it takes a higher dose to regain effective pain control.

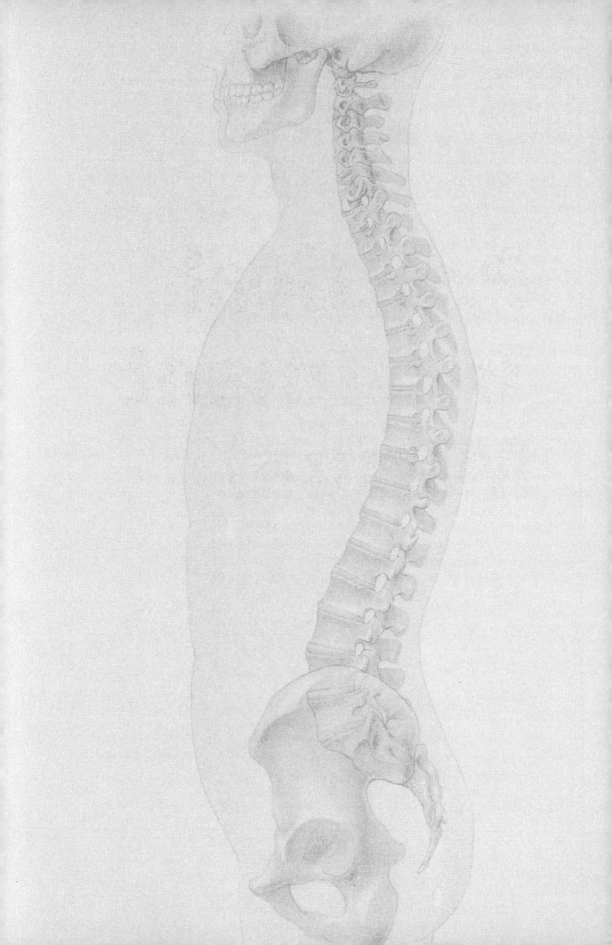

Practical Treatment Manual

Sudden Onset Back Pain

Quick Reference Chart

- Refer to the Quick Reference chart at the beginning the book and highlight or circle information relevant to your condition.

- Taking the Quick Reference chart to your doctor may help you both to arrive at an understanding of your condition and to work out an effective treatment plan.

'Red Flags'

Potentially Serious Causes of Back Pain

- Significant injury
- Symptoms of cauda equina syndrome
- Severe, unremitting night pain
- Fever
- History of cancer
- Rapid and unexplained weight loss
- History of osteoporosis or steroid medication

Individuals vary in their pain, their health, and their level of concern, so it is impossible to give universally applicable guidelines to all back conditions in all circumstances. Nevertheless, we can offer a treatment manual for most conditions in most circumstances. As you work through this section of the book, be sure to refer back to the discussion of the various treatment modalities provided in the previous section. If you are still worried about your condition, it is always advisable to seek medical attention.

Lumbar Strain

In the absence of any 'Red Flags' to indicate a more significant underlying cause, the term 'lumbar strain' is used to describe everything from a mild twinge to flat-out-on-the-couch incapacitating spinal discomfort. The term 'myofascial strain' is sometimes used to give the diagnosis a more 'medical' feel as it implies some accuracy with regard to the location of the strain. 'Myo' refers to muscle, 'fascial' to the surrounding fibrous tissue. While in some cases this may be an accurate assessment, most of the time the specific site of the injury remains unknown and would be unlikely to show up on even the most accurate MRI.

However, the specific anatomic diagnosis is not important in this case, as it does not affect management or outcome. The patient can be reassured that the pain will, with all likelihood, be gone in 4 to 6 weeks and that trying to search for a precise area of damage will only delay treatment and cause undue anxiety.

Symptoms

The characteristics of a lumbar strain include a history of minor trauma followed by development of back pain. Typically, there will be some inkling that an injury has occurred, although the degree of pain is usually mild. You may just feel a 'pull' or a 'catch' while changing position or lifting something heavy. You may continue to work or finish your game only partially aware that you have sustained any damage. In some instances, you may not even recognize a specific event, and only once the pain has developed a few hours later can you retrospectively recall a particularly heavy rock or aggressive tackle. Sometimes there is no memorable warning or likely precipitating event. The appearance of back pain in this instance can be particularly worrying to the affected individual.

The pain of a lumbar strain is felt predominantly in the back rather than the legs. The pain may be more to one side than the other and may radiate down to the back of the pelvis or buttock. There may be a dull ache, with sudden sharp, cramp-like pain on movement that subsides again slowly with rest. There is generally no numbness or weakness. The pain is intermittent, aggravated by movement, and relieved by certain resting positions.

Injury Sites

The specific site of injury in a lumbar strain can be hard to identify. Distinguishing features of a lumbar strain due to a muscle tear include localized swelling, tenderness, and bruising, usually only on one side of the spine. Next to muscle injury, facet strain is probably the second most common cause of acute low back pain. Injury to the posterior elements of the spine, including the facet joints, will generally cause pain worse on extension of the spine and relieved by flexion. Lumbar strain may also be caused by disc injury, specifically annular tears. By the age of 50, over 90% of lumbar discs show evidence of deterioration and development of acute annular tears is certainly a consideration. Unfortunately, the vast majority of tears are asymptomatic and concluding evidence of acute disc injury is therefore difficult. Unless there is rapid development of radicular leg pain (sciatica) with associated nerve dysfunction and findings to indicate a frank disc herniation, diagnosis of annular 'strain' remains conjectural. Injury to the anterior structures, which may include the intervertebral disc, may be implied by symptoms characterized by pain on flexing forward and relief by extending or arching backward.

Lumbar Strain Facts

"You've strained your back." Lumbar strain is the most common diagnosis made for the individual with acute low back pain.

Symptoms

- Rapid onset (within 36 hours).
- Often related to minor injury (fall, twisting, lifting).
- Predominantly back pain (possible radiation to buttocks).
- No numbness or weakness in legs.
- Pain aggravated by movement, eased with rest.
- No 'Red Flags'.

Lumbar Strain Diagnosis

The 'symptomatic' classification of lumbar strain is valuable as it helps direct treatment at a time when specific diagnosis is less important than pain relief and functional recovery.

Muscle Injury

While the original damage may be painless or felt as a simple 'pull', the subsequent chemical and cellular changes result in significant discomfort. This takes hours to develop and is the reason why the real pain from a lumbar strain injury is felt later on. Associated with this pain and inflammation is a decrease in the ability of the muscle to contract, resulting in weakness, increased fatiguability, and risk of further injury. Distinguishing features of a lumbar strain due to a muscle tear include localized swelling, tenderness, and bruising, usually only on one side of the spine.

Disc Injury

Disc injury is thought to be an uncommon cause of acute low back pain and is certainly almost never a factor in individuals under the age of 30 in whom disc degeneration has not established a foothold. By the age of 50, however, over 90% of lumbar discs show evidence of deterioration, and development of acute annular tears is certainly a consideration. Injury to the *anterior* structures, which may include the intervertebral disc, are characterized by pain on flexing forward and relief by extending or arching backward. This 'symptomatic' classification is valuable as it helps direct treatment at a time when specific diagnosis is less important than pain relief and functional recovery.

Facet Injury

The facets are joints, just like the knee or the shoulder, and are prone to injury. The surrounding capsule and ligaments can be stretched by movement or force beyond their tolerance, and the joint itself can become inflamed and swollen. The facet joint is a significant pain generator, often resulting in both local and referred pain, muscle spasm, reduced flexibility, and tenderness. Next to muscle injury, facet strain is probably the second most common cause of acute low back pain. As with disc injury, the specific diagnosis is less important than the symptoms in acute low back pain. Injury to the *posterior* elements of the spine, including the facet joints, will generally cause pain worse on extension of the spine and relieved by flexion. Again, this is a valuable modifier of treatment.

Lumbar Strain Treatment

Investigations are not indicated at this stage. If the pain is not improving, appears to be worsening, or new symptoms, such as sciatic-type leg pain or numbness, appear, then evaluation may be required. Referral for more formal rehabilitation is useful in some individuals who are having difficulty advancing the exercise component of their recovery.

Pain lasting over 4 to 6 weeks is an indicator for plain X-rays and a simple blood test (blood count and ESR). Pain for 3 months in a young individual, particularly 'rest' pain relieved by exercise, warrants evaluation for ankylosing spondylitis.

Acute Stage (onset to 48 hours)

Ice and Activity: The acute stage of a lumbar strain should be treated with ice (cryotherapy) and reduced activity. That does *not* mean complete bed rest! While some periods of recumbancy, or other such comfortable, pain-relieving position, may be required, effort should be made to remain as active as possible. Of course, this does not mean finishing the outdoor landscaping project that may have resulted in the original injury! It does mean walking, stretching, and simple daily activity. Whether or not you go to work depends on a number of factors, including your level of discomfort, type of work, and degree of motivation.

Exercise: Therapeutic exercise remains the mainstay of treatment during the initial stages of a lumbar strain. This involves a combination of comfortable postures with simple stretching and moderate aerobic activity. Achieving a comfortable posture is important in that it relieves pain and allows relaxation. Not only is this reassuring, by reducing pain input and muscle spasm, secondary pain sources and sensitization are reduced. Experimenting with posture and pillows is best. Reducing strain through the lumbar spine may help, for example, by lying with a pillow under your knees or on the floor with your hips flexed and lower legs resting on a low chair or sofa. If the lumbar strain involves the posterior part of the spine, then flexion will be more comfortable. Curling knees to chest either seated or lying may help, or pelvic tilts on all fours. In cases where flexion is painful, extension exercises such as the 'sloppy-push-up' or arching backward while standing with hands on hips may offer relief.

Simple stretches include knees to chest, lateral bending, hamstring and quads stretch and pulling back the shoulders and arching the back. As with all activity at this stage, these should be performed cautiously to avoid aggravation of the

Lumbar Strain Treatment Facts

In the absence of any 'Red Flags', a visit to the doctor is not generally required during the initial 4 to 6 weeks as long as you are making progress toward recovery.

Back Treatment Strategies

Refer to the previous section of this book for comprehensive discussions of these treatment strategies.

Recommended Acute Stage Treatments

- Ice and Reduced Activity

- Therapeutic Exercises:
  - Comfortable Postures
  - Cautious Stretching
  - Gentle aerobic Exercise

- Analgesics and Anti-Inflammatory Drugs

- Nutrient Supplements (Calcium/Magnesium, Essential Fatty Acids, Zinc)

- Herbal Supplements (Willow, Ginger, Devil's Claw)

- Spinal Manipulation (Chiropractic)

- TENS

- Acupuncture

- Decrease Dietary Inflammatories/ Increase Dietary Protein

Not Recommended
- Complete bed rest

- Heat

- Massage

- Back Braces and Lumbar Supports

pain. A good stretch should not be painful! Correcting postural trunk shifts to the left or right should be attempted but are not essential if they cause too much discomfort at this stage.

Aerobic exercise should be carried out within your pain tolerance. To start with this may be a simple as a short walk, but trying to increase this type of physical activity is desirable. Indeed, warming up muscles may make stretching more comfortable. Using a stationary bicycle or swimming is preferable to impact exercise such as jogging at this stage. Stair climbing requires a slightly flexed position and may therefore be tolerated in those individuals where flexion eases the pain.

Medications: Analgesics (pain killers) such as Tylenol and an anti-inflammatory such as Advil (assuming no contraindications to use) are valuable, but there is no proven role for muscle relaxants.

Manipulation: Spinal manipulation (chiropractic treatment) remains a highly popular treatment for all types of low back pain. However, its value remains controversial as good clinical studies to assess its effectiveness are lacking. If there is one area where chiropractic seems most beneficial, it is in the short-term management of acute low back pain or lumbar strain. Most positive research is in this area and anecdotally it has most support. Although the cynical may argue that the natural history of acute low back pain is for recovery regardless of treatment, there is some evidence that manipulation can ease or speed that process. Whether that is a direct result of spinal 'adjustment' or due to better education and personal interaction is irrelevant. As long as it is of benefit to the patient and has no significant side effects (as is true for lumbar spinal manipulation), then it should be considered valuable. It should not be used in the presence of radicular nerve pain (sciatica) with numbness or weakness.

TENS and Acupuncture: There may be some value to using TENS or acupuncture during the initial stages of an acute low back strain. Although predominantly applied for chronic pain, the analgesic effects of these modalities may promote faster rehabilitation and functional recovery.

Nutrition and Supplements: Keep well hydrated (drink lots of water), avoid caffeine and alcohol, and avoid foods that increase inflammation (dairy products, red meat, peppers, eggplant, and tomato). Increase protein intake for repair, particularly fish. Supplement with calcium/magnesium, essential fatty acids, and zinc. Use natural pain killers and anti-inflammatories such as willow, ginger, devil's claw, and arnica.

Contraindications: Heat is generally avoided for the first 48 hours of an acute strain. Massage is similarly avoided during the initial stage of muscle injury when inflammation is likely to be at its maximum. Back braces and lumbar supports are not recommended for lumbar strain because, although sometimes reducing discomfort, they detract from other modalities and instill a sense of disability or permanence to the condition.

Hamilton Hall's Recommendations for Acute Stage Care

Pattern 1
Fast responder (pain worse on flexion, eased by extension)
- Repeated back extensions.
- Lumbar roll to increase lumbar lordosis while seated.
- Rolled towel under low back at night.

Slow responder (pain worse on flexion, but also has pain on extension)*
- Less aggressive postures and movements.
- Start with limited flexion.
- Progress to extension as pain settles.
- Less lumbar lordosis correction.

Pattern 2
Pain worse on extension, relieved by flexion
- Repeated flexion exercises.
- Reduce postural lumbar lordosis (no lumbar roll/back support).

**Hamilton Hall points out that this group often needs more cautious and structured therapy to avoid aggravation of pain.

Sub-Acute Stage (beyond 48 hours)

The 'sub-acute' stage may last from a few days to a few weeks, its end being marked by complete resolution of the pain and restoration of motion. Getting to that point may require no more than time and simple exercise, but it may require more active and specialized treatment.

Heat and Ice: As the acute pain settles, heat can be introduced to promote healing, reduce spasm, and increase flexibility. Ultrasound may be used in the same way. Ice can still be used but after exercise or stretching is complete.

Sub-Acute Stage Facts

Pain from a muscle strain and inflammation may actually increase over the first 48 hours, which may lead to increased concern and a feeling that the pain is not going to resolve. However, in the absence of any 'Red Flags', persistence with physical activity and modalities will lead to improvement.

Sub-Acute Stage Treatments

- Heat and Ultrasound
- Ice After Exercise
- Exercises:
- Comfortable Postures
- More Advanced Stretches
- More Intense Aerobic Exercise
- Yoga and Tai Chi
- Manual Therapies:
- Massage
- Shiatsu
- Chiropractic
- ART
- Manual Physiotherapy
- Intermittent Use of Analgesics and Anti-Inflammatory Drugs
- Nutrient Supplements (Calcium/Magnesium, Essential Fatty Acids, Zinc)
- Decrease Pharmaceutical and Natural Analgesics and Inflammatories

Recovery Facts

It is important to recognize that as you recover from your lumbar strain, you will continue to feel back pain, albeit intermittent and less severe.

Posture and Exercise: Continued use of pain-relieving postures is useful during periods of rest, but overall the active components of rehabilitation should become increasingly prominent. More aggressive stretching (after an adequate warm-up) and longer periods of aerobic activity are recommended. At this stage, aggravation of the acute pain is less likely and feeling a little discomfort is an indicator that you are making progress without doing harm. If exercises are too easy, then you are likely not progressing forward. Gentle exercise that incorporates stretching, posture, and core conditioning such as Yoga and Tai Chi are useful at this stage.

Manual Therapy: Manual therapy at this stage may be useful. There is evidence that certain types of massage and myofascial treatment can induce plastic deformation of collagen, which, if used correctly, can help restore range of motion. Massage, shiatsu, chiropractic, ART, and manual physiotherapy techniques all possess the ability to reduce residual stiffness and restore motion and may be appropriate if recovery is progressing slowly. Resolution of pain with persistent restriction in range of motion would be an indication to consider one of these therapies.

Medications: Intermittent use of analgesics and anti-inflammatory medication may be helpful as activity increases but should be gradually tapered off.

Nutrition and Supplements: Continued hydration and calcium/magnesium supplementation is recommended along with protein, essential fatty acids, and zinc. Natural analgesics and anti-inflammatories should be tapered off.

Recovery

Due to the sensitization that occurs within the nervous system, the normally inconsequential ache or twinge associated with a stretch or muscle ache will trigger the same feelings of low back pain as the original injury. This explains in part why the resolution phase may take longer in some individuals than others and can foster the fear that the pain is never going to resolve.

A patient who has never practiced stretching and strengthening exercises will be unfamiliar with the discomfort associated with this process. In addition, trying to restore fitness to muscles and ligaments never previously conditioned is in itself an uncomfortable experience. This may explain why injuries such as a lumbar strain improve so much more rapidly in fitter, more athletic individuals.

What remains important during the recovery phase is that

you keep moving forward, doing a little more each day. Learning that 'hurt' does not always result in 'harm' is an essential psychological exercise as it helps overcome the sensitization that promotes so much residual pain from the low back. Patients often report that they still have pain at 6 or 8 weeks when they walk more than an hour or pick up something heavy. What they do not recognize, however, is the tremendous progress they have made. I ask how long they could walk 2 weeks previously or how much they could lift 3 weeks ago. Invariably, it is substantially less. If they were still functioning at that lower level, they would have no pain. Still, they are correct to increase their tolerance gradually.

Patients need to know that despite the pain, they have done no damage and overall are getting back to normal. Eventually they will have 'retrained' their back to its original level of strength and flexibility and they will no longer have discomfort with day-to-day chores.

Prevention

Low back strain is an opportunity to learn and improve so that it does not happen again. Many individuals expect their backs to perform at the level of a top sportsman or weightlifter without even a thought about the amount of training this would entail. They then seem surprised when an injury occurs. Prevention is about education, learning how to move, stand and lift correctly, and conditioning, ensuring adequate strength and flexibility in the spine to withstand daily traumas.

Education: Education can be as basic as a pamphlet on lifting technique to a formal 'Back School' program, employing physiotherapists and occupational therapists to teach posture, balance, and ergonomic theory. The results of such programs are variable and depend largely on the style of teaching and the population comprising the 'class'.

Conditioning: Conditioning of the spine involves a significant component of core stability combined with flexibility, lower limb strengthening, and aerobic conditioning. A maintenance program that can be continued beyond the formal sessions is vital, though instilling motivation to perform this is probably the hardest aspect of treatment.

Weight Management and Nutrition: As part of the prevention program, a weight-management diet may be incorporated if appropriate, along with ongoing supplementation. Active individuals need to maintain hydration, particularly at work, and ensure adequate calcium/magnesium and a balanced diet with sufficient protein and essential fatty acids.

Disc Herniation and Sciatica

Symptoms

There are a number of ways in which a disc herniation can present itself in terms of symptoms. An acute disc herniation may follow a sudden lift, twist or fall, or may be induced by a particularly vigorous cough or sneeze. Disc degeneration with disruption and herniation is an important cause of chronic or recurrent low back and leg pain. A large, slowly developing disc may lead to symptoms suggestive of spinal stenosis, further compromising a narrow spinal canal. Disc herniation may also cause no symptoms whatsoever, a finding that clearly demonstrates our ongoing failings when it comes to understanding and explaining this pathology!

Disc Herniation Facts

Symptoms

- Common in males age 30–50.
- Rapid onset (within 36 hours).
- Often related to minor injury (fall, twisting, lifting) or cough/sneeze.
- Predominantly leg pain.
- Possible numbness or weakness in legs.
- Pain aggravated by flexion.
- No 'red flags'.

'Red Flags'

Potentially serious problems requiring intervention

- Significant injury (e.g., fall from height).
- Symptoms of cauda equina syndrome.
- Rapid progression of numbness/weakness.
- Fever.
- History of cancer.

Disc Herniation and Sciatica

Presentations

Acute:	Young person with sudden onset of radicular leg pain often with numbness in a localized area. Can follow a sudden movement or even a cough or sneeze. May be preceded by episodes of low back pain. Rarely cauda equina syndrome.
Chronic:	Older person with chronic or recurrent low back and leg pain. Leg pain more referred than radicular. Localized numbness uncommon.
Stenosis:	Leg pain and numbness with activity. May be superimposed on long standing degenerative stenosis with a history of chronic back pain and leg symptoms with activity.

Diagnosis

The acute episode of pain from disc herniation occurs following a lifting or twisting injury or even a cough or sneeze. While there may be some associated back soreness, the predominant pain is in one or other leg depending on the side of the herniation. The pain radiates down the back of the leg to the calf, shin, or foot, where there may be a well-localized area of burning pain associated with numbness or tingling.

If this pattern in associated with more widespread loss of

feeling, weakness in the legs, inability to pass urine or loss of bowel control then cauda equina syndrome is suspected. Emergency attention should be sought.

Examination of the patient with an acute disc herniation will reveal a list to one side in an attempt to reduce pressure from the disc. Flexing forward increases pain and sitting is avoided. There will be protective spasm in the back muscles, and the affected leg will generally be held slightly flexed at the hip and knee to reduce tension on the sciatic nerve. It is difficult to get comfortable. There are often tender points in the muscles supplied by the irritated nerve. Testing will reveal evidence of nerve root irritation and possibly nerve dysfunction with reduced sensation and reflexes.

Due to the self-limiting nature of many cases of lumbar disc herniation, there is no absolute need for any tests within the first 6 weeks. Plain X-rays are of no value for assessing the disc, and unless there are 'Red Flags' that indicate an unusual cause for the symptoms or if urgent surgery is planned, CAT scan and MRI are not warranted. This may seem a little disturbing to the patient who is often quite incapacitated and concerned about possible 'nerve damage'. However, the natural history of uncomplicated disc herniation supports expectant management.

If symptoms persist beyond 6 weeks, then plain X-rays (performed as a routine screen and to correlate with MRI or CT) should be taken and a CAT scan or MRI arranged. If there is doubt as to the clinical symptoms of nerve compression or there is concern about peripheral nerve entrapment or generalized neuropathy (as found in diabetes, for example), EMG nerve testing may be appropriate. It is not, however, considered routine.

The role of these tests is to confirm diagnosis and plan surgical intervention in the event that conservative management fails. However, the results can also help direct other forms of less invasive therapy, such as epidural injection.

Disc Herniation Pain

Patients presenting with an acute disc herniation are usually in their thirties or forties and may have had some previous episodes of low back pain in the past. Typically, this pain would be aggravated by forward flexion, eased by extension (arching back), and possibly associated with vague referred leg pain.

Disc Herniation

Ability of Clinical Findings and Tests to Predict Condition:

Nerve dysfunction on clinical examination	55%
Positive Straight-leg-raise (SLR) test	66%
Nerve dysfunction + positive SLR test	86%
Nerve dysfunction + positive SLR + positive MRI/CT	95%

In the absence of any 'Red Flags', initial management of acute disc herniation is non-surgical.

Recommended Non-Surgical Treatments
• Heat
- May reduce spasm/pain
• Acupuncture
• Medications
- Analgesics and Anti-inflammatories
- Cautious Use of Narcotics
- Tricyclic Anti-Depressants (for pain)
• Natural Supplements
- Essential Fatty Acids
- B-Vitamins (particularly B-12)
- Manganese
- Glucosamine Sulphate and MSM
- Arnica, Ginger
• Exercises
- Alternate Short Periods of Activity and Rest
- Comfortable Postures
- Extension (Sloppy Push-Ups)

Not Recommended
• Complete Bed Rest
• Massage
• Chiropractic

Acute Disc Herniation Treatment

Non-Surgical Treatment

Activity: Bed rest is not recommended but in extreme cases may be required to overcome the initial pain. Beyond 48 hours, however, bed rest becomes detrimental to recovery and should not be encouraged.

Medications and Supplements: Immediate use of analgesics (including cautious use of narcotics) and anti-inflammatory medication is valuable to reduce pain and allow improved mobility. The use of muscle relaxants remains controversial. Pain-relieving anti-depressant medication such as amitriptyline can be used judiciously. Valuable supplements include essential fatty acids (for example, flaxseed oil), B-vitamins (particularly B-12) for nerve recovery, manganese, glucosamine sulphate and MSM for the disc, and arnica and ginger for inflammation. Physical modalities such as heat or ice may reduce discomfort, as will TENS and acupuncture.

Posture: Finding a comfortable posture involves a little experimentation. Lying with a roll under your low back to increase extension and supporting the affected leg in a flexed hip and knee position may work. Others find lying on their front with a pillow underneath the pelvis or arched back supported on the elbows beneficial. Periods of activity followed by shorter periods of rest reduce discomfort and maintain a certain level of activity and function.

Exercise: Exercises are difficult due to pain, at least during the first few days. However, a back extension program including the "sloppy-push-up" is useful to reduce pain and restore mobility. Flexion exercises should be avoided.

Traction: Traction is reported to be useful in reducing herniations and nerve compression but this is not born out by clinical study.

Contraindications: Chiropractic and massage therapy are not recommended during the acute phase.

Treating Unresolved Sciatic Pain

The estimated lifetime incidence of sciatica in the general population is around 40%, while the incidence of disc surgery is only 1% to 2%. Part of this difference relates to the fact that not all sciatica is due to a well-localized and identifiable disc herniation, but a significant factor is spontaneous resolution. The mechanism of non-surgical recovery involves resorption of the disc material, regression of the inflammation and swelling, along with recovery of the injured nerve.

Surgery: Identification of a specific, well-localized disc herniation in a young individual, where the pathology correlates with the clinical findings, may warrant early surgical intervention. Operating before 6 weeks is unusual, except in cases of cauda equina syndrome or progressive nerve loss with major muscle weakness, while evidence indicates a poor outcome once symptoms have been present for over 6 months. This may result from development of scarring around the nerve, chronic changes to the nerve itself, or persistent activation of central pain pathways.

Epidural Steroid Injection: In less clear-cut cases or where the patient is not keen to undergo surgery, consideration of epidural steroid injection should be made. There is sufficient research to support this procedure in specific instances with careful, X-ray guided technique. It can reduce pain significantly, allowing progression of activity and rehabilitation.

Minimally Invasive Procedures: Alternatives to surgical discectomy, the mainstay and accepted 'gold standard' of treatment, include minimally invasive procedures such as chemonucleolysis, percutaneous laser or suction discectomy, and arthroscopic discectomy.

Recovery

The natural history of disc herniation varies according to a number of factors, including the size, type, and location of the herniation, the existence of other pathology such as arthritis, and the time-frame of development. For the uncomplicated posterolateral lumbar disc herniation without other spinal pathology, nearly 50% of individuals will show significant improvement in 2 weeks, and 70% in 6 weeks. (Other studies have shown 40% by one month, 50% by 2 months, and 70% by 3 months). Only between 10% and 20% have persistent radicular symptoms.

Sciatic Pain Facts

Only a small percentage of individuals with 'sciatica' end up needing surgery. However, sciatic pain that fails to resolve or improve considerably within the first 4 to 6 weeks is an indication for investigational imaging and more aggressive treatment.

Prevention

Activity and Exercise: As the pain from a herniated disc settles, activity can gradually be increased. Bending, twisting and lifting should be avoided in the short term but overall activity and exercise should progress. A back extension program should be continued and the strengthening component increased. Once the pain has settled completely, a full core-conditioning program can be started, advancing slowly with particular caution applied to flexion exercises, which should be delayed if they cause any recurrence of the original pain. Improved aerobic conditioning and weight loss may also aid in prevention of recurrence. Incorporation of Yoga or Tai Chi into a daily routine can be considered. Long-term ergonomic changes in posture, lifting technique, and other strenuous activity can help reduce the risk of recurrence.

Supplements: Although ongoing supplementation with essential fatty acids and vitamin B can have more general health benefits, they can be stopped about 3 weeks after the sciatic pain has completely resolved. Glucosamine and MSM can be taken long term and may provide some protective effect, although this has only been demonstrated in arthritis.

Fractures

Normal Bone Strength and Excessive Force

Assessment of the patient with a possible spine fracture in the emergency room involves evaluation of injuries, stabilization, and resuscitation, if necessary. In a patient with numerous injuries, particular attention is paid to the neck and back because injuries or fractures here can go unnoticed.

Once stabilized and a through examination is completed, plain X-rays will provide the initial screen for a fracture of the spine. Until these are complete and the results known, strict spinal precautions are maintained. Depending on the results of plain X-rays, further tests such as CAT scan or MRI may be performed to evaluate the injury further. With compression fractures, the degree of compression is assessed by measuring the percentage loss of height at the front of the vertebra and the angle by which it is wedged.

Note: This section deals with treatments for compression-type fractures of the lumbar spine and not the extensive and complex classification and management of spinal trauma or spinal cord injury.

Fracture

Emergency Care

The presence of significant back pain after a fall or other such injury should ring mental alarm bells and immediate precautions need to be taken to protect the spine and prevent further damage:

- Avoid moving the injured individual and encourage him or her not to move.
- Call for emergency medical service.
- Transfer the patient to hospital with appropriate spinal immobilization including neck brace and rigid spine board. Emergency personnel have access to numerous devices that enable safe extrication from the place of injury. If the injury occurs in a sports setting, equipment should not be removed unless for resuscitation.

Treatment of Stable Compression Fractures

With less than 40% loss of height or less than 25 to 30 degrees wedging, a compression fracture is considered stable because there is no disruption of the posterior part of the spine.

Extension Brace: Management should include a rigid back extension brace for three to four months with serial X-rays to assess healing or progression of deformity. Although rare, increasing deformity or collapse despite brace usage or abnormal motion between vertebrae once healing is complete may indicate a need for surgical intervention.

Exercise: Patients should be encouraged to lie on their front and to avoid lying on their back on a soft mattress. Back extension exercises are performed once healing is considered complete.

Nutrition and Supplements: During the healing process, adequate calcium/magnesium supplementation is recommended along with vitamin D, boron and zinc. Caffeine and carbonated drinks should be avoided as much as possible as they leach calcium from bone.

Occupational Therapy: Persistent back pain following a compression fracture in a young person is common even in cases where the compression is just a few percent and healing is complete with no evidence of residual instability. Part of this likely relates to the soft tissue damage that accompanies the fracture, along with weakness and core deconditioning

Vertebral Compression Fractures

Symptoms

- Immediate or very rapid onset (within hours).
- Often related to injury such as a fall or sudden forward flexion.
- Predominantly well localized back pain (possible radiation to buttocks).
- No numbness or weakness in the legs.
- Pain aggravated by movement but present at rest.
- History of osteoporosis or steroid treatment.

'Red Flags'

Indications of potentially serious fractures

- Significant injury — fall from height, motor vehicle accident.
- Neurologic symptoms — numbness, weakness, or cauda equina syndrome.
- Severe pain.
- Other fractures sustained in same accident.

that results from prolonged brace use. This can make return to a strenuous occupation difficult. Management involves an active rehabilitation program with gradual increase in activity. Overcoming psychological barriers associated with the trauma and development of back pain in a young individual may need to be addressed.

Stable Compression Fractures

Treatments
- Rigid Back Extension Brace
- Serial X-rays
- Avoid Lying on Back
- Back Extension Exercises Once Healing Complete
- Supplement Diet with Calcium/Magnesium, Vitamin D, Boron, Zinc
- Avoid Caffeine and Carbonated Drinks

Normal Force but Weakened Bone

The most common presentation of a compression fracture in weakened bone is an elderly person presenting with sudden onset of back pain from a fall. Evaluation of sudden onset back pain in an elderly is generally given the 'Red Flag' treatment. Medical assessment and investigation is required to determine if the cause of the fall was due to a heart attack or stroke. The high incidence of osteoporosis increases the likelihood of compression fracture as a cause, and the pain is normally severely debilitating in these individuals. In addition, there is an increased risk of malignancy, a spread of cancer from the breast, kidney, lung, or prostate to the bone, another cause of pain and bony insufficiency leading to fracture. A patient with a history of cancer (possible spread) or steroid treatment (causes osteopenia) similarly should be treated with caution and investigated thoroughly.

Even the patient with osteoporosis may have a secondary cause for their new pain or compression fracture. MRI is probably the most valuable test for the assessment of a vertebral fracture with worrying features. It provides information about the bony quality at that level and at surrounding levels and can assess for associated soft tissue mass. Certain characteristics of the MRI image can indicate infection or tumor. A bone scan can screen for other areas of bone spread if tumor is suspected. In cases where a malignancy is a concern, a full workup is needed, including tests to locate a primary tumor if one is not already known. The details of such testing, however, are outside the scope of this book.

Cancers that Typically Spread to Bone

- Breast
- Prostate
- Lung
- Kidney
- Thyroid
- Lymph (immune cell): Myeloma, Lymphoma

Compression Fracture Facts

An estimated 600,000 vertebral compression fractures due to primary osteoporosis occur each year in the United States. One third of these develop chronic pain or deformity. Each fracture is associated with a 15% increase in mortality risk. These figures have prompted the trend toward more aggressive management.

Treatment of Osteoporotic Compression Fractures

Once assumed to be benign and of little consequence, the increasing frequency of these fractures in an aging population has led to the realization that they often lead to residual pain, functional decline, and psychosocial dysfunction.

In cases where the compression fracture is found to be secondary to osteoporosis, treatment is bi-directional in managing of the fracture and addressing the cause. The priority is management of the acute fracture, its associated pain, and functional impairment.

Conservative Management: Traditional conservative management of osteoporotic compression fractures is with analgesics, anti-inflammatory drugs, bracing, and rapid mobilization, often in an acute hospital or rehabilitation unit. Concurrent care with a geriatrician will improve management of medical and psychological issues, which can often be the most complicated aspect of the case. Many elderly people are living on the edge of independence and an injury such as this can 'push them over the edge' into requiring more long-term support.

Invasive Techniques: The need for rapid mobilization to reduce complications associated with bed rest and to avert psychological stressors such as loss of independence and removal from a familiar environment has led to the development of more invasive pain control techniques. These include local anesthetic nerve blocks, epidural anesthesia, and minimally invasive reconstructive procedures such as vertebroplasty and kyphoplasty.

Osteoporosis

Concomitant assessment and treatment of osteoporosis can be initiated along with pain control and medical stabilization. Diagnosis is based on risk history, blood tests of bone turnover, and bone densitometry (BMD) testing. This latter technique evaluates the density of bone and compares it to a healthy 25-year-old. The ratio determines the degree of 'thinning' and evaluates fracture risk as low, medium, or high. Treatment is summarized below.

Osteoporosis refers to the 'thinning' of bone, generally seen in older individuals. The bone has the same constituents, the same level of minerals, but there is less of it. Osteoporosis leads to fractures, particularly of the spine, hip, pelvis, and wrist. In the United States, 21% of post-menopausal women have osteoporosis, 16% have had a fracture. In women over 80

Osteoporotic Compression Fracture Facts

Treatments
- Analgesics and Anti-inflammatory Drugs
- Bracing
- Rapid Mobilization
- Anesthetic Nerve Blocks
- Epidural Anesthesia
- Vertebroplasty
- Kyphoplasty

Osteoporosis Facts

Risk Factors
- Female
- Post-Menopausal
- Family History (by far the greatest additional risk factor)
- Smoking
- Anorexia/ Malabsorption/ Underweight
- Lack of Exercise
- Steroid Use
- Kidney/Liver Problems

Osteoporosis Causes

Osteoporosis occurs when bone is resorbed too quickly, resulting in a reduction of bone density below a critical level, which increases risk of fracture.

This can happen in two situations:

- **High-turnover Osteoporosis:** Resorption is occurring at an excessively high rate such that new bone formation (remodeling) fails to keep up.

- **Low-turnover Osteoporosis:** New bone formation is impaired in the presence of normal resorption.

Cortisol Facts

While there have been no definitive studies linking chronic stress and osteoporosis, there is clearly a connection between bone mass, bone cell activity, and the production of cortisol. Reduction of stress is certainly one way of reducing your risk of osteoporosis and should be combined with other treatments.

years of age, 40% have had an osteoporosis-related fracture. In men, the risk occurs 10 years later.

Bone is an active living tissue composed of a structural framework made mostly of collagen fibers with protein and calcium phosphate to provide strength. It contains cells predominantly of two types: osteoblasts, which lay down new bone, and osteoclasts, which absorb it. The combination of the protein fibers of collagen and the hard calcium phosphate mineral give bone its unique characteristics of strength and flexibility. Bone is continually turning over, being resorbed by the osteoclasts and laid down by the osteoblasts.

Up to approximately age 30 more bone is laid down than resorbed. This point represents peak bone mass, a time at which there is maximum bone density and strength. Thereafter, the resorption of bone exceeds creation. For women in the first few years after menopause, the degree of resorption is extremely rapid.

Bone Mineral Densitometry (BMD) involves X-ray and comparison of bone density to a hypothetical same-sex individual at maximum bone mass (age 25). Those within 1 standard deviation of this value are normal, between 1 and 2.5 standard deviations are 'osteopenic', and beyond 2.5 standard deviations 'osteoporotic'.

Steroids and Stress

Cortisol

High levels of cortisol or other steroids are associated with osteoporosis. This is most clearly demonstrated in Cushing's disease (abnormal secretion of high levels of cortisol) and in certain diseases such a rheumatoid arthritis where prednisone (a medicinal form of cortisol) is administered by mouth for prolonged periods. Even subjects with mildly increased cortisol levels are found to have significantly increased bone loss compared to normal. Major depressive disorder is associated with a disruption of the hypothalamic-pituitary-adrenal axis and chronically elevated cortisol levels not responsive to endogenous or exogenous suppression or feedback. These individuals are at significantly higher risk of osteoporosis.

Osteoprotegerin is an important bone cytokine. It has the ability to bind the chemical messenger that normally induces bone cells to form new bone-absorbing osteoclasts. By this means it acts to reduce bone resorption. Cortisol significantly reduces the amount of osteoprotegerin, resulting in an increase in osteoclast formation and a shift in favor of resorption.

Osteocalcin is a protein molecule produced by osteoblasts during production of bone. It provides a marker for bone activity and is generally increased in osteoporosis associated with high bone turnover and reduced in the low-turnover type, such as malnutrition-associated osteoporosis. Cortisol impairs production of new bone by osteoblasts and thereby reduces levels of osteocalcin. Osteocalcin, in fact, shows a daily rhythm of activity similar to that seen with cortisol. Studies of patients with anorexia and Cushing's disease, in which cortisol levels are elevated, reveal a marked reduction in osteocalcin levels. Osteoporosis is common to both these conditions.

Thus, it would appear that cortisol induces osteoporosis through both high and low turnover mechanisms.

Leptin

Leptin is a hormone produced by fat tissue. Its primary effects are to reduce appetite and increase energy expenditure, part of the body's control mechanism to maintain a steady weight. During starvation, it allows conservation of energy by reducing metabolic rate, whereas in the well-fed state, its increased production by fat cells promotes calorie burning. Its daily cycle incorporates a peak at night, ensuring we continue to burn calories yet don't feel hungry. Leptin also appears to have a role in bone metabolism and osteoporosis, although its specific action remains elusive.

There is some evidence that it inhibits bone formation, likely through reduction of osteoblast recruitment and function. However, in starvation, a state with low leptin, osteoblast activity is reduced (as measured by osteocalcin). And, in obesity, associated with high leptin, osteoporosis is unusual. Both of these point to a role for leptin in the maintenance of bone mass. While chronic stress and cortisol stimulate leptin production, they induce leptin resistance and this may counteract any protective role the hormone may have in preserving bone stock.

Stress results in a reduction in gonadotrophin releasing hormone (GnRH) from the hypothalamus, with subsequent effects on the reproductive hormone levels in men and women. A reduction in estrogen or testosterone has a profound effect on bone mass. This likely represents another avenue through which cortisol increases osteoporosis risk.

Stress Solutions

For more information on stress and stress-related diseases, see *The Complete Doctor's Stress Solution* by Penny Kendall-Reed and Stephen Reed.

Osteoporosis

Prevention

Maximum bone mass is attained by age 30 and starts to decrease thereafter. Prevention aims to make sure your bones are as strong as possible at this stage and helps slow subsequent loss.

* Adequate Calcium (required amount varies with sex and age).
* Adequate Vitamin D (diet and sunlight).
* Exercise (stimulates bone formation).
* Stop Smoking (smoking increases bone loss).
* Alcohol (in excess increases osteoporosis risk).
* Reduce Caffeine and Carbonated Beverages.
* Stress Reduction.

Treatment

May also be employed as a preventive measure in 'at risk' individuals or in established cases.

* Nutrition (adequate protein, calcium, vitamin D).
* Exercise (remains important at any age).
* Medication:
  * Biphosphanates (Alendronate/Fosamax, Risedronate/Actonel) act to reduce bone resorption and may increase osteoblast activity.
  * SERMs (selective estrogen receptor modulators), e.g., Raloxifene/Evista, reduce bone resorption but should be used after menopause only.
  * Calcitonin (injectable/nasal spray form of bone hormone) acts to reduce bone resorption, may increase osteoblast activity, and useful for pain control.
  * Teriparatide (Forteo) injectable parathyroid hormone acts to increase bone formation.
  * Hormone replacement therapy acts to reduce bone resorption and may increase osteoblast activity but recent evidence cautions use due to side effects.
* Fall Prevention (balance training and home-proofing).
* Stress Reduction and Psychological Counseling.

Recurring Back Pain

Recurrent low back pain is defined as episodes of pain lasting less than 12 weeks that recur over time with significant pain-free intervals. While these terms may seem a little arbitrary, there is an important distinction here between recurrent and chronic low back pain. The dividing line is defined by the frequency and severity of the pain and the amount of disruption it causes to an individual's lifestyle. One or two episodes per year lasting a few days to a few weeks would be tolerable to most people, while pain recurring on a monthly basis is likely to be considered disabling. Clearly the definition of 'recurrent' as opposed to 'chronic' is individual. This chapter will try to deal with recurrent pain that is 'annoying' rather than disabling.

Recurrent low back pain is less likely than chronic pain to have any significant underlying pathology within the spine. It is less likely to result in significant, lasting disability or dysfunction. It is far less likely than chronic back pain to ever need surgical intervention. And, in most cases, it can be prevented or minimized by simple conservative management.

Recurrent Back Pain Facts

- Low likelihood of significant spine pathology.
- Less disability than chronic low back pain.
- Rarely considered for surgical intervention.
- Easily managed with conservative therapy.

 BACK FACTS

There is rarely a significant underlying spinal disease or condition in recurrent low back pain. This is one of the low back problems that does not require a specific anatomic or pathologic diagnosis. What is far more important is the pattern of symptoms and the treatment plan aimed at resolving them.

Symptoms

Some symptoms may point to a cause. For example, if you get back pain each time you shovel the driveway, the problem is likely a recurrent lumbar strain. A sudden sharp pain that catches you on standing up may indicate a facet joint injury. Regardless of the precise diagnosis, the pattern helps define treatment and directs a preventive program.

Thus, the question we should be asking is not "What causes the low back pain?" but "Why does it keep recurring?"

- Spinal deconditioning.
- Poor posture, biomechanics, ergonomics.
- Inadequate training for employment or sport.
- Overweight.
- Stress.

Individual Episode Facts

The individual episode of recurrent back pain can be treated like an acute lumbar strain and incorporate many of the recommendations, modalities, and therapies presented in the previous chapter.

There are a number of possible answers to this question and one or more may apply to a particular individual. Spinal deconditioning implies a combination of weakness, reduced flexibility, and poor aerobic fitness. Poor posture, both standing and sitting, has an adverse effect on the spine, as does unbalanced body biomechanics and inefficient ergonomic function (the way we carry out tasks). Being overweight adds its own set of problems to the low back in addition to reflecting conditioning. Inadequate training for employment and sports combines a number of these factors to influence back pain recurrence. And finally, there is increasing evidence that lifestyle stress can induce or prolong back pain. Fortunately, all these factors can be addressed without the need for a scalpel!

Managing recurrent low back pain involves two phases: first, treatment of the individual episode; and second, instituting changes to prevent recurrence.

Treating the Individual Episode

Most of the time, recurrent low back pain will involve separate episodes of 'acute low back pain'. The majority of these episodes are termed 'lumbar strains' and may result from injury to any one of a number of structures, although the specific diagnosis is far less relevant than the pattern of the pain. Acute disc herniation results in leg pain rather than back pain, and is unlikely to become a recurrent problem. Similarly, compression fractures, if recurrent, need a far more aggressive treatment plan to address medical issues such as osteoporosis and recurrent falls.

There is one significant advantage with recurrent low back pain — the benefit of experience! Recurrent back pain sufferers are in a far better position than first timers. They know what to expect, they know what works and what does not, and, most importantly, they know they are going to get better!

Use all this to your advantage. Rather than descending into negativity and feeling sorry for yourself, think, "I've beaten this before, I can do it again," only this time plan to do it faster and more easily. Your low back has disrupted your life enough in the past. Minimize its impact this time. A positive mental attitude is vital. Buoy your spirits with the knowledge learned from your past episodes. You may have seen a doctor before and have undergone to a number of tests that proved negative. You were probably told there was nothing terribly wrong with your spine and that in all likelihood the pain would resolve. And it did!

On a practical level, you know the most comfortable positions, the right balance of medication, and whether to use heat or ice. You know if the chiropractor or the massage therapist helped last time. Recurrent episodes tend to follow the same pattern, so treat them in the same way and they will resolve.

Diagnosis Trap

Do not fall into the 'diagnosis trap'. There is a tendency with recurrent back pain to go in search of a final 'answer'. A distinct problem in your spine that means you get pain while your neighbor does not. It helps rationalize the condition and gives you a reason to suffer. Unfortunately, in most cases, not only does a diagnosis have no bearing on the pain, it just adds fear and anxiety to your symptoms. Just because a plain X-ray shows 'mild arthritis' or an MRI shows a 'bulging disc', this does not mean that is the cause of your back pain. Findings such as these are extremely common and are likely present on your pain-free neighbor's X-rays as well. These diagnoses appear non-treatable, so linking your back pain to them immediately ruins your chances of recovery — an outcome that is both negative and unfounded.

Hamilton Hall's Recommendations for Acute Stage Care

Pattern 1
Fast responder (pain worse on flexion, eased by extension)
- Repeated back extensions.
- Lumbar roll to increase lumbar lordosis while seated.
- Rolled towel under low back at night.

Slow responder (pain worse on flexion, but also has pain on extension)*
- Less aggressive postures and movements.
- Start with limited flexion.
- Progress to extension as pain settles.
- Less lumbar lordosis correction.

Pattern 2
Pain worse on extension, relieved by flexion
- Repeated flexion exercises.
- Reduce postural lumbar lordosis (no lumbar roll/back support).

*Hamilton Hall points out that this group often need more cautious and structured therapy to avoid aggravation of pain.

Treatment for an Individual Episode
- Ice and Reduced Activity

- Therapeutic Exercises:
- Comfortable Postures
- Cautious Stretching
- Gentle Aerobic Exercise

- Analgesics and Anti-Inflammatory Drugs

- Nutrient Supplements (Calcium/Magnesium, Essential Fatty Acids, Zinc)

- Herbal Supplements (Willow, Ginger, Devil's Claw)

- Spinal Manipulation (Chiropractic)

- TENS

- Acupuncture

- Decrease Dietary Inflammatories/ Increase Dietary Protein

Sometimes Useful
(particularly if you have found them beneficial in previous episodes)
- Heat

- Massage

- Back Braces and Lumbar Supports

Not Recommended
- Complete Bed Rest

Preventing Recurrence

Spinal Conditioning

It is quite easy to determine the degree of fitness in your arm or leg. Not only can one side be compared to the other, range of motion at each joint is easy to measure and strength testing relatively straightforward. Muscle bulk in a limb can be measured with a tape, and with more advanced equipment, response and endurance can be evaluated. Unfortunately, this is not the case with the spine. The low back offers few insights into its function from simple observation and movement, and even less information regarding its degree of 'fitness' to perform anything from daily chores to heavy construction duties. However, there is no doubt that, as with any musculoskeletal unit, pain, injury, lack of use, and immobility lead to a reduction in joint mobility, muscle weakness with loss of endurance, impaired feedback, and limited functional ability.

The basis behind exercise as a treatment for recurrent and chronic back pain is the biomechanical theory that improved control and stability, along with strength and endurance, will restore the ability of muscular support to protect the spine. If pain is due to repeated mechanical irritation of pain-sensitive structures, then preventing that irritation will reduce pain and improve mobility. In addition, there is ample evidence to support a change in muscle control and coordination in those with both acute and chronic low back pain. While this may in part be secondary to the sensation of pain itself affecting muscle function, it is undoubtedly a two-way street, with altered function contributing to pain, particularly its persistence.

Core Conditioning: Deconditioning in the spine involves a number of elements, all of which need to be addressed in a rehabilitation and preventative program. Central to this program is 'core' conditioning, which recognizes the importance of both lumbar paravertebral and abdominal muscles in support of spinal function. These muscles need components of tone, strength, and endurance in order to provide optimum protection.

Deconditioned Components in the Lumbar Spine

- Spinal and abdominal muscle strength, endurance, and tone.
- Posture maintenance and adjustment.
- Trunk flexibility.
- Hip, pelvis, and leg flexibility and strength.

Spinal Conditioning Exercises

- Yoga, Tai Chi.
- Progressive aerobic exercise, particularly swimming.
- Trunk flexibility, hamstring, quads, gluteal and calf stretch.
- Core stability program.
- Lower limb strength program.
- Adequate warm-up, preparation for activity.

Note: See the 'Exercise Treatments' in 'Back Treatment Strategies' section for a detailed guide to back exercises. Some individuals may need more formal education as part of a structured physiotherapy program.

Posture: Linked to core conditioning is posture maintenance and adjustment, which requires endurance and strength, along with positional feedback and balance. Flexibility is essential to allow adequate maneuverability and reduce risk of strain. The hips, pelvis, and legs, part of the biomechanical linkage by which the spine interacts with the environment, need to be equally as strong and flexible. Correct posture, both standing and sitting, can reduce forces across the low back and minimize the likelihood of injury.

Biomechanics and Ergonomic Function

Yoga, Tai Chi, and the Alexander Technique can be valuable in the development of improved movement and posture, particularly when combined with aspects of conditioning mentioned above. More advanced programs establish beneficial patterns of movement and function that optimize the biomechanical function of the spine for everything from getting out of bed to job or sport-specific actions. Understanding how the spine moves and works and working within its parameters can reduce the risk of injury caused by exceeding its capabilities.

Improving ergonomic function can be as simple as learning how to bend and lift correctly or as complex as adjusting your golf swing. Changing the way you do things on a long-term basis such that stress across the lumbar spine is minimized, particularly when combined with improved strength and flexibility, will greatly reduce back pain recurrence.

Biomechanics and Ergonomic Improvement

- Yoga, Tai Chi, Alexander Technique.
- Improved sitting posture, use of footstool, lumbar support.
- Improved standing posture, footstool, regular hamstring stretch.
- Correct lifting technique.
- Know your strength limitations.
- Improved sports technique (e.g., golf swing).

Lifting Ergonomics

- Do not lift awkward or unbalanced loads and avoid sudden movements. When lifting, always face the task.
- Do not twist and lift.
- Keep the object as close to your body as possible, and if that is not possible due to awkward shape or position, then ask for help.
- Bend your knees and keep your back straight while lifting. Looking up rather than at the object will help with this, as will keeping it close.
- To change direction, turn your feet rather than your shoulders. Reverse the process when setting the object down.

Note: See the 'Exercise Treatments' chapter in the 'Back Treatment Strategies' section for more information on posture, biomechanics, and ergonomics.

Work and Sport Facts

Recurrent back pain, particularly when related to work or sport, is a 'wake-up call'. You need to ensure your back is prepared for the physical insults you may throw at it.

Adequate Training for Employment or Sport

The level of fitness in individuals involved in heavy work such as construction or manufacturing and in amateur and professional sports is astounding. Here are people expecting their bodies, day after day, to jump, climb, bend, twist, lift, and pull. However, weekend handymen and weekend warriors often fail to maintain a sufficient level of fitness to do the job or play the game safely.

This involves back conditioning, discussed above, aerobic fitness, along with adequate nutrition and supplementation. In addition, you may need training to learn skills that improve your efficiency in the workplace or on the sports field in order to minimize injury.

Smoking

Stopping smoking is an important part of back health and preventing recurrence. There is ample evidence to show that smoking is an additional risk factor in the development and recurrence of low back pain. Not only does it appear to increase the risk of disc herniation, it is can also accelerate disc degeneration by compromising the blood supply and nutrition of this important structure.

Weight Loss

There is sufficient evidence that being overweight increases the incidence of low back pain to recommend a weight management program as part of an overall plan to prevent low back pain recurrence.

Although it is generally accepted that there is an association between excess body weight and low back pain, the clinical evidence as to whether this is a causative relationship has been conflicting. The difficulty with study design along with numerous confounding variables, such as nutrient intake, smoking, social status, job-related stress, exercise, and access to therapy, has made establishing a clear link difficult. However, a number of epidemiologic studies have found weight to be a significant factor in recurrent low back pain.

A simple, effective weight loss and management program, such as the naturopathic diet, also improves overall medical health.

Naturopathic Diet Plan

Stage One: Weight Loss
This stage lasts about 8 weeks.
- Protein per meal 15–25 grams.
- Unlimited salads and most other vegetables.
- Two pieces of fruit per day maximum, no bananas.
- No grains, rice, pasta, or starches.
- Very limited high carbohydrate, low protein foods such as chickpeas and lentils
- Limited portions of dressings and condiments.
- No alcohol.
- Increased fluid levels by drinking more water.

Stage Two: Maintenance
Once dietary balance is achieved, this stage becomes a constant weight management program.
- Continue 15–25 grams of protein per meal.
- Continue unlimited salad/vegetable.
- Reintroduce carbohydrates:
    Type: Follow reintroduction order below.
    Amount: Slowly introduce carbohydrates at a ratio of 3:1 protein to carbohydrate.
    Increase: Slowly increase this ratio to 1:1.
    Adjust: If symptoms of hyperinsulinemia return, reduce carbohydrate to the point where no symptoms occur.

Stage Two Carbohydrate Reintroduction Order
- Fruits
- Whole Grains, Breads, Cereals
- Pasta
- Rice
- Potatoes and Squash
- Candy and Alcoholic Beverages

Note: See the "Weight Management" chapter in the 'Back Treatment Strategies' section for more information about the Naturopathic Diet.

Reducing Stress

The role of stress as a deleterious factor in all aspects of health is the subject of a rapidly expanding field of research. Its importance as a significant risk factor in the development and recurrence of low back pain is becoming increasingly recognized. A study published in *The American Journal of Public Health* in 2001 found that individuals who experienced significant psychological stress in their early twenties were over two and a half times as likely to develop low back pain in their thirties as similar stress-free subjects. This finding accounted for other factors such as smoking and social status. In one study, disc injections into control subjects with no prior back pain resulted in only temporary discomfort with no lasting pain. Similar injections in subjects with abnormal psychometric testing (and no prior back pain) resulted in 40% having chronic significant back pain. Psychological factors appear to be better predictors of low back pain than MRI findings.

Simple Stress Management

• Deep Breathing

• Meditation

• Regular Massage

• Lavender Oil Baths

• Yoga/Pilates/Tai Chi

• Regular Exercise

• No Caffeine or Alcohol

Stress in day-to-day life and especially in the workplace increases risk of both the development and recurrence of low back pain. To examine this, in one study, subjects were required to perform a lifting task with or without additional psychological stress. Shear and compression forces across the spine increased substantially in the presence of mental stress, a finding the authors propose might be due to reduced muscle coordination and impaired ergonomics.

A stress reduction program should include deep breathing exercises. Yoga, meditation, physical exercise, and massage in a daily routine can have a profound effect on stress and cortisol (our stress hormone) levels. Alterations to diet, addition of supplements, visualization, psychotherapy, and other more intensive management techniques can be included in a more advanced program.

Persistent (Chronic) Back Pain

What if your back pain does not go away? The first thing to recognize is that we are all different — physically, mentally, and emotionally — so our recovery period from acute or recurrent back pain may not always follow 'textbook' generalizations. If a lumbar strain resolves in most people by 6 weeks and you are better in 3 days, you are unlikely to be too concerned or upset. This is just as much a variation of 'normal' as if the pain continues for 8 weeks. You may have seen your doctor or had an X-ray, but as long as there are no serious findings, you can assume you are at the far end of the recovery curve. Like recovery periods, the level of pain experienced varies among individuals. While some people may accept and live with a regular 'twinge' or ache in their low back, others find the pain intolerable and functionally disabling.

Persistent Back Pain

Causes
- Disc Degeneration
- Spinal Arthritis
- Spinal Stenosis
- Spondylolisthesis (instability)

 BACK FACTS

Unfortunately in some situations, back pain does not always resolve in a reasonable timeframe, resulting in an ongoing source of concern, irritation, and possible dysfunction. Sometimes the cause of this pain is disc degeneration, spinal arthritis, spinal stenosis, or spondylolisthesis (instability). There may also be mental and emotional factors at play to account for 'chronic pain' in a small number of patients where no clear musculoskeletal cause for their pain can be identified and where all treatment modalities have failed.

Degenerative Disc Disease

Degenerative disc disease (DDD) is probably the most controversial topic in the field of back pain care. While touted as a significant cause of low back pain, it is present in most spines, regardless of symptoms. One study found disc degeneration on X-rays of 80% of adults, with over half having no complaints of back pain. Another found evidence of degeneration in 90% of all discs at autopsy in people aged 50 and above. The fact that this condition is often termed 'idiopathic

DDD and Chronic Pain

About 10% of low back pain sufferers go on to develop chronic pain, and of these, about 40% are found to have disc degeneration on clinical and MRI testing. Whether disc degeneration is the cause of the chronic pain remains a controversial question.

low back pain' accentuates the paradox of disc degeneration as 'idiopathic' means 'of unknown cause'.

The correlation of internal disc derangement (IDD) as seen on MRI and back pain is poor. Some individuals with minimal evidence of degeneration have severe chronic pain, while others with apparently horrendous deterioration experience little or no discomfort at all. Clearly, despite the fact that both the frequency of diagnosis and the incidence of surgical treatment for this condition are increasing, there still remains much we do not understand.

Degenerative Disc Disease (DDD) is a low back condition defined by clinical features. Internal Disc Derangement (IDD) is an abnormality found on MRI indicative of disc degeneration.

Diagnosis

Unfortunately, unlike many of the diagnoses discussed in this book, the diagnosis of DDD remains rather nebulous. Despite attempts to define it more clearly as a clinical entity, the condition tends to be a catch-all for back pain that is persistent yet fails to fall into any other pathologic category. This results in considerable over-diagnosis and likely over-treatment, creating one of those situations where finding a diagnosis for diagnosis's sake in order to placate the patient and reassure the physician can have far-reaching consequences. What is most important here is to identify that small group of patients in whom the DDD is definitely responsible for their pain rather than trying to find an answer for everyone. Having done that, specific treatment options may be considered.

The patient with DDD will typically have back-dominant pain, although referred pain in the legs, as far as the knees, is common. This referred pain should be distinguished from radicular pain, normally associated with nerve root irritation, which is uncommon in this clinical setting. Pain is usually worse with repeated or prolonged forward flexion and reduced by arching backwards. There is often a 'catch' of pain when moving from a standing, flexed-at-the-waist position to a fully erect posture. Prolonged sitting, particularly in a vehicle, is aggravating.

Examination often reveals quite marked low back tenderness, a feature associated with the marked sensory sensitization in this condition. There is no detectable sensory or motor nerve loss, and tests of nerve irritation, such as the straight-leg-raise (SLR), produce only back pain.

Unfortunately, despite these guidelines, there are no truly specific symptoms or findings for DDD and most of the above descriptors can equally be applied to any number of low back conditions.

X-ray and MRI Tests

Plain X-rays are of little help in diagnosing DDD. While 'narrowing of the disc space' is often heralded as an indicator of disc deterioration, most often this is due to variations in X-ray technique. There is no definitive measurement to support this feature as having diagnostic value. By the time severe narrowing, osteophytes (bony nodules), and instability appear, it is more likely that the problem is degenerative arthritis or spondylosis.

The advent of MRI has certainly added to the popularity of DDD as a diagnosis and cause of low back pain. MR imaging allows visualization of changes within the intervertebral discs that can be correlated with age (IDD). These changes appeared on the MRIs of patients with back pain, so the pathologic association is made. However, these changes are almost ubiquitous, with little relationship between the clinical picture and those on the MRI screen. Numerous studies have attempted to correlate MRI disc findings with pain using discography (injection into a disc to create pain) as a test. Despite claims of up to 86% predictive value for MRI findings such as the 'high intensity zone' (HIZ), most research has found little reliability. In one study, over 20% of discs classified as 'normal' on MRI produced pain on discography, while a significant proportion of 'degenerate' discs were painless.

Discography

Discography involves the placement of a needle using X-ray guidance into an intervertebral disc followed by injection of radio-opaque dye and saline (salt water) under pressure. The role and value of discography remains controversial, yet it remains the only available test to determine whether or not a disc is actually a source of low back pain. Although this is probably the most useful test we have to confirm an association between IDD seen on MRI and the clinical picture of DDD, it still has significant limitations. Several factors can increase the value of this test in predicting which discs are responsible for the pain and may improve selection of patients for surgery. Discography should only be used in a patient who has failed conservative treatment and is being considered for surgery. It should not be used if a disc appears normal on MRI.

Diagnosis

Clinical Picture:
- Patient age 20–50 years.
- Male more often than female.
- Heavy job, driving.
- Smoker.
- Overweight.
- Diabetes.

Pain:
- Persistent or frequently recurrent low back pain.
- Referred pain to legs (a far as the knee).
- Pain aggravated by flexion (bending forward).
- Pain reduced by extension (arching backward).
- Worse with prolonged sitting.
- Tender low back.

Tests:
- Plain X-rays usually normal.
- MRI shows degeneration – IDD, possible high intensity zone (HIZ).

Degenerative Disc Disease

Treatment

Conservative
- Exercise
  - Core Stability
  - Trunk Flexibility
  - Limited Flexion Exercises (in early stage)
  - Aerobic Fitness
- Weight Loss
- Ergonomic Modification
- Supplements
  - Glucosamine Sulphate, MSM
  - Vitamins A, C, E and Selenium (anti-oxidants)
- Acupuncture
- Postural Program: Yoga, Alexander Technique
- Medication: NSAIDS (on intermittent basis)

Minimally Invasive
Consider after 6 months of adequate conservative care and after careful patient selection through clinical and imaging evaluation.
- Epidural Steroid Injection
- Botox Therapy
- Intradiscal Electrothermal Coagulation

Surgical
Consider after 6 months of adequate conservative care, after failure of minimally invasive therapy (if appropriate), and after careful patient selection through clinical and imaging evaluation.
- Spinal Fusion
- Disc Replacement (currently in research stage)

Discography Facts

Factors Increasing Predictive Value
- Experienced practitioner.
- X-ray or CT guidance.
- Comparison across multiple levels.
- Use of 'control' blocks.
- Awake patient with minimal sedation.
- 'Familiarity' of pain produced by injection.
- No underlying patient psychological factors.

Treatment of DDD

It may not be immediately apparent whom to treat for this condition and what exactly should be treated. However, once other causes of persistent back pain have been ruled out, a reasonable management protocol can be outlined regardless of whether a specific disc is 'degenerate' or responsible for symptoms. Only when conservative treatment has failed does this become important.

Conservative Treatments

Conservative treatment remains the primary management of DDD. Unless an individual has had at least 6 months of an adequate program, nothing more invasive should be considered.

Exercise: Central to this protocol is an active exercise regimen to build trunk strength and flexibility. Core stability is essential but abdominal strengthening may have to be achieved without aggressive flexion exercises, which are likely to aggravate symptoms in the early stages. Aerobic fitness with avoidance of impact exercise is vital and can be combined with a weight management program if needed.

Supplements: Supplements to help maintain and rebuild collagen and matrix may be beneficial along with anti-oxidants to reduce the inflammation and degradation within the disc.

Other: Passive treatments are not generally recommended, although in the early stages massage and acupuncture may help alleviate pain. Yoga, Tai Chi, and the Alexander Technique, along with ergonomic modification (altering the way you move, twist, and lift), provide both exercise and postural adjustment.

Minimally Invasive Options

Failure of an adequate conservative program occurs in about 30% of cases. Persistent pain at his stage may be an indicator to proceed with investigation and more invasive treatment. However, 6 months is just a guideline — there is no harm in continuing for longer as improvement may still occur at 12 or even 18 months. This is not life or death situation, nor will waiting result in your being confined to a wheelchair or deteriorating beyond the point where invasive treatments surgery can help.

Epidural Steroid Injections: Epidural steroid injections are controversial but may have a role in the non-surgical management of DDD. This procedure is principally recommended for disc herniation with radiculopathy and is probably most useful during the acute phase rather than in chronic pain.

Botox Injections: Botox injections are a relatively new form of treatment. Their use in chronic low back pain aims to treat muscle pain and spasm rather than the disc pathology itself. By reducing forces across the disk and limiting nerve sensitization, these injections may be useful in DDD.

Intradiscal Electrothermal Coagulation: Intradiscal electrothermal coagulation is a new, minimally invasive procedure specifically for DDD. Initial results look promising but further research is needed to determine its role.

Surgery for DDD

The current mainstay of surgical treatment is spinal fusion or arthrodesis, a procedure in which the involved disc is resected and the two adjacent vertebrae fused together with bone. By removing motion at this segment, there can be no further pain — at least that is the theory. In effect, some degree of pain persists, although markedly reduced in most cases. Surgical selection is rigorous and involves examination, MRI, and discographic evaluation, as this seems to be the only way to enhance the predictability of this procedure.

Artificial disc replacement or spine arthroplasty is currently at the research stage and not available as an option for most individuals, except in a carefully monitored clinical trial. However, this may be the future of disc surgery.

Osteoarthritis (Degenerative Joint Disease)

Arthritis Fact

In the vast majority of people, the presence of arthritis in their lumbar spine causes no pain, stiffness, or loss of function.

For most individuals with osteoarthritis or lumbar spondylosis, the symptoms related to arthritis in the low back will be tolerable, occasionally bothersome, and rarely disabling. Learning to live with this discomfort involves an ongoing program to minimize severity and recurrence. Aggravating activities should be identified and avoided. Keeping a diary of your pain, its ups and downs, things that seem to irritate it and those that give relief, is a useful exercise. Accept your diagnosis and realize it is exceedingly unlikely to ever progress to a stage where you need surgery or are confined to bed or a wheelchair. In fact, over time it will likely improve as your spine adjusts and stabilizes, the inflammation settles, and your desire for vigorous pursuits diminishes.

Dangers of Diagnosis

With unfortunate frequency, patients with back pain are sent for X-rays, which show a degree of 'degenerative arthritis' and are told that this is the cause for their pain. Arthritis cannot be cured so they are then stuck with a condition likely to cause them pain for the rest of their lives. The alarm and stress this causes to the patient is tremendous. The doctor, however, is relieved to have found something to explain the pain and can recommend simple treatment that may or may not work. The truth is that a very high percentage of patients, particularly over the age of 40 will show some evidence of 'wear and tear' in the spine on X-ray. More sensitive tests such as bone scan or MRI may even pick up changes in people in their twenties and thirties. The fact is, however, that in almost all of these cases, the findings are incidental and not related to any back pain the person might be experiencing.

Treatment of Lumbar Spine Osteoarthritis

There are, however, some individuals in whom arthritis is a major cause of their low back pain, and in these people the pain is likely to persist, progress, or recur with great frequency. Pain tends to be back-dominant and associated with stiffness and is likely to follow the pattern of arthritis in other areas with pain-free periods and gradual step-wise deterioration. There may be evidence of arthritis in joints or tissues remote from the spine and, apart from ankylosing spondylitis and some rheumatoid patients, this is generally an affliction of the older individual (over 60 years).

For individuals with no symptoms, reassurance is all that is required. In a younger individual with low back pain, arthritis on X-ray is likely an incidental and non-contributory finding. Standard conservative treatments and rehabilitation will resolve the acute or recurrent pain. Similarly, for those patients considered to have only mild symptoms of stiffness or pain, a simple non-invasive management plan should be instituted. This can include heat, massage, trunk strengthening and flexibility, weight-loss if appropriate, supplements such as glucosamine, and exercise, including Yoga or Tai Chi.

Other Presentations of Lumbar Osteoarthritis

Besides lumbar spondylosis discussed above, which generally causes little or no significant pain or disability, osteoarthritis in the low back can present with narrowing of the spinal canal (stenosis) or slippage of one vertebra upon another (instability or degenerative spondylolisthesis). These conditions can cause far more severe symptoms and require more aggressive treatment, including surgery.

Osteoarthritis Facts

As opposed to degenerative disc disease, lumbar spine osteoarthritis (also called lumbar spondylosis) tends to affect multiple levels rather than one or two and involves all anatomic components of the spine, including discs, facets, and ligaments.

Osteoarthritis (Lumbar Spondylosis)

Treatment
- Heat Pack, Whirlpool, Shower Massage
- Lumbar Back Support
- Exercise
  - Low back, buttock and hamstring stretches
  - Abdominal and back muscle strengthening (core conditioning)
  - Cycling
  - Yoga, Tai Chi
- Hands on Treatments
  - Massage
  - Shiatsu
- Diet
  - Manage weight
  - Increase essentially fatty acids
  - Reduce meat intake, increase fish
  - Reduce nightshades (potatoes, peppers, tomatoes, eggplant)
  - Supplements:
    - Glucosamine sulphate, chondroitin sulphate, MSM
    - Ginger
    - Devil's Claw
    - Capsicum topical cream

Spinal Stenosis

The symptoms of spinal stenosis can often be obscure and misleading, which results in a failure of diagnosis. These symptoms usually resolve with rest and leaning forward. The extended posture further compromising the already tight spinal canal leads to the various neurologic sensations in this condition. Flexing forward tends to increase space, so individuals with this condition have to bend forward or sit in addition to just stopping activity. Flexing forward prolongs endurance, and patients can often delay the onset of symptoms by walking bent over a shopping cart, for example. Some people find they have no difficulty cycling or walking uphill as the body is bent forward, whereas going downhill is unbearable. In some cases, only lying and bringing the knees to the chest will provide enough flexion to relieve pain.

Rarely, spinal stenosis will present as an acute cauda equina syndrome requiring emergency treatment.

Diagnosis

Besides the typical history, diagnosis in spinal stenosis relies on diagnostic imaging. Clinical examination should rule out a vascular cause, but otherwise clinical tests may well be negative in the resting state. Occasionally, it is useful to get the patient to exercise until the pain or numbness develops, and then test power, reflexes, and other aspects of nerve function.

Plain X-rays are valuable as they best show the overall alignment of the spine and identify any slippage or instability between vertebrae. They do not, however, give any insight into the dimensions of the spinal canal or neural foraminae. The most valuable tests for this are CAT scan and MRI. These imaging modalities allow accurate assessment and measurement of available space, while confirming the anatomic structures responsible for the stenosis.

A canal diameter between 10 and 12 millimeters is considered 'relative stenosis', while less than 10 is called 'absolute'. These figures are, however, based on average values across populations and this varies tremendously with age. As with all imaging studies (and tests in general), the findings need to be taken in clinical context. Finding a canal diameter of 11 millimeters in a patient with intermittent back pain and no leg symptoms is likely to be of no relevance in the management of that patient. In addition diagnosing the patients with 'spinal stenosis' will only cause unnecessary concern.

Treatment of Spinal Stenosis

The natural history of spinal stenosis is poorly defined. The fact that many individuals with severely narrowed spinal canals have few or no symptoms, while others with marginal stenosis present with classic findings makes predication of outcome impossible.

It does appear that over time the spinal cord and nerves have some ability to adjust to the tighter environment with a subsequent reduction in symptoms. A trial of conservative treatment is warranted in most cases. Careful monitoring for progression of symptoms should be carried out. Individuals who are increasingly disabled or not improving with a level of dysfunction or pain they are unable to live with should be considered for surgical treatment.

There are a large number of non-operative treatment options in spinal stenosis (excluding cauda equina syndrome).

Posture and Exercise: Simple postural adjustments to increase flexion can improve walking and standing tolerance. Improving abdominal muscle tone, stretching the hamstrings

---

Spinal Stenosis Facts

Symptoms

- Pain in the lower back and/or buttocks — develops during walking or other activities.
- Pain radiating into one or both thighs, calves, or feet.
- Numbness, weakness, pins-and-needles, or hot/cold feelings in the legs.
- Clumsiness, frequent falls, 'foot-slapping' gait.
- Symptoms relieved by bending forward, sitting, or lying down.

Treatment in Addition to Osteoarthritis Therapies

- Postural Adjustments
- Exercise
- Flexion Exercises
- Hamstring Stretch
- Cycling
- Weight Loss
- Stop Smoking
- Supplements
- Essential Fatty Acids
- Vitamin B complex
- Anti-inflammatory Medication
- Epidural Cortisone Injection
- Decompression Surgery

and decreasing anterior pelvic tilt will reduce lumbar extension and thus improve stenosis. Intermittent rests, again with a flexed posture will allow longer periods of activity. Exercises will help improve posture and aerobic fitness as well as contributing to weight loss. Cycling is often a good option as it is performed in a flexed position. Walking uphill on a treadmill may also be tolerable.

Weight Loss: Weight loss has a number of benefits, including a reduction in forces across the spine and reversal of the back extension that goes along with a protuberant abdomen. Smoking is known to both accelerate disc degeneration and hamper the formation of new blood vessels, both of which will limit your ability to heal.

Supplements and Medications: Supplements can be used to address the arthritic component of the spinal stenosis as well as promoting nerve recovery and blood flow. Anti-inflammatory medications not only reduce the pain of arthritis but may decrease any inflammation-related swelling around the nerves that is contributing to the stenosis. A similar rationale is used for lumbar epidural steroid injection.

Instability from Arthritis (Degenerative Spondylolisthesis)

Instability due to arthritic changes within the lumbar spine is most common in the older female where wear and tear in the disc and facet joints typically allow the L4 vertebrae to slide forward on L5, resulting in narrowing of the spinal canal. This results in low back pain and leg pain made worse by walking, a result of the stenosis caused by this slippage. For many individuals, the symptoms are manageable and there is no indication for any aggressive intervention. Conservative measures are all that is required. For others, however, in whom pain affects quality of life, surgical decompression with fusion may be considered.

Treatment of Degenerative Spondylolisthesis
The treatment of degenerative spondylolisthesis follows similar guidlelines to those for spinal stenosis and incorporates general therapies for osteoarthritis. Surgical treatment, however, always requires spinal fusion in addition to decompression in order to address the issue of instability.

Degenerative Spondylolisthesis Facts

Treatment in Addition to Osteoarthritis Therapies
- Postural Adjustments
- Exercise
- Flexion Exercises
- Hamstring Stretch
- Cycling
- Weight Loss
- Stop Smoking
- Supplements
- Essential Fatty Acids
- Vitamin B complex
- Anti-inflammatory Medication
- Epidural Cortisone Injection
- Decompression Surgery with Fusion

Rheumatoid Arthritis

The diagnosis of rheumatoid arthritis can be difficult and elusive. A referral to a rheumatologist is recommended. A careful history, examination, blood tests, and X-rays can help clarify the diagnosis. In addition, removal of fluid from a joint for testing or sampling of the joint lining and examination under the microscope can also be used to aid diagnosis if it is unclear.

Rheumatoid Arthritis

Symptoms
- Morning stiffness (stiffness of joints lasting at least 1 hour in the morning).
- 3 or more joint areas involved.
- Hand joints involved (wrist and knuckle joints).
- Symmetrical joint involvement (same joints on both sides of the body).
- Rheumatoid nodules (nodules under skin, generally at elbows).
- Rheumatoid factor in blood.
- X-ray changes typical for rheumatoid arthritis.

Treatment
- Heat
- Dietary Modifications
  - Reduce animal protein, nightshades
  - Check food allergies/sensitivities
- Supplements
  - Glucosamine Sulfate, Chondroitin Sulfate
  - Devil's Claw
  - Boswellia
  - Essential Fatty Acids
- Massage Therapy
- Yoga/Tai Chi
- Medical Treatments
  - Simple Analgesics (Tylenol)
  - NSAIDS (non-steroidal anti-inflammatory drugs)
  - DMARDS (disease modifying anti-rheumatic drugs):
    - corticosteroids, prednisone
    - anti-malarials, gold, penicillamine, methotrexate
  - Biologic Response Modifying Drugs:
    - Infliximab (Remicaide)
    - Etanercept (Enbrel)
    - Antibiotic Therapy

Much like its presentation, the course of rheumatoid arthritis is variable. Among patients, 15% to 20% run an intermittent cause, showing frequent, partial, or complete remissions without the need for ongoing medical therapy. About 10% show similar long clinical remissions but require ongoing treatment. The largest group of 65% to 70%, show progressive disease, which may follow a rapid or slow course. They require ongoing medical and often surgical treatment. The outcome in rheumatoid arthritis is likely to be poor if rheumatoid factor is present in the blood tests from the outset, if rheumatoid nodules are present in the skin, or if the patient develops the disease after the age of 60. The good news is that effective and structured treatment involving a number of modalities can help slow the progress of disease, alleviate discomfort, and prolong function.

Ankylosing Spondylitis

Diagnosis of ankylosing spondylitis relies on the characteristic symptoms, presenting in an at-risk individual, plus findings of limited spinal mobility and chest expansion, alteration of posture, along with irritation of the sacroiliac joints. The spinal vertebrae gradually fuse together in a flexed position, causing straightening of the normal lumbar curve and increased arch in the upper back. In addition, the neck assumes a rigid, flexed position, making it difficult for the affected individual to look ahead. X-rays of the sacroiliac joints and the spine often reveal classic findings helping with the diagnosis of the disease. Blood tests include ESR, Hemoglobin, and HLA B-27.

The outlook for ankylosing spondylitis is variable, but considered better than for rheumatoid arthritis. The disease can be mild and self-limited. Evidence indicates that life expectancy is not reduced in the majority of patients. Many patients continue to function well, and one-third may become pain free. For most patients, the disease runs a mild course with little involvement of tissues outside the musculoskeletal system.

The mainstay of treatment for ankylosing spondylitis is an ongoing exercise program to maintain mobility and strength. Rarely is surgery required in the lumbar spine to correct severe deformity.

Ankylosing Spondylitis

Symptoms
- Low back pain of at least three months duration improved by exercise and not relieved by rest.
- Limitation of lumbar spine movement.
- Reduced chest expansion.
- Bilateral sacroilitis (irritability of the sacro-iliac joint at the back of the pelvis).
- Unilateral sacroilitis.

Characteristics
Five factors differentiate inflammatory back pain induced by spondylitis from back pain of other causes:
- Onset of back discomfort before age 40 years.
- Insidious onset.
- Persistence for at least three months.
- Associated with morning stiffness.
- Improvement with exercise.

Psoriatic Arthritis

In general, psoriatic arthritis causes much less disability than rheumatoid arthritis and ankylosing spondylitis. Only between 5% and 15% of all patients affected will progress to the severely destructive form of the arthritis with subsequent disability. Many more have a mild course with frequent remissions.

Psoriatic Arthritis

Symptom Patterns
- Arthritis of the DIP joints (redness and swelling of the end joints of the hand).
- Destructive arthritis with involvement of all the joints of hand and marked deformity.
- Symmetrical arthritis of a number of joints similar to rheumatoid arthritis.
- Asymmetric arthritis involvement of various joints with no specific pattern in the hand.
- Spondyloarthropathy predominately involvement of the spine and sacroiliac joints.

Other features include development of foot pain related to plantar fasciitis (heel spurs) and inflammation of the Achilles' tendon or heel cord.

Psoriatic Arthropathy

The diagnosis of psoriatic arthropathy is based primarily on clinical examination and presentation. Positive blood tests are rare, as with ankylosing spondylitis, although HLA testing may be beneficial. If positive, radiographs of the spine, sacroiliac joints, or fingers may show distinctive signs of psoriatic arthritis (so-called 'pencil in cup' abnormality).

Spondyloarthropathies (Ankylosing Spondylitis, Psoriatic Arthritis, Psoriatic Arthropathy)

Treatments
- Education, physiotherapy and occupational therapy.
- Acupuncture and massage.
- Supplements:
  - Glucosamine, chondroitin, MSM, ginger and curcumin.
  - High-dose essential fatty acids.
  - Quercitin (natural anti-histamine) for skin lesions.
  - Zinc for skin repair.
- Diet:
  - Remove or reduce animal products from the diet.
- Medical Treatments:
  - Simple Analgesics (Tylenol).
  - NSAIDS (non-steroidal anti-inflammatory drugs).
  - DMARDS (Disease modifying anti-rheumatic drugs): corticosteroids, prednisone, anti-malarials, gold, penicillamine, methotrexate
  - Biologic Response Modifying Drugs
  - Infliximab (Remicaide)
  - Etanercept (Enbrel)
- Radiotherapy: Controversial and currently little-used modality to reduce the rate of spinal fusion.
- Surgery: Rarely performed to correct deformity in the lumbar spine.

Other Types of Lumbar Spine Instability

Instability secondary to degenerative arthritis was discussed above. There are, however, other causes of instability or spondylolisthesis that tend to present in younger individuals. Many of these are incidental findings with no clinical symptoms, but occasionally they require treatment.

Spondylolytic Spondylolisthesis (Spinal Stenosis Due to Instability)

The majority of adults with spondylolytic spondylolisthesis are completely asymptomatic. Unfortunately, low back pain is so common that once in a while someone with this abnormality does develop symptoms and subsequent X-rays reveal what appears to be the cause, a vertebral slip. Of course, this is a misplaced assumption. While occasionally adults may develop symptoms from their spondylolisthesis, most of the time the back pain is unrelated and due simply to a lumbar strain or other benign condition. As such, except in circumstances where there is evidence of spinal stenosis or neurologic deficit, these patients should be treated just like anyone else with back pain.

In cases where back pain is persistent or recurrent, or when there is evidence of nerve root compromise, further investigation is warranted to determine the role for the spondylolisthesis in the overall clinical picture. CAT scan and MRI can be used to image the defect and identify stenosis or nerve root compression. EMG studies are helpful in localizing specific nerve root involvement. Discography and nerve root blocks will help localize the source of pain. Local anesthetic injection into the pars defect causing the slip is possible under X-ray guidance and will reveal whether this is contributing to the discomfort.

Treatment of Spondylolisthesis

In most cases of adult spondylolisthesis non-operative treatment is all that is required. Resolution of the acute phase is followed by an ongoing program to maintain trunk core stability, particularly extension strength, and avoid hamstring tightness. Weight control is important to reduce translational stress across the level of instability. Progression of symptoms and radiculopathy may be treated with epidural injections or nerve root blocks. Failure to improve with conservative measures and ongoing unacceptable back and leg pain or spinal stenosis symptoms is an indication for surgical evaluation.

Adult Spondylolisthesis Facts

Treatment

- Exercises:
  - Core Stability
  - Extension Strength
- Weight Management
- Epidural Injections
- Nerve Blocks
- Surgery

Adolescent Spondylolisthesis

Adolescents and children with spondylolisthesis often develop symptoms quite rapidly, with pain, numbness or weakness, and occasionally cauda equina syndrome. A far higher percentage of these children develop symptoms and require surgery. Interestingly, this type of spondylolisthesis does not predispose a person to low back pain in later life.

Adolescent Spondylolisthesis

Characteristics
* Majority are 'lytic' related to a defect in the pars (part of the bony vertebral arch) between L5 and S1
* Present in 5–6% boys, 2–3% girls
* Majority remain asymptomatic
* Associated with American football, weightlifting, gymnastics
* Only a small minority show progressive slip
* Slip and symptoms may progress in 30s and 40s or during pregnancy

Symptoms
* Tight Hamstrings
* Back Pain
* Nerve Root Irritation (typically L5)

Treatment
* Treatment involves hamstring stretching and analgesics/NSAIDS for acute episodes.
* Surgery considered if slip progresses or symptoms unresolved.

Glossary

Absorption The selective taking-in or abstraction of water or other materials from the alimentary canal (digestive tract) into the blood or lymphatic system.

Acidosis An accumulation of hydrogen in body fluids due to increased production as seen in a diabetic coma or failure of normal elimination by the kidney or excessive administration of acids.

Active Compound A chemical agent that directly kills a pest. A constituent in a pesticide.

Active Release Therapy Therapeutic treatment that mobilizes, stretches, and releases abnormalities in the soft tissues of the body.

Acupuncture The process of inserting needles into specific points along meridians on the body to increase flow of Qi or energy and promote healing.

Adenosine Triphosphate (ATP) A compound containing three phosphates that when broken down produces energy and enables muscles and organs to function.

Adrenaline The catecholamine released by the adrenal medulla in response to stress. It is short acting and causes activation of the adrenergic receptors.

Adrenal Cortex The portion of the adrenal gland that secretes corticosteriod hormones such as cortisol in response to stress.

Adrenal Gland The small gland that sits above the kidneys. It is divided into the adrenal medulla and adrenal cortex.

Adrenal Medulla The portion of the adrenal gland that secretes the catecholamines such as adrenaline and noradrenaline in response to stress.

Adrenocorticotropic Hormone The hormone produced by the anterior pituitary gland that interacts with the adrenal glands and forces them to secrete cortisol and other corticosteroids.

Adipose Tissue The layer or distribution of fat found between the muscle and skin.

Afferent Pertaining to the nervous system, a nerve fiber going from a receptor in the body to the spinal cord or brain.

Alexander Technique A therapy designed to integrate every muscle and cell in each body movement as one unit in order to restore body harmony.

Alpha Waves One of the natural electrical rhythms of the brain observed on an EEG (electroencephalogram) of a relaxed yet awake individual.

Amino Acid An inorganic nitrogen rich acid that forms the basic subunit of protein. Each subunit or amino acid is linked to another though a peptide bond. There are 8 essential amino acids (9 for infants) and 13 (or 12) non-essential acids for adults and children, respectively.

Analgesics (painkillers) The first line in the medicinal treatment of pain.

Ankylosing spondylitis A type of inflammatory arthritis associated with the gene HLA-B27, most commonly presenting with back pain.

Anorexia A condition of being without or having lost the appetite for food leading to severe weight loss and associated with amenorrhea, and psychological or physiological issues.

Antibody: A protein produced by the immune system that binds to an antigen to neutralize or destroy it.

Antigen: A substance recognized as foreign to the body inducing antibody formation against it.

Anti-oxidant A substance that neutralizes free radicals in the body. This aids the body in faster recover and promotes stronger, healthier tissues.

Arteriosclerosis A common blood vessel disorder characterized by calcified yellow plagues, lipids and debris that line the walls of the arteries.

Arthritis Inflammation of a joint. Several different forms exist.

Arthralgia Literally means pain in a joint. While arthritis does present with arthralgia, not all arthralgia is arthritis. Arthralgia is common in illness such as influenza.

Arthrodesis A fusion of the joint such that no movement is allowed following the surgery.

Arthrography Radiological technique in which dye is injected into a joint prior to the taking of X-rays.

Arthropathy Damage or dysfunction within a joint.

Arthroplasty Creation of a new joint. Most commonly refers to the replacement of a damaged joint (total joint replacement arthroplasty).

Arthroscopy A minimally-invasive surgical technique used to evaluate and treat problems within certain joints. It is now the most commonly performed orthopaedic procedure.

Articular Relating to a joint.

Articular Cartilage The smooth cartilage covering the end of a bone at a joint.

Auto-immunity An immune response produced by the body against one of its own cells or tissues.

Autonomic Nervous System The part of the nervous system that is not under conscious or voluntary control. It is responsible for functions such as blood pressure, heart rate, sweating, etc.

Avascular Necrosis A condition in which the blood supply to an area of bone is lost, resulting in bone death and collapse.

Basal Metabolic Rate The rate at which the body expends energy for maintenance activities such as organ function and breathing.

Basophil A type of white blood cell that produces histamine.

Beta Waves An electrical rhythm of the brain seen on EEG of an individual who is awake, alert and with open eyes.

Bioavailability The ability of ingested nutrients to pass through the digestive tract into and through the bloodstream to its destination cells to be used.

Biochemical Reactions The chemical activities associated with life as exhibited in humans and other living organisms. These are the reactions that drive all bodily functions.

Bioflavanoid (also known as Vitamin P) A group of plant pigments that provide the colors to many plants and flowers. In humans they play a role in combating pain and inflammation, histamine, absorption of certain nutrients, and many other health benefits.

Biomechanics The study of the way in which the body is constructed and moves.

Biotin (also known as Vitamin H) A necessary vitamin for the body and is an essential co-factor in many enzymatic reactions.

Blood Pressure The pressure of the blood measured against the walls of the arteries. Normal is considered 120/80.

Bone Bruising A recent injury identified at the joint surface. The injury is seen only by MRI examination of the joint following trauma.

Bone Scan This test measures 'bone cell activity'. It involves injection of a (non-harmful) radioactive marker into a vein in the hand, followed, two hours later, by a scan of the whole body or a specific area. Active areas show up as 'hot spots'.

Boron A trace mineral that was only recently discovered as helpful to humans in the repair of bone and joints. It is found widely in fruits and vegetables.

Boswellia A small tree native to India that has a gummy resin. This resin contains potent anti-inflammatory properties.

Botulinum Toxin (Botox) The product of a bacterium Clostridium botulinum used to prevent muscle contraction and spasm.

Bromelain Contains enzymes naturally found in pineapple. Several beneficial results have been achieved by using these proteolytic enzymes as anti-inflammatory agents.

Brown Fat Fatty deposits found in particular places on the body such as in between the shoulder blades. This is the type of fat that generates heat, particularly in hibernating animals.

Bulimia Perpetual and voracious appetite for large quantities of food to a morbid degree. It is usually associated with vomiting the food after consumption and psychological issues.

Bursa One of the many protective sacks that occur throughout the body. The bursa is a slippery sack lined with the same tissue that lines a joint synovial membrane. They provide cushioning and lubrication between structures.

Bursitis Inflammation of a bursa.

Calcium An essential mineral to the body necessary for bone strength, cardiac function, muscle regulation, and much more.

California Poppy A plant used therapeutically for the control of pain, anxiety and spasm.

Calorie A unit that characterizes the amount of energy available from food.

Capsicum Found in the chili pepper, red pepper, or cayenne pepper it is one of the oldest spices. Now used therapeutically for its anti-inflammatory effects.

Carbohydrate An organic compound in nature consisting of carbon, hydrogen and oxygen that is used by the body as a potential fuel source. This includes starches, sugars, fiber, cellulose, and gums.

Carnitine An amine that is often considered an amino acid that helps to transport fat to the mitochondria to be burned for energy.

Cartilage A complex composite connective tissue that covers the surfaces of bone (articular cartilage), providing strength and shock absorption to a joint. Other forms of cartilage exist throughout the body.

CAT Scan CT or computer tomography uses X-rays from different angles to give a 3-dimensional image of the body.

Catecholamine A generic term used to describe the stress neurotransmitters adrenaline and noradrenaline.

Cauda Equina Syndrome A syndrome comprising an inability to pass urine, full bladder with leaking, loss of bowel continence, loss of feeling in legs, and loss of feeling between legs due to compression of nerve roots at the bottom of the spinal cord.

Centralization Centralization phenomenon describes the change in location of pain from the foot or leg towards the midline of the spine.

Cerebellum The part of the brain behind the pons that controls the fine motor movements of the body.

Cerebral Cortex The outer layer of the cerebellum, the most sophisticated and highly developed area of the brain.

Chemonucleolysis (Chymopapain injection) A technique whereby an enzyme is introduced into the intervertebral disc via needle and guided X-ray to dissolve the nucleus pulposus.

Chiropractic Treatment The gentle movement of joints and the surrounding musculature for therapeutic purposes.

Cholecystokinin A hormone formed in the presence of dietary fat that stimulates the contraction of the gall bladder and a sensation of satiation.

Cholesterol A waxy substance present in all cell membranes that is important for the transportation and absorption of substances in and out of cells. Cholesterol is widely manufactured by the body and many dangers arise when it is produced in excess.

Chondrocyte A mature cartilage cell.

Chondroitin A mixture of hydrolyzed GAGs (glycosaminoglycans) and sugars. Its function is to inhibit the enzymes that break down collagen and provide building materials for cartilage.

Chondrogenic Potential to promote cartilage growth or regeneration.

Chondromalacia Refers to deterioration in the quality of the articular cartilage that overlies the end of a bone at a joint.

Chromium An essential mineral for the body that helps to stabilize blood sugar levels.

Circadian Rhythm The body's natural wake-sleep cycle controlled via the hormone melatonin.

Co-enxyme A substance that must be present with an enzyme to allow that enzyme to function. Coenzymes are mandatory for the use of vitamins and minerals in the body.

Collagen Long, chain-like, structural protein that provides strength to many tissues including cartilage.

Collagenase An enzyme that breaks down collagen.

Complex Carbohydrate A carbohydrate that also contains fibre and has a slower release of sugar into the blood stream than a simple carbohydrate.

Compression Fracture A break in the vertebral bone that occurs when the force compressing the front part of the vertebral body is greater then the strength of the bone.

Conjugated Linoleic Acid An essential fatty acid that helps prevent muscle wasting.

Constipation A condition in which stools are passed infrequently and with difficulty.

Contrast Treatment Alternating application of heat and cold. Contrast baths are particularly effective at reducing tissue swelling.

Copper Copper is an essential trace mineral that is part of several important enzyme reactions in the body. It is the third most abundant mineral in the human body.

Coronal View from the front plane.

Cortico-releasing Hormone (CRH) Produced in the hypothalamus in response to stress, and stimulates the pituitary to release ACTH (see above).

Corticosteroids A group of hormones synthesized in the adrenal glands. They have a multitude of effects, including control of the absorption and movement of fluids in the body, metabolism of glucose, and the control of inflammatory reactions in the body.

Cortisol The body's major stress hormone produced in the adrenal glands in response to stimulation from ACTH from the pituitary glands. This is the longer lasting stress hormone.

Cortisone (injection) A long acting form of the anti-inflammatory medicine used for injection into a joint.

COX Acronym referring to cyclo-oxygenase enzymes that initiate inflammation through the production of different chemicals.

Cryotherapy Treatment with cold or ice.

Curcumin Curcumin or tumeric is a perennial herb native to Southern Asia and grown extensively in the Carribean. It is a member of the ginger family and has similar anti-inflammatory properties.

Cyclo-oxygenase Essential enzymes involved in the production of prostaglandins and other chemicals that mediate inflammation.

Cytokines Molecules released during inflammation that act to modulate the immune response by acting on numerous cell and tissue types. Include interleukins (ILs) and tumor necrosis factor (TNF).

Debridement Procedure refers to the evaluation of a joint with arthroscopy and the treatment of damaged areas within the joint. It can be considered a 'spring clean up' or 'lube, oil and filter'.

Decompression The surgical removal of pressure on nerves in the spinal cord.

Degenerative Joint Disease (DJD) Synonymous with arthritis.

Delta Waves A natural wave pattern of the brain observed on EEG of a sleeping individual.

Demyelination The loss of the protective insulation that covers nerves.

Derangement Syndrome The most common McKenzie classification of back pain due to mechanical deformation of soft tissues as result of internal alterations of fluid, tissue, and bone.

Detoxification The process of ridding the body of poisonous chemicals, carcinogens, and other toxins.

Devil's Claw Devil's claw or *Harpago phytum* is a herbaceous plant native to South Africa. It possesses anti-inflammatory qualities and is used in the treatment of arthritis.

Dexamethasone A drug that mimics cortisol.

Dexamethasone Suppression Test A test whereby dexamethasone is injected into a subject to observe the reaction of the hypothalamic-pituitary-adrenal axis reaction.

Diabetes A disorder characterized by excessive urine excretion and thirst with oscillations between hypoglycemia and acidosis.

Diarrhea The frequent passage of unformed liquid stools.

Diathermy A physical modality of treatment providing deep heating to tissues.

Disc The supportive structure between two vertebra consisting of a tough outer shell and a gel like core.

Discectomy Surgical removal of the herniated nucleus pulposus fragment of the intervetebral disc.

Disc Herniation A painful condition whereby the jelly like matrix leaks out of the disc and inflames the nearby nerves. Also known as ruptured discs.

Discography The placement of a needle with X-ray guidance into an intervertebral disc, followed by injection of a radio-opaque dye under pressure.

Diuretic A substance that causes increased urine output by forcing the kidneys to excrete more salt, potassium and water.

Dimethyl Sulfoxide (DMSO) A bi-product from the wood industry. Once in the body, it is converted into MSM and is used for the repair and health of cartilage.

DMARD (disease modifying anti-rheumatic drug) Any one of a number of medications used in inflammatory arthritis to modify the immune response.

Double-blind Study A type of clinical trial in which neither the subjects nor the examiner know which product is being taken in order to reduce bias in results.

Dysfunctional Syndrome A McKenzie classification of back pain where pain results from the stretching of structures that have become sensitive and shortened.

Dysplasia An abnormal formation or development in the body.

Edema Fluid retention in the body resulting in swelling and bloating in the skin and other tissues.

Efferent A nerve fiber leaving the brain or spinal cord, going to muscles or glands of the body.

Eicosapentaenoic Acid (EPA) An omega-3 fatty acid that is also known as an essential fatty acid found in fresh water fish.

Electroencephalogram (EEG) A machine designed to monitor the signal produced by electrical activation of the cerebral cortex.

Electrolytes The ionized salts in the blood. A specific ratio known as the electrolyte balance is essential for proper bodily function.

Endocrine System The collection of glands that produce and secrete hormones and chemical messengers in the body and deliver them to the blood.

Enzyme One group of proteins produced in cells that are capable of greatly accelerating chemical reactions in the body without being broken down or consumed themselves.

Epidural Steroidal Injection Steroid injected into the space that surrounds the nerve root and nerve sheath to reduce local inflammation swelling and pain.

Essential Fatty Acids (EFAs): Fatty acids that the body cannot manufacture and therefore have to be obtained from diet, e.g., linoleic acid and arachidonic acid.

Essential Nutrients Substances that the body can not produce itself and are necessary for survival.

External Fixation A rigid device that is surgically placed on two parts of a bone to hold the bone together.

Extra-articular Outside or surrounding a joint.

Extracellular Outside the cell.

Facet (zygoapophyseal) Joint Block A procedure whereby a steroid or anesthetic is injected into the facet joint capsule to decrease pain or help diagnose the source of the pain.

Fat Cell A cell that stores fatty acids for energy.

Fatty Acids Fats and lipids that are nutritional, yet in high quantity can be harmful. These include cholesterol, triglycerides, prostaglandins, lecithin, choline, and more.

Fiber Plant compounds that are indigestible to the human digestive tract.

5-HTP A brain neurotransmitter that is readily converted into serotonin.

Fracture A break in any bone.

Free Radical A highly reactive molecule that is known to injure cell membranes, damage DNA, and contribute to aging and degenerative illnesses.

Free Radical Scavenger A substance, like an anti-oxidant, that seeks out and destroys free radicals in the body.

Frozen Shoulder Also called adhesive capsulitis, this condition causes the shoulder to become painful and stiff.

Fructose A simple carbohydrate or sugar that comes from fruits and is absorbed and utilized by the body at a slower rate than glucose.

Garcinia Cambogia A herb that helps to suppress an appetite and prevents lipogenesis.

Genistein An isoflavone found in soy products (see Isoflavone).

Ginger Ginger or Zingiber is an herb with therapeutic use in digestion and inflammation.

Glucocorticoids Steroidal hormones that are secreted by the adrenal glands that affect the metabolism. Cortisol is one of them.

Glucagon A polypeptide hormone secreted by the pancreas in response to hypoglycemia. It is responsible for raising blood sugar levels when they fall too low.

Gluconeogenesis The synthesis of glucose by the liver and kidneys from non-carbohydrate sources like amino acids and fatty acids.

Glucose A simple carbohydrate or sugar that is the end product of carbohydrate metabolism and the main energy source for all living organisms.

Glucosamine Sulfate Glucosamine sulfate is a combination of glutamine and sulfate. It is used in the manufacture of GAGs to increase the strength and structure of cartilage, maintain synovial fluid, and inhibit damaging enzymes.

Glutamine An amino acid that has been shown to increase the rate of muscle growth in humans and decrease fat production.

Glycemic Index A scale used to measure the amount of glucose present in different foods.

Glycogen The main storage form of glucose, manufactured by and largely stored in the liver and muscles.

Glyconeogenesis The breakdown of glycogen stores in the liver to produce glucose in response to low blood sugar levels.

Glycosaminoglycans (GAGs) Chemical building blocks for cartilage that also help to attract water to maintain cushioning and resilience.

Gout A form of crystal arthritis caused by a deposition of uric acid crystals.

Gonadotropic Hormone (GnRH) A hormone from the hypothalamus that controls the release of FSH and LH from the pituitary gland.

Growth Hormone A polypeptide hormone secreted by the anterior pituitary gland. It acts on bone and muscle growth, and on carbohydrate and nitrogen metabolism.

High-density Lipoproteins (HDL) Complexes of lipids and proteins that are important in structural and catalytic activities in cell membranes. These are the good lipids that help prevent the bad lipids (LDLs) from building up in the arteries.

Hippocampus Part of the limbic system responsible for coordinating the 'fight or flight' response.

Histamine A substance released from the mast cells and basophils that increases inflammation, edema, redness, and pruritis.

Hormone A chemical substance formed in one part of the body and transported to a different area where it has a regulatory effect on different functions.

Homeostasis The steady state of the body where all 'things' lie within their natural and normal levels.

Hops A natural supplement that contains resinous compounds that have hypnotic and sedating effects.

Hyaluronic Acid (hyaluronan) The most important GAG in articular joint cartilage and joint fluid.

Hydrotherapy The external use of water-based modalities for treatment of back pain.

Hypercholesterolemia An excess of cholesterol in the blood.

Hyperglycemia An excessive amount of sugar in the blood.

Hyperinsulemia An excess of insulin secretion, resulting in low blood sugar levels or hypoglycemia.

Hyperlipidemia A condition in which lipids are present in excess in the blood.

Hypertension Persistently high arterial blood pressure, usually diagnosed after three consecutive readings of 140/100 or more on three different dates.

Hypertrophic Arthritis Arthritis in which the body produces extra bone or cartilage.

Hypoglycemia A low blood sugar concentration.

Hypothalamus The region of the brain that controls the release of hormones from the pituitary gland. Receives signals from almost all other areas of the body.

Immune System The system of the body that recognizes and attempts to destroy foreign material such as bacteria, viruses, tumors, and allergens.

Immunoglobulin Anti-body protein molecules in which one end is used for the recognition of foreign material (antigens) and the other end activates an immune response.

Inflammation A complex interaction of chemicals and cells forming a pathway that results in pain, swelling, stiffness, and tissue damage.

Inflammatory Arthritis Arthritis in which there is an identifiable, immune-based, inflammatory response, which results both in arthritis and damage to other tissues.

Interferential Bio Electrical Stimulation Treatment that uses the application of two 'interfering' medium frequency alternating currents to help control pain, swelling, and muscle wasting.

Intradiscal Electrothermal Coagulation (IDET) A technique whereby a heating probe is introduced into the disc under X-ray guidance to cauterize or close off the nerve fibers supplying the annulus to decrease pain.

Isoflavone A type of phytoestrogen (plant estrogen) found in soy products. (see Phytoestrogen).

Isotope Scan (Technetium) A scan that measure bone cell activity.

Insulin A protein hormone formed and secreted by the pancreas in response to a rise in blood sugar level. It promotes lipid synthesis as it stores the sugar from the blood as fat.

Insulin Resistance A condition in which the body is insensitive and even resistant against the effects of insulin. In most cases the body responds by producing even more insulin.

Interleukins Molecules in the cytokine group, released during inflammation and acting to modulate the immune response by activating numerous cell and tissue types.

Intra-articular Within a joint.

In vitro Existing outside of a living cell or body. Pertaining to an artificial or manufactured environment.

In vivo Existing within a living cell or body, either animal or plant in nature.

Ketone Body An acidic substance produced by the rapid metabolism of fatty acids.

Ketosis The presence of excessive ketone bodies in the tissues, usually the result of starvation or diabetes mellitus.

Kyphoplasty A surgical procedure involving the insertion of an inflatable balloon into the vertebral body under X-ray to restore height and correct structural deformities in the vertebra.

Kyphosis Curvature of the spine with the apex backwards or away from the body as seen in the thoracic spine.

Lavender A plant that used to enable sleep, promote relaxation, prevent depression, and improve moods.

Leptin A hormone produced by the fat that decreases appetite and increases energy expenditure or metabolism.

Leukotrienes Arachidonic acid metabolic products, which, along with prostaglandins, act to mediate the inflammatory response.

Ligament Bands or cords of strong fibrous collagen that join bones together.

Limbic System The extensive neuronal circuitry of the brain that controls emotion, behavior, and motivation.

Lipogenesis The formation of fat, and the transformation of non-fat materials into body fat.

Lipoprotein Lipase The enzyme involved in the chemical reaction that stores fat in the body.

Liver The central organ of metabolism of carbohydrates, proteins, and fats. It stores glycogen and takes part in regulating blood sugar levels and other essential substances such as vitamins blood clotting factors. It is also the chief detoxifying organ of the body, rendering toxic or foreign substances innocuous.

Lordosis Curvature in the spine with the apex forward or towards the front of the body, as seen in the cervical and lumbar regions of the spine.

Low Density Lipoproteins (LDLs): Complexes of lipids and proteins found in the blood that contribute to heart disease and high cholesterol when produced in great concentrations.

Lymphocyte A type of white blood cell that is involved in specific immune reactions.

Macronutrient The nutrients that are required daily by the body in large amounts such as ounces and grams. They include protein, carbohydrates, lipids, and water.

Macrophage A type of white blood cell derived from monocytes that engulfs and digests foreign materials.

Magnesium An essential mineral for the body that plays a role in metabolism and muscle maintenance. Required for many enzymatic reactions in the body.

Magnetic Resonance Imaging (MRI) Changing magnetic field used to examine different structures in the body.

Magnetotherapy The use of magnets as a physical therapy.

Manganese A mineral that is essential to the growth and repair of skeletal abnormalities.

Manipulation The mobilization of joints and soft tissues to improve range of motion.

Massage Therapy The technique of manual manipulation of the soft tissue of the body. It is used to increase circulation, decreases pain and spasticity, and promotes healing.

Matrix The molecular 'mesh' composed of glycosaminoglycans (GAGs) that attracts water in cartilage.

Medial Branch Neurotomy An injection of a chemical substance adjacent to a nerve while under the guidance of an X-ray to disrupt the nerves pathways that carry pain sensation from facet joints, thus relieving pain.

Menopause The cessation of spontaneous periods.

Metabolic Syndrome (Syndrome X) A disease characterized by obesity, high blood pressure, increased insulin resistance, increased cholesterol, and increased risk of heart disease and stroke.

Metabolism The chemical processes of every living cell in which energy is produced, tissues are built up (anabolism), and tissues are degraded (catabolism).

Methylsulfonylmethane (MSM) MSM is a naturally occurring sulfur containing compound used as structural building material for cartilage.

Metalloproteases Enzymes that break down cartilage matrix.

McKenzie Method A system that involves assessment, treatment, and prevention of common back problems.

Micro-discectomy Discectomy performed through a very small incision.

Micronutrient Nutrients that are necessary in the diet in small amounts, generally measured in milligrams or micrograms. They include vitamins, minerals, and herbs.

Mineral An inorganic substance found in the earth.

Mitochondria The cell components that produce the energy required for metabolism. Also called fat burners or power house cells.

Monocyte A type of white blood cell.

Mosaicplasty Involves the resurfacing of a damaged area of joint surface with good cartilage from another area that is not subject to loading during normal movement.

Myalgia Pain in the muscles. Often associated with unaccustomed exercise or, as in arthralgia, associated with influenza.

Natural Killer Cells Cells within the immune system that are responsible for identifying and destroying cancer cells.

Naturopathy Medical practice using clinical nutrition, traditional Chinese medicine, homeopathy, and natural substances (herbs, vitamins, minerals, etc) to stimulate the body's innate healing response and produce therapeutic effects.

Neurogenic Claudication Pain in lower legs and feet with a burning sensation due to nerve root compression.

Neuropathy A disease process characterized by the disintegration or destruction of specialized tissue in the nervous system. Resulting symptoms include numbness and tingling, pain, muscle weakness, and visual disturbances.

Neuron A nerve cell.

Neurotransmitter A chemical messenger released by a neuron that activates specific receptors, muscle cells, or glands to initiate a message, action, or emotion.

Neutrophil A white blood cell that, like macrophages, can ingest and destroy bacteria.

Nociceptors Pure pain sensors found all through the body.

Noradrenaline A catecholamine released from the adrenal glands in response to stress.

NSAID (non-steroidal anti-inflammatory drug) Medications that include ASA and have a specific effect at controlling inflammation through inhibition of the prostaglandin pathway.

Obesity An excessive accumulation of fat in the body, mainly deposited in the subcutaneous tissues. It is generally considered 30% above normal body weight.

Occupational Therapy A therapy that involves activity modification, pacing, and postural retraining to minimize discomfort and maximize function. Design and manufacture of splints and aids.

Orthopedics The division of surgery that deals with ailments of the locomotor system. Includes joints, muscles, ligaments, and tendons from the toes to the skull.

Orthotics Inserts within footwear designed to aid the foot during walking and improve biomechanics.

Osteoarthritis Chronic arthritis or inflammation of a joint that is degenerative in nature. It is usually but not always associated with aging and obesity, and is not accompanied by involvement of remote tissues or organs (cf. Inflammatory Arthritis).

Osteoporosis Loss of bone mass.

Osteotomy Refers to the realignment of a bone above or below a joint in order to change the forces across the joint. Generally, the procedure is carried out to unload a damaged area of the joint.

Pancreas The organ or gland in the body which secretes insulin and glucagan upon differing metabolic demands to help regulate blood sugar levels.

Parasympathetic Nervous System One of the two major divisions of the autonomic nervous system that controls digestion, resting, sleep, etc.

Phosphate A mineral that is essential to the body as it is exists in tissue, blood, bone, and chemical reactions in the body.

Phospholipases A group of enzymes that degrade the structural phospholipid layer that surrounds cells.

Physiological Pertaining to all the reactions and systems in the body and how they connect together to function as a whole.

Physiotherapy A therapy that incorporates education, passive and active stretching, strengthening, mobilization, posture and balance, as well as many physical modalities.

Phytoestrogen A type of phytosterol that mimics endogenous estrogen in the body (see Phytosterol).

Phytosterol A plant property similar to our own endogenous hormones.

Placebo An inactive substance used as a comparison in clinical tests.

Pituitary Gland An endocrine gland that is located below the hypothalamus and secretes six hormones, including ACTH, FSH, LH, TSH, GH, and prolactin.

Pons The region of the brainstem that is located between the medulla and the midbrain.

Postural Syndrome A McKenzie classification of back pain attributed to mechanical deformation of soft tissues.

Polyarticular Involving a number of joints.

Potassium A mineral that is essential for the body and is found in high concentrations in tissues. It is necessary to maintain proper electrolyte balances in the body through its ionic charge and is used to excite or enhance action potential reactions.

Prostaglandins Arachidonic acid metabolic products, which, along with leukotrienes, act to mediate the inflammatory response.

Protein A class of organic nitrogen-based compounds, essential structural components of all cells and the basis of the majority of active molecules in the body.

Protein Kinase A generic term for an enzyme that phosphorylates (adds a phosphate to) protein.

Proteinase Enzyme that breaks down protein.

Proteoglygans A component of the extra cellular matrix or 'ground substance' of cartilage.

Pseudogout An inflammatory arthritis of the joints caused by crystals of calcium pyrophosphate. Also known as calcium pyrophosphate deposition disease (CPDD).

Psoriatic Arthritis A type of inflammatory arthritis associated with the skin condition psoriasis.

Psychology The branch of science/medicine that deals with the mind and all mental processes.

Radicular Pain Nerve pain in the leg, rather than the back, burning in nature, often associated with numbness or tingling.

Rapid Eye Movement (REM) The phase of sleep characterized by the desynchronized brain activity and dreaming. This is a paradoxical form of sleep as it is non restful.

Receptors Membrane-bound molecules with specific sites for other molecules such as neurotransmitters to bind into.

Replacement A surgical technique to replace a 'real' disc with an artificial one to restore strength to the spine.

RDA (Recommended Daily Allowance) The dosage of vitamins, minerals, and other nutrients as suggested by the FDA.

Rheumatoid Arthritis One of a number of inflammatory diseases that diffusely affect tissues and joints throughout the body.

Rosen Method A physical therapy that treats both the mind and the body as one in order to regain an optimal homeostatic state.

S-Adenosylmethionine (SAM-e) Formed from the amino acid methionine and ATP, it increases proteoglycan production.

Saggital View from the side plane.

Saturated Fats A fatty acid that has every possible bond filled with hydrogen atoms and is therefore less reactive. They tend to be solid at room temperature and generally are from an animal origin.

Sensory Receptors A type of pain receptors that carry impulses such as touch and pressure.

Serotonin A neurotransmitter that regulates depression and plays a role in sleep patterns.

Shortwave Diathermy Diathermy involves passage of a high frequency current with no nerve stimulation. The rapid vibration induces deep heat in the tissues.

Sciatica Pain primarily in the back with radiation to the buttocks and back of thighs.

Shiatsu Therapeutic body treatment that apples finger pressure on specific points of the body along 'energy meridians'.

Simple Carbohydrate A simple form of sugar such as glucose, lactose, and fructose that is rapidly absorbed into the bloodstream. These foods are the sugars and starches like potatoes and candy.

Soy A leguminous plant with many medicinal properties.

Spondyloarthritis Osteoarthritis of the spine.

Spondylolithesis: Vertebral slipping.

St John's Wort A herbal supplement that prevents the re-uptake of serotonin, GABA, and dopamine, used in the treatment of depression and anxiety.

Stabilization: A surgical fusion procedure in the spine to regain strength and structure.

Starvation A condition induced by continuous lack of sufficient food, causing renal failure, muscle cramping, and fatigue.

Stenosis A condition of the spine defined by a group of symptoms caused by any spinal pathology that results in inadequate space for the neural elements (spinal cord, nerve roots etc) to function properly.

Straightening A surgical procedure using bone grafts and metal hardware to recreate the normal spinal alignment.

Strengthening A surgical technique using injection bone cement to increase the integrity of bone. Also known as vertebroplasty.

Subchondral Refers to the bone layer just beneath the cartilage in a joint.

Substance P A neuroactive peptide or chemical messenger that is released from pain fibers.

Superoxide Dismutase An enzyme produced in the body to scavenge free radicals that decreases oxidation and inflammation.

Sympathic Nervous System One of two divisions of the autonomic nervous system that is activated during stress responses.

Synapse The junction between two neurons or between a nerve cell and a muscle cell.

Synovium The tissue that lines every synovial joint, producing synovial fluid.

Synovial Fluid The viscous lubricating fluid within a joint.

Synovectomy Removal of the synovial lining from a joint.

Tai Chi A moving form of yoga that works all joints in their full range of motion.

Tendonitis Inflammation of a tendon.

Tenosynovitis Inflammation of the sheath that surrounds a tendon.

Thalamus An area in the brain that integrates sensory information.

Thermogenesis The production of heat or energy through an increase in metabolism above normal levels.

Theta Waves The low frequency waves seen on an EEG of an individual who is in Stage 1 sleep.

Thymus An organ in the lymphathic system that produces the T-lymphocytes.

Traction The mechanical treatment that uses longitudinal distraction force along the length of the spine.

Transcutaneous Electrical Nerve Stimulation (TENS) The application of electrical stimulation to nerves and muscles for therapeutic use.

Triglyceride A combination of glycerol and a fatty acid such as oleic or stearic acid. Most animal and vegetable fats are triglyceride esters and the major storage molecules of the diet. High levels in the blood greatly increase the risk for heart disease.

Trypsic Hydrolysate Milk Peptide An extract from milk that binds into GABA receptors to promote relaxation and anxiolytic properties.

Tyrosine Kinase The enzyme that governs cell growth and differentiation.

Tumeric Tumeric or curcumin is a perennial herb. It is a member of the ginger family and has similar anti-inflammatory properties.

Tumor Necrosis Factor A chemical messenger within the immune system.

Ultrasound Mechanical energy in the form of high frequency vibration, transmitted to tissues as a form of physical therapy.

Valerian A natural supplement that interacts with the GABA receptor and prevents the break down of GABA to promote relaxation and sedation.

Vascular Claudication Pain and cramping in the calf muscles due to inadequate blood supply to exercising muscles.

Vasoconstriction The narrowing of a blood vessel that decreases blood flow and increases the pressure within it.

Vasodilation The relaxation or expansion of the blood vessels which increases blood and decreases blood pressure.

Vertebra The bony components of the spine.

Vertebroplasty Surgical injection of bone cement in to the vertebra to increase bone strength.

Vitamin A constituent of the diet other than protein, carbohydrate, fat, and inorganic salts that is necessary for the growth and repair of the body.

Vitamin B Complex A group of water soluble B vitamins that aid in nerve control and repair, fat metabolism, regulation of the nervous system and several enzyme reactions in the body.

Vitamin C (also known as ascorbic acid) A water-soluble vitamin with anti-oxidant properties. Also acts as a co-enzyme in several reactions in the body.

Vitamin E (also known as tocopherol) A fat-soluble vitamin with anti-oxidant properties.

Water Soluble Ability to dissolve in water.

White Fat The fat that is subcutaneous and found around the internal organs. Changes in size and is lost during weight loss.

Willow Willow or salix is a well-known herb also known as aspirin.

Yoga The physical practice that uses strengthening and stretching to bring balance and healing to all aspects of the body, the emotional, mental, and physical.

Zinc A mineral present in every cell in the body. It is a component in over 200 enzyme reactions and is used for several functions such immune, prostate, and bone.

Selected References

Andersson GBJ, Lucente T, Davis AM, et al. A comparison of osteopathic spinal manipulation with standard care for patients with low back pain. N Eng J Med 1999;341: 1426-31.

Andersson, GBJ. Intervertebar disc: Clinical aspects. In Musculoskeletal Soft Tissue Aging: Impact on Mobility. Buckwalter JA, Goldberg VM, Woo SL-Y, eds. AAOS 1993.

Axelsson P, Johnsson R, Stromqvist B, Andreasson H. Temporary external pedicular fixation versus definitive bony fusion: A prospective comparative study on pain relief and function. Eur Spine J 2003 Feb;12(1):41-47. Epub 2002 Sep 19.

Bao QB, Yuan HA Prosthetic disc replacement: The future? Clin Orthop 2002;394:139-45.

Barr JD, Barr MS, Lemley TJ, et al. Percutaneous vertebroplasty for pain relief and spinal stabilization. Spine 2000;25:923-28.

Bener A, Alwash R, Gaber T, Lovasz G. Obesity and low back pain. Coll Antropol 2003 Jun;27(1):95-104.

Bermond P. Therapy of side effects of oral contraceptive agents with vitamin B-6. Acta Vitaminol enzymol 1982;4(1-2):45-54.

Bernet F, Montel V, Noel B, Dupouy JP. Diazepam-like effects of a fish protein hydrolysate on stress responsiveness of the rat pituitary-adrenal system and sympathoadrenal activity. Psychopharmacology 2000 Mar;149(1):34-40.

Bigos S, Bowyer O, Braen G, et al. Acute Low Back Problems in Adults. Clinical Practice Guideline, Quick Reference Guide Number. 14. Rockville, MD: U.S. Department of Health and Human Services, Public Health Service, Agency for Health Care Policy and Research, AHCPR Pub. No. 95-0643. December 1994.

Borman P, Keskin D, Bodur H. The efficacy of lumbar traction in the management of patients with low back pain. Rheumatol Int 2003 Mar;23(2):82-86.

Brady LH, Henry K, Luth JF 2nd, Casper-Brunett KK. The effects of shiatsu on lower back pain. J Holistice Nurs 2001 Mar;19(1):57-70.

Bush K, Hillier S. A controlled study of caudal epidural injections of triamcinolone plus procaine for the management of intractable sciatica. Spine 1991;16:572-75.

Byrns G, Agnew J, Curbow B. Attributions, stress, and work-related low back pain. Appl Occup Environ Hyg 2002 Nov;17(11):752-64.

Carey TS, Garrett J, Jackman A, et al. The outcomes and costs of care for acute low back pain among patients seen by primary carte practitioners, chiropractors, and orthopaedic surgeons. The North Carolina Back Pain Project. N Engl J Med 1995;333:913-17.

Carey TS, Motyka TM, Garrett JM, Keller RB. Do osteopathic physicians differ in patient interaction from allopathic physicians? An empirically derived approach. J AM Osteopath Assoc 2003;103:313-18.

Carette S, Leclair R Marcoux S, et al. Epidural corticosteroid injections for sciatica due to herniated nucleus pulposus. N Engl J Med 1997;336:1634-40.

Carette S, Marcoux S, Truchon R, Grondin C, Gagnon J, Allard Y, Latulippe M. A controlled trial of corticosteroid injections into facet joints for chronic low back pain. N Engl J Med 1991 Oct 3;325(14):1002-07.

Carragee EJ, Paragioudakis SJ, Khurana S. Lumber high intensity zone and discography in subjects without low back problems. Spine 2000;25:2987-92.

Carragee EJ, Chen Y, Tanner CM, Hayward C, Rossi M, Hagle C. Can discography cause long-term back symptoms in previously asymptomatic subjects? Spine 2000 Jul 15;25(14):1803-08.

Cheing GL, Hui-Chan CW. Transcutaneous electrical nerve stimulation: Nonparallel antinociceptive effects on chronic clinical pain and acute experimental pain. Arch Phys Med Rehabil 1999 Mar;80(3):305-12.

Chrubasik S, Thanner J, Kunzel O, Conradt C, Black A, Pollak S. Comparison of outcome measures during treatment with the proprietary Harpagophytum extract doloteffin in patients with pain in the lower back, knee or hip. Phytomedicine 2002 Apr;9(3):181-94.

Cherkin DC, Eisenberg D, Sherman KJ, et al. Randomized trial comparing traditional Chinese medical acupuncture, therapeutic massage, and self care education for chronic low back pain. Arch Intern Med 2001 Apr 23;161(8):1081-88.

Cohen SP, Larkin T, Abdi S, Chang A, Stojanovic M. Risk factors for failure and complications of intradiscal electrothermal therapy: A pilot study. Spine 2003 Jun 1;28(11):1142-47.

Coghill RC, McHaffie JG, Yen YF. Neural correlates of interindividual differences in the subjective experience of pain. Proc Natl Acad Sci USA 2003 Jun 24.

Cooper G, Lutz GE, Hong HM. Intradiskal electrothermal therapy for treatment of chronic lumbar diskogenic pain: A minimum 2-year clinical outcome study: Michael S. Lee, MD (Hospital for Special Surgery, New York, NY). Arch Phys Med Rehabil 2003 Sep;84(9):E10.

Cott JM. In vitro receptor binding and enzyme inhibition of Hypericum perforatum extract. Pharmacopsychiatry 1997;30(suppl 2):108-12.

Davis KG, Marras WS, Heaney CA, Waters TR, Gupta P. The impact of mental processing and pacing on spine loading: 2002 Volvo Award in biomechanics. Spine 2002 Dec 1;27(23):2645-53.

Derby R, Klein G, Schwarzer A, et al. Relationship between intradiscal pressure and pain provocation during discography. Orthop Trans 1995;19:59-60.

Devor M. Pain arising from the nerve root and dorsal root ganglion. In Low Back Pain – A Scientific and Clinical Overview. Weinstein JN, Gordon SL, eds. American Academy of Orthopedic Surgeons 1996.

Diamond TH, Champion B, Clark WA. Management of acute osteoporotic vertebral fractures: A nonrandomized trial comparing percutaneous vertebroplasty with conservative therapy. Am J Med 2003 Mar;114(4):257-65.

Diamant, D. Diagnosing zygapophysial joint-mediated pain is more effectively done via comparative anesthetic (and saline placebo) blocks and exacting and demanding process. Spine 2002 Feb 1;27(3):328-29.

Diego MA, Jones NA, Field T, Hernandez-Reif M, Schanberg S, Kuhn C, McAdam V, Galamaga R, Galamaga M. Aromatherapy positively affects mood, EEG patterns of alertness and math computations. Int J Neurosci 1998;96(3-4):217-24.

Difazio M, Bahman J A focused review of botulinum toxins for low back pain. Clin J Pain 2002;18:S155-62.

Dolan AL, Ryan PJ, Arden NK, et al. The value of SPECT scans in identifying back pain likely to benefit from facet joint injection. Br J Rheumatol 1996;35:1269-73.

Donelson R, Grant W, Kamps C, Medcalf R. Pain response to sagittal end-range spinal motion: A prospective, randomized, multicentered trial. Spine 1991;16: S206-12.

Donelson R, Silva G, Murphy K. The centralization phenomenon: Its usefulness in evaluating and treating referred pain. Spine 1990;15:211-15.

Dreyfuss P, Halbrook B, Pauza K. Efficacy and validity of radiofrequency neurotomy for chronic lumbar zygoapophyseal joint pain. Spine 2000;25:1270-77.

Ernst E, White AR, Wider B. Acupuncture for back pain: Meta-analysis of randomized controlled trials and an update with data from the most recent studies. Schmerz 2002 Apr;16(2):129-39.

Faraj AA. External fixation in lumbar segmental instability. Acta Orthop Belg 2003;69(1):9-12.

Fassoulaki A, Paraskeva A, Patris K, Pourgiezi T, Kostopanagiotou G. Pressure applied on the extra 1 acupuncture point reduces bispectral index values and stress in volunteers. Anesth Analg 2003;96(3)885-90.

Foster L, Clapp L, Erickson M, Jabbari B. Botulinum toxin A and chronic low back pain: A randomized, double-blind study. Neurology 2001;56:1290-93.

Fransen M, Woodward M, Norton R, Coggan C, Dawe M, Sheridan N. Risk factors associated with the transition from acute to chronic occupational back pain. Spine 2002;27(1):92-98.

Friede M, Henneike von Zepelin HH, Freudenstein J. Differential therapy of mild to moderate depressive episodes (ICD-10 F 32.0: F32.1) with St John's Wort. Pharmacopsychiatry 2001;34(suppl 1):38-41.

Geenen R, Jacobs JW, Bijlsma JW. Evaluation and management of endocrine dysfunction in fibromyalgia. Rheum Dis Clin North Am 2002;28:389-404.

Gehweiler JA, Daffner RH. Low back pain: The controversy of radiologic evaluation. Am J Roentgenol 1983;140:109-12.

Gibson JN, Waddell G, Grant IC. Surgery for degenerative lumbar spondylosis. Cochrane Database Syst Rev 2000;(3):CD001352.

Golf SW, Happel O, Graef V, Seim KE. Plasma aldosterone, cortisol and electrolyte concentrations in physical exercise after magnesium supplementation. J Clin Chem Clin Biochem 1984 Nov;22(11):717-21.

Grob D, Humke T, Dvorak J Degenerative lumbar spinal stenosis: Decompression with and without arthrodesis. J Bone Joint Surg 1995;77A;1036-41.

Gura ST. Yoga for stress reduction and injury prevention at work. Work 2002;19(1):3-7.

Hall, H. The New Back Doctor. Toronto: Macmillan of Canada, 1980.

Hall, H. A Consultation with the Back Doctor. Toronto; McClelland & Stewart, 2003.

Han TS, Schouten JS, Lean ME, Seidell JC. The prevalence of low back pain and associations with body fatness, fat distribution and height. Int J Obes Relat Metab Disord 1997 Jul;21(7):600-07.

Heary RF. Intradiscal electrothermal annuloplasty: The IDET procedure. J Spinal Disord 2001 Aug;14(4):353-60.

Hernandez-Reif, Field, T, Krasnegor J, Theakton H. Lower back pain is reduced and range of motion increased after massage therapy. Int J Neurosci 2001;106(3-4):131-45.

Hertsman-Miller RP, Morgenstern H, H Hurtwitz, et al. Comparing the satisfaction of low back pain patients randomized to receive medical or chiropractic care: Results from the UCLA low back pain study. Am J Public Health 2002 Oct;92(10):162-63.

Hirsch C, Ingelmark BE, Miller M. The anatomical basis for low back pain: Studies on the presence of sensory nerve endings in ligamentous, capsular and intervertebral disc structures in the human lumbar spine. Acta Orthop Scand 1963;33:1-17.

Hodges PW. Core stability exercise in chronic low back pain. Orthop Clin North Am 2003;34:245-54.

Hudson S. Yoga aids back pain. Aust Nurs J 1998 Apr;(9):27.

Hurwitz EL, Morgenstern H, Harber P, et al. A randomized trail of medical care with and without physical therapy and chiropractic care with low back pain: 6-month follow-up outcomes from UCLA low back pain study. Spine 2002 Oct 15;27(20):193-204.

Jackson RP, Jacobs RR, Montesano PX. 1988 Volvo award in clinical sciences. Facet joint injection in low-back pain. A prospective statistical study. Spine 1988 Sep;13(9):966-71.

Jarvik JG, Hollingworth W, Martin B, Emerson SS, Gray DT, Overman S, Robinson D, Staiger T, Wessbecher F, Sullivan SD, Kreuter W, Deyo RA. Rapid magnetic resonance imaging vs radiographs for patients with low back pain: A randomized controlled trial. JAMA 2003;289:2863-65.

Jellema P, van Tulder MW, van Poppel MN, Nachemson AL, Bouter LM. Lumbar supports for prevention and treatment of low back pain: A systematic review within the framework of the Cochrane Back Review Group. Spine 2001 Feb 15;26(4):377-86.

Johnston JM, Landsittel DP, Nelson NA, Gardner LI, Wassell JT. Stressful psychosocial work environment increases risk for back pain among retail material handlers. Am J Ind Med 2003 Feb;43(2):179-87.

Johnsson KE, Uden A, Rosen I. The effect of decompression on the natural curse of spinal stenosis: A comparison of surgically treated and untreated patients. Spine 1991;16:615-19.

Kahn RS, Westenberg HG, Verhoeven WM, Gispen-de Wied CC, Kamerbeek WD. Effects of a serotonin precursor and uptake inhibitor in anxiety disorders; a double-blind comparison of 5-hydroxytrytophan, clomipramine and placebo. Netherlands, Int Clin Psychopharmacol 1987;2(1):33-45.

Kahn RS, Westenberg HG. L-5-hydroxytrytophan in the treatment of anxiety disorders. J Affect Disord 1985;8(2):197-200.

Kamei T, Toriumi Y, Kimura H, Ohno S, Kumano H, Kimura K, Decrease in serum cortisol during yoga exercise is correlated with alpha wave activation. Japan 2000;90(3 pt 1):1027-32.

Karasek M, Bogduk N. Twelve-month follow-up of a controlled trial of Intradiscal Thermal Annuloplasty for back pain due to Internal Disc Disruption. Spine 2000;25(20):2601-07.

Keen CL, Zidenberg-Cherr S. Manganese. Present Knowledge in Nutrition, 6th ed. Brown ML, ed. International Life Sciences Institute, Washington, DC, 1990:279-86.

Keitel W, Frerick H, Kuhn U, et al. Capsium pain plaster in chronic non-specific low back pain. Arzneimittelforschung 2001 Nov;51(11):896-903.

Kelsey JL, Golden AL. Occupational and workplace factors associated with low back pain. Occup Med 1988:3:7-16.

Kilpikoski S, Airaksinen O, Kankaanpaa M, Leminen P, Videman T, Alen M. Interexaminer reliability of low back pain assessment using the McKenzie method. Spine. 2002 Apr 15;27(8):E207-14.

Kim DJ, Yun YH, Wang JM. Nerve-root injections for the relief of pain in patients with osteoporotic vertebral fractures. J Bone Joint Surg Br 2003 Mar;85(2):250-53.

Kim YS, Chin DK, Yoon DH, Jin BH, Cho YE. Predictors of successful outcome for lumbar chemonucleolysis: Analysis of 3000 cases during the past 14 years. Neurosurgery 2002 Nov;51(5 Suppl):123-28.

Koh TC. Tai Chi and ankylosing spondylitis – a personal experience. Am J Chin Med 1982; 10(1-4):59-61.

Koes BW, Assendelft WJ, van der Heijden GJ, Bouter LM. Spinal manipulation for low back pain. An updated systematic review of randomized clinical trials. Spine 1996;21:2860-71.

Koes B, Scholten R, Mens, J, et al. Epidural steroid injections for low back pain and sciatica: an updated systematic review of randomized clinical trials. Pain Digest 1999;9:241-47.

Koltzenberg M, Torebjork HE, Wahren LK. Nociceptor modulated central sensitization causes mechanical hyperalgesia in acute chemogenic and chronic neuropathic pain. Brain 1994;117:579-91.

Kumar V, Singh PN, Bhattacharya SK. Anti-stress activity of Indian Hypericum perforatum L. Indian J Exp Biol 200;39(4):344-49.

Leboeuf-Yde C, Kyvik KO, Bruun NH. Low back pain and lifestyle. Part II — Obesity. Information from a population-based sample of 29,424 twin subjects. Spine 1999 Apr 15;24(8):779-83; discussion 783-84.

Leboeuf-Yde C. Body weight and low back pain. A systematic literature review of 56 journal articles reporting on 65 epidemiologic studies. Spine 2000 Jan 15;25(2):226-37.

Lee CK, Vessa P, Lee JK. Chronic disabling low back pain syndrome caused by internal disc derangements: The results of disc excision and lumbar interbody fusion. Spine 1995;20:356-61.

Lee KS, Doh JW, Bae HG, Yun IG. Diagnostic criteria for the clinical syndrome of internal disc disruption: Are they reliable? Br J Neurosurg 2003;17:19-23.

Loisel P, Vachon B, Lemaire J, et al. Discriminative and Predictive Validity Assessment of the Quebec Task Force Classification. Spine 2002;27:851-57.

Long AL. The Centralization Phenomenon: Its usefulness as a predictor of outcome in conservative treatment of chronic low back pain (a pilot study). Spine 1995;20:2513-21.

Lord S, Barnsley L, Wallis B. Percutaneous radiofrequency neurotomy for chronic cervical zygoapophyseal joint pain. N Engl J Med 1996:335:1721-26.

Lord SM, Barnsley L, Bogduk N. The utility of comparative local anaesthetic blocks versus placebo-controlled blocks for the diagnosis of cervical zygoapophyseal joint pain. Clin J Pain 1995;11:208-13.

Louis M, Kowalski SD. Use of aromatherapy with hospice patients to decrease pain, anxiety, and depression and to promote an increased sense of well-being. Am J Hosp Palliat Care 2002;19(6):381-86.

Lutz G, Vad V, Wineski R Fluoroscopic transforaminal epidural steroids: An outcome study. Arch Phys Med Rehab 1998;79:1362-66.

Louwaege A, Goubau J, Deldycke H, Brugman E, Friberg J, Gheysen F, Deryckere P, Herpels V. Efficiency of discography followed by chemonucleolysis in the treatment of sciatica. J Belge Radiol 1996 Apr;79(2):68-71.

MacDonald RS, Bell CM. An open controlled assessment of osteopathic manipulation in nonspecific low-back pain. Spine 1990 May;15(5):364-70. Erratum in: Spine 1991 Jan;16(1):104.

McKenzie RA. The lumbar spine: Mechanical diagnosis and therapy. Spinal Publication Limited, Waikanae, New Zealand, 1981.

McKenzie RA: Treat your own back. Spinal Publication Limited, Waikanae, New Zealand, 1985.

McMorland G, Suter E. Chiropractic management of mechanical neck and low-back pain: A retrospective outcome-based analysis. J Manipulative Physiol Ther 2000;23:307-11.

Marchand S, Charest J, Li J, et al. Is TENS purely a placebo effect? A controlled study on chronic low back pain. Pain 1993;54:99-106.

Medcalf R, Aprill C A, Donelson RG, Grant WA, Incorvaia K. Discographic outcomes predicted by pain centralization and "directional preference": A prospective, blinded study. Presented at annual meeting of the North American Spine Society, Washington, DC, October 1995.

Mender-Huber KB. Orgotein in the treatment of rheumatoid arthritis. Eur J Rheumatol Inflam 1981;4:201-11.

Meng CF, Wang D, Ngeow J, Lao L, Peterson M, Paget S. Acupuncture for chronic low back pain in older patients: A randomized, controlled trial. Rheumatology (Oxford) 2003 Jul 30.

Milne S, Welch V, Brosseau L, Saginur M, Shea B, Tugwell P, Wells G. Transcutaneous electrical nerve stimulation (TENS) for chronic low back pain. Cochrane Review 2001; The Cochrane Library Issue 4.

Molsberger AF, Mau J, Pawelec DB, Winkler J. Does acupuncture improve the orthopedic management of chronic low back pain — a randomized , blinded, controlled trial with 3 months follow up. Pain 2002 Oct;99(3):579-87.

Moneta GB, Videman T, Kaivanto K, Aprill C, Spivey M, Vanharanta H, Sachs BL, Guyer RD, Hochschuler SH, Raschbaum RF, et al. Reported pain during lumbar discography as a function of anular ruptures and disc degeneration. A re-analysis of 833 discograms. Spine 1994 Sep 1;19(17):1968-74.

Muller WE. Current St. John's wort research from mode of action to clinical efficacy. Pharmacol Res 2003 Feb;47(2):101-09.

Nakamura SI, Takahashi K, Takahashi Y, et al. The afferent pathways of discogenic low back pain. Evaluation of L2 spinal nerve infiltration. J Bone Joint Surg (Br) 1996;78:606-12.

Nordby EJ, Wright PH, Schofield SR. Safety of chemonucleolysis: Adverse effects reported in the United States 1982-91. Clin Orthop 1993;293:122-134.

Nordby EJ, Javid MJ. Continuing experience with chemonucleolysis. Mt Sinai J Med 2000 Sep;67(4):311-13.

Pedersen HE, Blunck CFJ, Gardner E. The anatomy of lumbosacral posterior rami and meningeal branches of spinal nerves (sinu-vertebral nerves): With an experimental study of their function. J Bone Joint Surg 1956;38A:377-91.

Phillips FM, Pfeifer BA, Lieberman IH, Kerr EJ 3rd, Choi IS, Pazianos AG. Minimally invasive treatments of osteoporotic vertebral compression fractures: Vertebroplasty and kyphoplasty. Instr Course Lect 2003;52:559-67.

Phillips FM, Ho E, Campbell-Hupp M, McNally T, Todd Wetzel F, Gupta P. Early radiographic and clinical results of balloon kyphoplasty for the treatment of osteoporotic vertebral compression fractures. Spine 2003 Oct 1;28(19):2260-65.

Power C, Frank J, Hertzman C, Schierhout G, Li L. Predictors of low back pain onset in a prospective British study. Am J Public Health 2001 Oct;91(10):1671-78.

Prateepavanich P, Thanapipatsiri S, Santisatisakul P, Somshevita P, Charoensak T. The effectiveness of lumbosacral corset in symptomatic degenerative lumbar spinal stenosis. J Med Assoc Thai 2001 Apr;84(4):572-76.

Raoul S, Faure A, Robert R, Rogez JM, Hamel O, Cuillere P, Le Borgne J. Role of the sinu-vertebral nerve in low back pain and anatomical basis of therapeutic implications. Surg Radiol Anat 2003 Feb;24(6):366-71. Epub 2003.

Razmjou H, Kramer JF, Yamada R. Intertester reliability of the McKenzie evaluation in assessing patients with mechanical low-back pain. J Orthop Sports Phys Ther 2000 Jul;30(7):368-83; discussion 384-89.

Report of the Quebec Task Force on Spinal Disorders. Scientific approach to the assessment and management of activity-related spinal disorders. A monograph for clinicians. Spine 1987 Sep;12(7 Suppl):S1-59.

Riew KD, Yin Y, Gilula L, et al. The effect of nerve-root injections on the need for operative treatment of lumbar radicular pain: A prospective, randomized, controlled, double-blind study. J Bone Joint Surg Am 2000;82:1589-93.

Rolland A, et al. Behavioural effects of the American traditional plant Eschscholzia californica: Sedative and anxiolytic properties. Planta Med 1991 June;57(3):212-16.

Rosa GD, et al. Regulation of superoxide dismutase by dietary mangaese. J Nutr 1980; 110: 795-804.

Ross MC, Bohannon AS, Davis DC, Gurchiek L. The effects of a short-term exercise program on movement, pain and mood in the elderly. Results of a pilot study. J Holist Nurs 1999;17(2):139-47.

Saal JA, Saal JS. Introdiscal electrothermal treatment for chronic discogenic low back pain. Spine 2000;25(20) 2622-27.

Seelig MS. Consequences of magnesium deficiency on the enhancement of stress reactions; preventive and therapeutic implications (a review). J Am Coll Nutr 1994 Oct;13(5):429-46.

Shekelle PG. A critical appraisal of the use of medications and spinal manipulation for idiopathic low back pain. In Low Back Pain: A Scientific and Clinical Overview. Weinstein JN, Gordon SL, eds. AAOS 1995.

Shekelle PG, Adams AH, Chassin MR, Hurwitz EL, Brook RH. Spinal manipulation for low-back pain. Ann Intern Med 1992 Oct 1;117(7):590-98.

Sengupta DK, Herkowitz HN. Lumbar spinal stenosis. Treatment strategies and indications for surgery. Orthop Clin North Am 2003 Apr;34(2):281-95.

Shekelle PG, Adams AH, Chassin MR, Hurwitz EL, Brook RH. Spinal manipulation for low-back pain. Ann Intern Med 1992 Oct 1;117(7):590-98.

Schulz H, Jobert M. Effects of hypericum extract on the sleep EEG in older volunteers. Journal of Geriatric Psychiatry and Neurology 1994;7(suppl 1):39-43.

Schwarzer AC, Aprill CN, Derby R, et al. The prevalence and clinical features of internal disc disruption in patients with chronic low back pain. Spine 1995;20:31-37.

Schwarzer AC, Wang SC, O'Driscoll D, Harrington T, et al. The ability of CT to identify a painful zygapophyseal joint in patients with chronic low back pain. Spine 1995:20:907-12.

Schwarzer AC, Derby R, Aprill CN, et al. Pain from the lumbar zygoapophyseal joints: A test of two models. J Spinal Disord 1994;7:331-36.

Sheen K, Chung JM. Signs of neuropathic paindepend on signals from injured nerve fibres in a rat model. Brain Res 1993;610:62-68.

Suseki K, Takahashi Y, Takahashi K, et al. Sensory nerve fibres from intervertebral discs pass through rami communicantes. A possible pathway for discogenic low back pain. J Bone Joint Surg (Br.) 1998;80:737-42.

Szpalski M, Gunzberg R, Mayer M. Spine arthroplasty: A historical review. Eur Spine J 2002;11 Suppl 2:S65-84.

Tesio L, Merlo A. Autotraction versus passive traction: an open controlled study in lumbar disc herniation. Arch Phys Med Rehab 1993;74:871-76.

Threlkeld AK. The effects of manual therapy on connective tissue. PhysTher 1992; 72:893.

Tile M, McNeil SR, Zarins RK, et al. Spinal stenosis: results of treatment. Clin Orthop 1976;115:104-08.

Toda Y, Segal N, Toda T, Morimoto T, Ogawa R. Lean body mass and body fat distribution in participants with chronic low back pain. Arch Intern Med 2000 Nov 27;160(21):3265-69.

Toda Y. Impact of waist/hip ratio on the therapeutic efficacy of lumbosacral corsets for chronic muscular low back pain. J Orthop Sci 2002;7(6):644-49.

Tournade A, Patay Z, Tajahmady T, Braun JP, Million S, Schmutz G. Contribution of discography to the diagnosis and treatment of lumbar disc herniation. J Neuroradiol 1991;18(1):1-11.

Truumees E. Medical consequences of osteoporotic vertebral compression fractures. Instr Course Lect 2003;52:551-58.

Tsuritani, I, Honda R, et al. Impact of obesity on musculoskeletal pain and difficulty of daily movements in Japanese middle-aged women. Maturitas 2002 May 20;42(1):23-30.

Turner JA, Ersek M, Herron L, et al. Surgery for lumbar spinal stenosis: Attempted meta-analysis of the literature. Spine 1992;17:1-8.

Vanitallie TB. Stress: A risk factor for serious illness. Metabolism 2002 Jun;51(6 Pt 2):40-45.

Volz HP, Murck H, Kasper S, Moller HJ. St John's Wort extract (LI 160) in somatoform disorders: Results of a placebo-controlled trial. Psychopharmacology 2002;164(3):294-300.

Watts RW, Silagy CA. A meta-analysis on the efficacy of epidural corticosteroids in the treatment of sciatica. Anaesth Intensive Care 1995;23:564-69.

Weiner B, Fraser R Foraminal injection for lumbar disc herniation. J Bone Joint Surg Br 1997;79:804-07.

Weishaupt D, Zanetti M, Boos N, Hodler J. MR imaging and CT in osteoarthritis of the lumbar facet joints. Skeletal Radiol 1999:28:215-19.

Williams NH, Wilkinson C, Russell I, et al. Randomized osteopathic manipulation study (ROMANS): Pragmatic trial for spinal pain in primary care. Fam Pract 2003;20:662-69.

Wittenberg RH, Oppel S, Rubenthaler FA, Steffen R. Five-year results from chemonucleolysis with chymopapain or collagenase: A prospective randomized study. Spine 2001 Sep 1;26(17): 1835-41.

Wolsko PM, Eisenberg DM, Davis RB, Kessler R, Phillips RS. Patterns and perception of care for treatment of back and neck pain: Results of a national survey. Spine 2003 Feb 1;28(3):292-97.

Yeung AT. The evolution of percutaneous spinal endoscopy and discectomy: State of the art. Mt Sinai J Med 2000;67:327-32.

Yong-Hing K, Kirkaldy-Willis WH. The pathophysiology of degenerative disease of the lumbar spine. Orthop Clin North Am 1983 Jul;14(3):491-504.

Kirkaldy-Willis WH, Burton CV. Managing Low Back Pain. 3rd ed. New York: Churchill Livingstone, 1992.

Yoshida H, Fujiwara A, Tamai K, et al. Diagnosis of symptomatic disc by MRI: T2-weighted and gadolinium-DTPA-enhanced T1-weighted MR imaging. J Spinal Disord Tech 2002;15:193-98.

Yoshizawa H, O'Brien JP, Smith WT. The neuropathology of intervertebral discs removed for low back pain. J Pathol 1980;132:95-104.*The Complete Doctor's Healthy Back Bible*

Index

A

acetaminophen, 175, 200-201
acidophilus, 204
active release therapy (ART), 128-129, 295
acupuncture, 8, 9, 33, 125-128, 205, 295
   for acute disc herniation, 262
   for ankylosing spondylitis, 292
   for degenerative disc disease, 282-283
   for lumbar strain, 256
   and naturopath's role, 28
   and pain gates, 78
   for psoriatic arthritis, 292
   for psoriatic arthropathy, 292
   for recurring back pain, 273
   and Tai Chi, 130
   and TENS, 113
acute back pain, 9, 45, 46, 140, 155, 228, 238
acute onset back pain, 19, 20, 47
Alexander Technique, 134, 275, 282, 283, 295
aloe vera gel, 204
amino acids, 162, 170, 295
analgesics. *See* painkillers
anatomy, 10-15, 30, 38, 40, 44-46, 51, 53, 57-69, 81, 90, 96, 103, 105, 120, 127, 271, 285, 287
ankylosing spondylitis, 43, 55, 81, 83, 89, 96, 99-101, 214, 285, 290-292, 295
anorexia, 267, 269, 295
annulus, 57, 62, 82-83, 87, 88, 216
annulus fibrosis (AF), 84, 214
antibiotics, 195, 207, 223, 289
anxiety, 34, 36, 47, 76, 105, 124, 128, 131, 135, 187, 191, 210, 239, 241-242, 252, 273
   supplements for, 195-199
arching, 22, 88, 141, 147, 253-255, 261, 280-281

arnica, 173, 256
arthritis, 18-21, 28, 29, 32, 33, 36, 37, 44, 46-48, 50-53, 55, 67, 68, 77, 81, 85, 87, 93, 96, 97, 100, 102, 103, 114, 115, 118, 121, 127, 129, 140, 158, 170, 172, 175, 179, 180, 182, 184, 186-188, 193, 194, 200, 201, 204, 207, 219, 263, 264, 273, 284, 285, 288, 291, 295. *See also* degenerative arthritis; facet joint arthritis; gout; hypertrophic arthritis; inflammatory arthritis; lumbar spine arthritis; osteoarthritis; pseudogout; psoriatic arthritis; rheumatoid arthritis; spinal arthritis; spinal osteoarthritis; spondyloarthritis
   definition, 97, 295
artificial disc replacement, 230-231, 284
ASA, 185, 200-202
assertiveness training, 242, 247
autonomic nervous system, 70-72, 105, 246, 296

B

back braces, 117-118, 256, 257, 273
back pain syndrome, 20, 33, 107, 196
back pain vs. leg pain, 21
back supports, 117-118, 257, 273, 286
bed rest, 8, 18, 110, 135, 255, 256, 262, 267, 273
behavior modification, 247
bending, 22, 30, 84, 88, 144, 147, 157, 255, 264, 281, 286
biofeedback, 242, 246
biologic response modifying drugs, 207, 289, 292
biomechanics, 30, 60, 115, 118-119, 230, 272, 275, 296
blood tests, 9, 27, 55, 96, 97, 101, 255, 267, 289, 290, 292

body fat percentage, 158, 160
body-mass index (BMI), 158-159
bone, cancers that typically spread to, 266
bone mineral densitometry, 267-268
bone spurs, 82, 99, 219, 220
bone strength 95, 96, 264-267. *See also* calcium, vertebroplasty
bony vertebrae, 45, 65, 88, 95-96, 219, 294
boron, 8, 172, 175, 265, 266, 296
Botox (botulinum toxin) injections, 213, 282, 284, 296
bromelain, 173, 186-187, 296
bulging disc, 82-83, 273

C

cabbage, 204
calcium 55, 170, 172-173, 256, 258, 259, 265, 266, 268, 270, 273, 296. *See also* pseudogout
California poppy, 173, 187, 296
cancer 8, 18, 19, 25, 26, 36, 40, 47, 49, 121, 125, 175, 190, 195, 199, 203, 252, 260, 266. *See also* natural killer cells
canes, 31, 117-118
capsicum, 172, 183-184, 286, 296
carbohydrates 161, 165-168, 170, 189, 277, 297
cascara sagrada, 204
CAT (computerized axial tomography) scan, 9, 48, 49, 51-52, 54, 209, 261, 264, 287, 294, 297
cauda equina syndrome, 22, 23, 25, 26, 37, 52-54, 85, 104, 260, 261, 263, 287, 294
chemonucleolysis (chymopapain injection), 214-215, 263, 297
chiropractic treatment, 31-32, 120-124, 128, 256, 258, 262, 273, 297
chondroitin sulfate, 172, 178-179, 289
chronic back pain, 9, 19, 20, 25, 46, 113, 125, 135, 157, 158, 172-174, 245, 248, 260, 271, 274, 279, 279-294
chronic pain management, 234-249
chronic pain specialist, 33
chronic pain syndrome, 33, 41, 238-239, 248
chymopapain injection. *See* chemonucleolysis

classification
    of arthritis, 97
    of clinical back pain, 20
    of symptoms, 38-46, 88, 254
Clinical Practice Guideline (Seriousness), 40
coenzymes, 170, 192, 297
cold treatment. *See* cryotherapy
cortisol, 268-269
cortisone steroid injections, 210
coughing, 23
cross innervation, 90
cryotherapy, 8, 26, 31, 111, 112, 114, 141, 212, 255-258, 262, 273, 298
curcumin, 172, 184-185
cyanocobalamin. *See* vitamin B-12

D

decompression 208, 218-221, 224-227, 229, 287, 288, 298. *See also* surgery
degenerative arthritis, 45, 103, 180, 281, 285, 293
degenerative disc disease, 96, 140, 158, 172, 228-230, 279-284
degenerative joint disease 98, 298. *See also* arthritis
degenerative spondylolisthesis, 221, 225, 227, 228, 285, 288
depression, 105, 124, 128, 170, 174, 189, 191, 203, 241, 242, 244, 248
    medication for, 205-206
    supplements for, 195-199
derangement syndrome, 42, 43, 298
devil's claw, 9, 182-183, 256, 273, 286, 289, 298
diagnosis 18, 20-24, 26, 27, 29, 30, 33, 34-59
    of ankylosing spondylitis, 100, 290
    of annular strain, 88
    benefits of, 34-35
    of chronic pain syndrome, 238-239
    classification of symptoms during, 28-46
    of degenerative disc disease, 228, 280-282
    of disc herniation and sciatica, 260-261
    of disc injury, 88
    of facet injury, 89

injections for, 56-59
of lumbar strain, 252-254
and medical examination, 36-38
and medical history, 35-36
of neurogenic vs. vascular claudication, 102
of osteoarthritis (degenerative joint disease), 284-285
of osteoporosis, 267
psoriatic arthropathy, 292
quick reference guide, 8-9
of recurring back pain, 271-273, 280
of rheumatoid arthritis, 289
of spinal stenosis, 102, 286-287
of stress, anxiety, and depression, 195
diagnostic tests, 30, 47-59, 211
diet, 25, 28, 169, 170, 175, 176, 194, 242, 278
  advice, 160
  and lumbar strain, 256, 259, 266
  naturopathic, 163-168, 276, 277
  and osteoarthritis (lumbar spondylosis), 286
  and osteoporosis, 270
  and recurring back pain, 273
  and rheumatoid arthritis, 289
  and spondyloarthropathies, 292
  and stable compression fractures, 266
  trends, 161-162
disc degeneration, 9, 21, 51, 57, 67, 68, 82-84, 86-88, 99, 180, 216, 223, 229, 230, 254, 260, 276, 279, 280, 288
disc herniation, 8, 84-86, 172-173, 260-264, 298
  and anatomic or pathologic classification, 45
  and back pain, 18-21
  and CAT scan, 51
  chemonucleolysis for, 214-215
  and classification of symptoms, 38
  common characteristics, 84
  diagnosis, 260-261
  and disc injury, 88
  and epidural steroid injections, 208-209, 283
  and facet joint injections, 211
  and family doctor, 27
  and Hamilton Hall's pain patterns, 44

and injury sites, 253
and local inflammation, 93
and massage, 33
and medical examination, 37
and MRI scan, 53-54
and muscles, 66-67
and nerves, 70, 92
in normal pain-free individuals, 54
prevention, 264
recovery, 263
red flags, 260
and sciatica, 85, 260-264
and slipped disc, 85
and smoking, 276
and stretching, 140
and supplements, 172-173
and surgery, 217, 218, 220-223, 228
symptoms, 260
and traction, 119
and treating episodes, 272
disc injury, 44, 88, 89, 253, 254
disc replacement, 217, 219, 230-231, 282, 284
discectomy 214, 221-223, 263, 298. *See also* micro-discectomy
discography
  and degenerative disc disease, 228-229, 281-282
  and disc herniation, 54
  and facet joint blocks, 58
  and localizing pain source, 56
discography, 9, 57, 298
disease modifying anti-rheumatic drugs (DMARDs), 207, 289, 292
duration of
pain, 19-20, 36, 39-41, 56, 100, 122, 123, 214, 215, 236, 291
dysfunction syndrome, 42, 43

E

emergency care, 26-27, 265
employment, 36, 248, 272, 276
enzymes, 55, 86, 93, 98, 112, 126, 161, 168, 170, 174, 176, 178, 181, 182, 184-187, 189, 190, 192, 196, 201, 210, 214, 299
epidural steroid injections, 208-210, 263, 282, 283, 288, 299

ergonomics, 8, 9, 30, 31, 61, 118-119, 259, 264, 272, 275, 278, 282, 283
essential fatty acids, 170, 173, 192-194, 204, 256, 258, 259, 262, 264, 273, 287, 288, 289, 292, 299
exercise, 25, 30, 31, 135-157. *See also* weight training
  and acute low back pain, 110
  and adult spondylisthesis, 293
  and ankylosing spondylitis, 100, 290-291
  basics, 136
  benefits of, 135
  and calcium, 173
  cardiovascular, 141-143, 154, 155
  and chiropractic treatment, 32
  and cold packs, 111
  cool-down, 139, 142, 143
  and decompression, 225
  and decompression with fusion, 227
  and degenerative disc disease, 282, 283
  and degenerative spondylolisthesis, 288
  and derangement syndrome, 42
  and disc herniation, 262, 264
  and Hamilton Hall's acute stage care, 257, 273
  and Hamilton Hall's pain patterns, 44
  and hydrotherapy, 114
  and lumbar strain, 255-256, 258
  and magnesium, 174-175
  and osteoarthritis, 286
  and osteopathic treatment, 32
  and osteoporosis, 267, 270
  and quick reference guide to treatment, 8, 9
  and recurring back pain, 273, 274
  and rheumatological symptoms, 29
  and self-managing chronic pain, 249
  and spinal stenosis, 287-288
  and spine anatomy, 60
  and spondylolytic spondylolisthesis, 227
  and stable compression fractures, 265-266
  and stress management, 278
  and sub-acute stage, 257
  and Tai Chi, 130-131
  and TENS, 113
  terminology, 136, 144

  and vascular claudication, 38
  warm-up, 138, 142
  and weight loss, 276
  and yoga, 129-130
extension, 8, 9, 22, 23, 45, 46, 89, 118, 144, 145, 147, 150-154, 172, 211, 212, 253-255, 257, 261, 262, 264-266, 273, 281, 288, 293
extension brace, 265, 266
external fixation, 233, 299

F

facet injury, 89, 90, 254
facet joint arthritis, 51, 52
facet joint blocks, 56
facet joint injections, 211-212
facet joint pain, 88-89
family doctor, 8, 26, 27, 34, 121
fight or flight response, 75, 76, 78, 107, 239
5-HTP, 197-198, 299
fractures, 264-267, 299
  and back braces, 117
  and calcium, 172
  compression, 8, 36, 95-96, 99, 220, 227, 231, 232, 265-267, 272, 297
  and diagnostic tests, 49-52
  and disk injury, 88
  emergency care, 265
  and location of back pain, 21
  and medical history, 36
  and osteoarthritis, 98
  and osteoporosis, 268
  and pain definition limitations, 234
  and pain-tension-anxiety cycle, 243
  and pathologic causes of low back pain, 81
  and self-managing chronic pain, 249
  and spinal stenosis, 103
  and surgery, 28-29, 219, 220, 227, 231-233
  and timeframe of back pain, 19
  and ultrasound, 112
functional spinal unit (FSU), 12, 62

G

gate control theory, 78-79
ginger, 9, 172, 181-182, 184, 185, 205, 256, 262, 273, 286, 292, 299

glucosamine sulfate, 172, 176-179, 262, 264, 282, 285, 286, 289, 299

gout, 185, 200, 235, 299

group therapy, 245, 247

H

Hamilton Hall, 43-44, 257, 273

heart rate, 71, 119, 131, 142-143

heat treatment, 8, 9, 31, 80, 111-112, 114, 125, 141, 190, 191, 212, 256-258, 262, 273, 285, 286, 289

herbs, 170, 181-187, 195, 199, 204-206

herniated disc, 53, 58, 84, 87-88, 214, 215, 219, 222, 264

hops, 173, 199, 300

hyaluronic acid (HA), 9, 172, 177, 179, 180, 300

hydrotherapy, 9, 114, 300

hyperglycemia, 163-164, 300

hyperinsulemia, 167-168, 300

hypertrophic arthritis, 98, 300

hypnosis, 235, 246

hypoglycemia, 163-164, 300

I

ice treatment. *See* cryotherapy

inflammatory arthritis, 25, 43, 45, 48, 55, 81, 98, 99, 101, 200, 207, 211, 300

injection therapy, 208-216

insidious onset back pain, 19-20, 100, 291

instability

    and arthritis, 81, 288

    and catching pain, 23

    and chemonucleolysis, 215

    and diagnostic tests, 47, 48, 49, 281, 287

    and disc degeneration, 86

    and herniation, 81

    and infection, 81

    and Kirkaldy-Willis degenerative cascade, 46

    and location of pain, 21

    and lumbar spondylosis, 99

    and muscle tear, 81

    and occupational therapy, 265

    and osteoarthritis, 285

    and pathological causes of low back pain, 81-82

    and recurrence of pain, 20

and rheumatoid arthritis, 99

and seeking medical attention, 25

spinal stenosis due to, 102-104, 293-294

and spondylolisthesis, 82, 279

and supplements, 172-173

and surgery, 224, 225, 227, 229

insulin resistance, 162, 164-165, 167, 178, 300

intensity of pain, 19, 24

interferential bio electrical stimulation, 112, 300

intervertebral disc, 64-65, 222

    anatomy and pain pathology of, 11-12

    and chemonucleolysis, 214

    and disc injury, 254

    and discography, 57, 281

    and functional spine units, 62

    and injury sites, 253

    and Kirkaldy-Willis degenerative cascade, 46

    and mattresses, 118

    and MRI scan, 53

    and non-specific origins of pain, 105

    normal, 82

    pain, 84-88

    and pain-tension-anxiety cycle, 243

intradiscal electrothermal coagulation (IDET), 216, 282, 284, 300

isotope scan (technetium), 49-51, 300

K

ketosis, 162, 300

Kirkaldy-Willis Degenerative Cascade, 45-46

kyphoplasty, 232-233, 267, 300

L

lavender, 173, 195-196, 278, 301

leg pain, 8, 9, 23, 35, 38, 40, 43, 45, 46, 58, 84, 85, 88, 96, 141, 209, 214, 218-224, 253, 255, 260, 272, 288, 293. *See also* sciatica

leptin, 269, 301

lifting, 22, 30, 38, 61, 91, 147, 260, 264. *See also* weight training

    and bone strength, 96

    and disc degeneration, 84, 280

    and disc injury, 88

and ergonomics, 119, 275
and herniation, 84, 260
and lumbar strain, 253
and muscles, 66, 91
and quick reference to symptoms and prevention, 8-9
and stress, 278
ligament pain, 89-91
ligaments, 10, 12, 65, 301
limbic system, 76-77, 301
location of pain, 19, 20-22
lumbar roll, 257, 273
lumbar spine arthritis, 96, 103
lumbar spine instability, 293-294
lumbar spondylosis, 96, 98-99, 284, 285, 286. *See also* lumbar spine arthritis; osteoarthritis
lumbar strain, 8, 33, 46, 90, 91, 96, 111, 140, 169, 172, 252-259, 271, 272, 279
  diagnosis, 254
  treatment, 255-257
lumbar vertebra, 10, 11, 15, 48, 61, 63

M

magnesium, 172, 174-175, 301
magnetotherapy, 114-115, 301
manganese, 172, 176
manipulation. *See* chiropractic treatment
manual therapy, 258
marshmallow, 204
massage therapy, 33, 123-125, 283, 301
mattresses, 118
McKenzie Classification, 41-43, 301
medial branch neurotomy, 212, 301
medical care, guidelines for seeking, 24-25
medical examination, 36-38
medical history, 35-36
medication, 200-216
  anti-depressant, 205-206
  for disc herniation, 262
  for lumbar strain, 256, 258
  for spinal stenosis, 288
methylsulfonylmethane (MSM), 172, 179-180, 301
micro-discectomy 221-223, 225, 301. *See also* discectomy
minerals, 170, 172-176, 301
movement, 19, 22-23

MRI (magnetic resonance imaging) scan, 52-54, 281, 301
muscle injury, 91, 254
muscle pain, 89-91
muscle relaxants, 205
muscle tear, 91
muscles, 13, 66-67
myelogram, 54

N

narcotics, 203
narrowing disc, 82-83
natural killer cells, 302
naturopathic diet, 163-168, 276-277
naturopathy, 27-28, 302
nerve damage, 22, 59, 84, 85, 92, 189, 192, 261. *See also* sciatica
nerve pain, 33, 92-95, 121, 126, 127, 189, 194, 206, 208, 256. *See also* sciatica
nerve paths, 70
nerve root, 11, 12, 14, 15, 21, 22, 23, 37, 38, 40, 41, 42, 54, 56, 58, 70, 73, 81, 85, 86, 87, 92, 93, 94, 95, 102, 103, 208, 209, 210, 214, 220, 222, 223, 261, 280, 293, 294
nerve root blocks, 56, 58-59, 293
nerve sensitivity, causes, 94
nerve tests, 55-56, 261
neurogenic claudication, 37-38, 102, 302. *See also* spinal stenosis
niacin. *See* vitamin B-3
NSAIDs (non-steroidal anti-inflammatory medications), 8, 9, 171, 177, 183, 185, 187, 201-202, 204, 205, 207, 211, 230, 282, 289, 292, 294, 302
nutrition
  and fitness, 276
  and insulin resistance, 164
  and lumbar strain, 256, 258, 259
  and naturopath, 28. *See also* naturopathic diet
  and nerve pain 92
  and osteoporosis, 269, 270
  and smoking 276
  and spinal fusion for degenerative disc disease, 230
  and stable compression fractures, 265

O

obesity, 118, 160, 162, 178, 216, 236, 269, 302. *See also* weight gain, as a symptom; weight management
occupational therapy, 31, 265, 266, 302
onset, 19-20
orthopedic surgeon, 28-29
orthotics, 115, 302
osteoarthritis, 9, 36, 63, 83, 89, 97-101, 104, 127, 177, 179, 184, 187, 188, 284-285, 287, 288, 302. *See also* degenerative disc disease
    diagnosis, 285
    treatment, 285-286
osteopath, 32
osteopathy, 122-123
osteoporosis, 267-270, 302
    causes, 268
    prevention, 270
    risk factors, 267
    treatment, 270
osteoporotic compression fractures, 267

P

pain
    acute vs. chronic, 236-237
    catching, 23
    causes of, 60-107
    good vs. bad, 141
    intervertal disc, 84-88
    limitations of definition, 234-235
    non-specific origins of, 105
    non-spinal causes, 81
    pathologic causes, 81
    peripheral, 21-22
    psychic, 105-107
    sciatica, 94-95, 263
    sensation and control, 72-80
    specific origins of, 81-107
    types of, 77-78
    words for, 24
pain clinics, 245
pain gates, 78-79
pain pathways, 73-75, 77, 106, 209, 263
pain receptors, 73
pain scales, 24
pain-tension-anxiety (PTA) cycle, 241-244

painkillers, 110, 120, 123, 200-205, 207, 256, 258, 262, 267, 273, 289, 292, 294
parasympathetic nervous system, 71-72, 302
pathologic classification, 44-46
peppermint, 205
peripheral pain, 21-22
peripheral sensitization, 80
peripheral symptoms, 23
persistent back pain. *See* chronic back pain
physiotherapy, 30-31, 245, 302
positions, 22-23
postural syndrome, 41, 42, 43, 302
posture, 144-146
    for disc herniation, 262
    for lumbar strain, 258
    prolonged, 23
    for spinal stenosis, 287-288
posture improvement, 115-117
pressure thresholds, 90
prevention, quick reference guide, 8-9
protein, 165, 303
pseudogout, 320
psoriatic arthritis, 29, 99-101, 291-292, 303
psoriatic arthropathy, 292
psychic pain, 105-107
pyridoxine. *See* vitamin B-6

Q

Quebec Task Force Classification, 40-41

R

radicular leg pain. *See* sciatica
radiofrequency neurotomy, 212
recurrence, 19, 20
recurring back pain, 9, 172-173, 271-278
    causes, 272
    preventing, 274-278
    symptoms, 271-272
    treatment for episode, 272-273
referred pain, 94
relaxation training, 245-246
reticular formation, 75
rheumatoid arthritis, 29, 36, 89, 97, 99-101, 188, 200, 207, 268, 289-291, 303
    medication for, 207
    symptoms, 29, 289-290
    treatment, 289-290

riboflavin. *See* vitamin B-2
Rosen Method, 132-133, 303
ruptured disc, 82-83

S

sacroiliac joint injections, 213-214
sciatic nerve, 15
sciatica, 84-86, 94-95, 194, 260-264, 303
selenium, 173
self-confidence, 248
self-help, 248-249
senna, 204
sensitization, 80, 84, 86, 87, 89, 90, 91, 93, 94, 107, 120, 121, 184, 208, 211, 213, 255, 258, 259, 280, 284
sex therapy, 248
sexual intercourse, 156-157
shiatsu, 127-128, 303
short-wave diathermy, 112
slipped disc, 62, 84, 85
slippery elm, 204
smoking, 276
sneezing, 23
sensory field widening, 90
SPECT scan, 49-51
spina bifida occulta, 48
spinal arthritis, 279
spinal conditioning, 274-275
spinal cord, 12, 14, 23, 48, 53, 54, 61, 63, 65, 69-75, 78-82, 88, 90, 92-94, 99, 102, 105, 107, 122, 183, 192, 211, 212, 217, 219, 234, 264, 287
spinal fusion, 229-230
spinal movement. *See* chiropractic treatment
spinal nerves, 15
spinal osteoarthritis, 9
spinal stenosis, 9, 83, 102, 194, 286-288
    causes, 102-103
    diagnosis, 287
    due to instability (spondylolisthesis), 103-104
    surgery, 224
    surgery for, 220
    symptoms, 286
    treatment, 287-288

spine
    anatomy, 60-69
    deconditioned components in lumbar, 274
    functions of, 61
spine curves, 68-69
spondyloarthritis, 303
spondyloarthropathies. *See* ankylosing spondylitis; psoriatic arthritis; *and* psoriatic arthropathy
spondylolisthesis, 83, 103-104, 293-294, 303
spondylolytic spondylolisthesis, 227-228, 293-294
spondylosis, 104
sports, training for, 276
spouse groups, 247
St John's Wort, 198, 303
strengthening, 140-141. *See also* strength training
steroid injections, 208-210
straightening, 22, 149-153, 303
stress
    reducing, 277-278
    supplements for, 195-199
stress response, 239-241
stretch thresholds, 90
stretching, 96, 117, 137-140, 144-148
    benefits of, 137
    types of, 138-140
sub-acute back pain, 20
sudden onset back pain, lumbar strain, 8, 172-173
sudden onset back pain, 252-270
supplements, 168, 169-199, 176-180
    basic terms, 170
    for degenerative disc disease, 283
    for disc herniation, 262, 264
    liver support and minor allergic reaction, 206
    for lumbar strain, 256, 258
    quality, 171
    safety, 171
    selecting and combining, 171
    for spinal stenosis, 288
    for stable compression fractures, 265
    for stress, anxiety, and depression, 195-199

surgery, 217-233
    candidates for, 220-221
    for degenerative disc disease, 284
    elective, 219
    indications for, 217-218
    procedures, 217, 219
    techniques, 221-233
    for unresolved sciatic pain, 263
sympathetic nervous system, 71-72, 304
symptoms
    associated, 19, 22-23
    classification of, 38-46
    neurogenic claudication, 38
    quick reference guide, 8-9
    rheumatologic, 29
    vascular claudication, 38

T

Tai Chi, 130-132, 274, 283, 304
technetium. *See* isotope scan
temporal classifications, 39
TENS (transcutaneous electrical nerve
    stimulation), 113, 256, 304
thiamin. *See* vitamin B-1
traction, 119, 262, 304
training, for employment or sports, 276
treatment
    for degenerative disc disease, 282-284
    hands-on physical, 120-134
    non-invasive, 110-119
    quick reference guide, 8-9
trypsic hydrolysate milk peptide, 196-197,
    304
twisting, 22, 64, 84, 253, 260, 264

U

underweight, 267. *See also* anorexia;
    weight loss, as a symptom
ultrasound, 31, 38, 57, 102, 111, 112, 257,
    258, 304

V

valerian, 173, 187, 199, 304
vascular claudication, 37-38, 102, 304
vertebroplasty, 8, 219, 231-233, 267, 304

vertebral column, 10-11, 95
vertebrae (bones), 63-64
vibration, 9, 22, 37, 66, 67, 78, 84, 112, 280
vitamins, 170, 188-192
    B complex, 173, 189-192, 287, 288, 304
    B-1 (thiamin), 169, 189
    B-2 (riboflavin), 169, 190
    B-3 (niacin), 190-191, 197
    B-6 (pyridoxine), 191-192, 197
    B-12 (cyanocobalamin), 192
    C, 173, 188-189, 194, 304
    E, 173, 188, 194, 304
vocational counseling, 248

W

weight, 9, 62, 119, 174, 241, 242, 249, 267,
    272, 280, 281
weight gain, as a symptom, 9, 91, 176, 236,
    241, 249, 242, 272, 280, 281. *See also*
    obesity
weight loss, as a symptom, 8, 19, 23, 25,
    26, 36, 47, 49, 236, 241, 249, 252,
    267
weight management, 8, 9, 135, 142, 143,
    158-168, 190, 259, 264, 269, 276-277,
    282, 283, 285, 286, 287, 288, 293
weight training, 103, 136, 140-141, 152,
    153, 259, 294
willow, 173, 185-186, 256, 273, 304

X

X-rays, 8, 9, 39, 47-49, 50, 51, 52, 54, 57,
    96, 97, 99, 103, 229, 255, 261, 264,
    265, 266, 273, 279, 281, 285, 287,
    289, 290, 293

Y

yoga, 8, 9, 60, 116, 129-130, 145, 258, 264,
    274, 275, 278, 282, 283, 285, 286,
    289, 304

Z

zinc, 8, 204, 256, 258, 265, 266, 273, 292,
    304
zygoapophyseal joints. *See* facet joints